Exercise, Nutrition, and Energy Metabolism

Editors:

Edward S. Horton, M.D.

Professor and Chairman of Medicine
Director of Endocrinology, Metabolism, and Nutrition
University of Vermont College of Medicine
Burlington, Vermont

Ronald L. Terjung, Ph.D.

Professor of Physiology
State University of New York
Health Science Center
Syracuse, New York

Exercise, Nutrition, and Energy Metabolism

Macmillan Publishing Company

New York

Collier Macmillan Canada, Inc.

Toronto

Collier Macmillan Publishers

London

Macmillan Publishing Company
866 Third Avenue, New York, New York 10022.

Collier Macmillan Canada, Inc.
Collier Macmillan Publishers • London

Library of Congress Cataloging-in-Publication Data

Exercise, nutrition, and energy metabolism.

   Includes bibliographies and index.
   1. Exercise—Physiological aspects. 2. Nutrition.
3. Energy metabolism.   I. Horton, Edward S.   II. Terjung,
Ronald L.   [DNLM: 1. Energy Metabolism. 2. Exertion.
3. Nutrition. QU 125 E96]
QP301.E968   1988   612'.04   87-22083
ISBN 0-02-357190-X

Printing: 1 2 3 4 5 6 7 8   Year: 8 9 0 1 2 3 4 5 6

PREFACE

A characteristic of all living organisms is the requirement to assimilate nutrients from the environment and convert them to energy for the wide variety of biochemical and biophysical reactions that are necessary for survival. In the animal kingdom, the ability to move and perform physical work is critical; of the various components of energy expenditure, that required for physical exercise is quantitatively the most variable among individuals. Whereas the resting metabolic rate is fairly constant (comprising 60 to 75% of total daily energy expenditure in relatively sedentary humans), as is processing of consumed food (which may require about 10% of the ingested calories), the energy requirements for physical exercise can vary from as low as 100 kcal/day in an individual at bed rest to as high as 18,000 kcal/day in one who runs continuously for 24 hours. For most of us, however, daily energy expenditures of 500 to 2000 kcal/day for physical exercise are common. Therefore, it is of great scientific and practical interest to understand how the body assimilates, stores, and converts food energy to make it available to power muscular contractions in the finely regulated and coordinated fashion required for performance of physical work.

The purpose of this book is to provide the professional with an in-depth view of the broad range of nutritional and metabolic implications imposed by exercise. After reviewing the available works in the field, we found that there was real need for an authoritative text that would bring together under a single cover the current knowledge of the relationships among nutrition, energy metabolism, and physical exercise, with particular emphasis on normal human physiology, the effects of physical training, and the impact of exercise and nutrition on selected disease states.

In this book, exercise will generally be considered to mean rhythmical whole-body physical activity such as walking, running, cycling, and swimming, although in some instances more specific definitions will be given. In considering the influence of exercise, we have adopted a rather broad definition of nutrition to include the assimilation, distribution, and particularly the utilization of nutrients. This latter emphasis, by necessity, includes a consideration of substrate oxidation, the control of energy metabolism within muscle, and the integration of substrate supply during exercise. In addition, we felt it important to consider the overall impact of exercise on metabolic processes during the subsequent nonexercise period. We hope this approach will develop for the reader an understanding of the special nutrient demands created by exercise. When possible, special sections have been included that develop current information on important nutritional requirements. Unfortunately, extensive information about the interaction between exercise and specific nutrient requirements is often lacking. We hope that future research will eliminate this void.

Each chapter has been written by one or more experts in the subject covered. An attempt has been made to provide a concise, yet authoritative, review and synthesis of the topic and a selected bibliography for those who wish to consult the original literature or read more detailed reviews. The book is divided roughly into two parts. The first deals with the basic metabolism and physiology of exercise and the effects of physical training. The second considers a variety of clinically related topics, focused on nutrient requirements and the interrelationships between nutrition and exercise in the prevention and management of common diseases such as cardiovascular disease, diabetes mellitus, hypertension, and obesity.

We hope the book will serve as a text and reference source for a wide range of professionals requiring knowlege about interactions between nutrition and physical exercise. This may include such groups as exercise physiologists, nutritionists, graduate students in the basic sciences, and medical students. In addition, scientists and clinical practitioners working in different but related disciplines may find this book a useful source of information to supplement knowledge in their own field of interest.

Edward S. Horton, M.D.   Ronald L. Terjung, Ph.D.
Burlington, Vermont   Syracuse, New York

CONTRIBUTORS

Richard A. Anderson, Ph.D. Lead Scientist, Beltsville Human Nutrition Research Center, U.S. Department of Agriculture, BARC East, Building 308, Room 224, Beltsville, MD 20705

Robert B. Armstrong, Ph.D. Professor of Physical Education, Department of Physical Education, University of Georgia, Athens, GA 30602

Per-Olof Åstrand, M.D. Professor of Physiology, Emeritus, Department of Physiology III, Karolinska Institute, Lidingovagen 1, Stockholm S-114 33, Sweden

Ola Björkman, Ph.D. Associate Professor of Clinical Physiology, Department of Clinical Physiology, Huddinge University Hospital, Huddinge, Sweden

Alexander Bortoff, Ph.D. Professor of Physiology, Department of Physiology, State University of New York, Health Science Center at Syracuse, 766 Irving Avenue, Syracuse, NY 13210.

David Costill, Ph.D. Professor and Director, Human Performance Laboratory, Ball State University, Muncie, IN 47306

Philip D. Gollnick, Ph.D. Professor of Physiology, Department of Anatomy, Pharmacology and Physiology, College of Veterinary Medicine, Washington State University, Pullman, WA 99164.

Michael N. Goodman, Ph.D. Associate Professor of Medicine, Division of Endocrinology, Medical Center, Sacramento, University of California at Davis, 4301 X St., Bldg. FOLB II-C, Sacramento, CA 95817

Helene N. Guttman, Ph.D. Associate Director, Beltsville Human Nutrition Research Center, U.S. Department of Agriculture, BARC East, Building 308, Room 224, Beltsville, MD 20705.

William L. Haskell, Ph.D. Associate Professor of Medicine, Stanford Center for Research in Disease Prevention, Stanford Medical School, 730 Welch Road, Palo Alto, CA 94304

John O. Holloszy, M.D. Professor of Medicine, Department of Internal Medicine, Washington University School of Medicine, 4566 Scott Avenue, St. Louis, MO 63110

Eric Hultman, M.D. Professor of Clinical Chemistry, Department of Clinical Chemistry II, Huddinge University Hospital, Huddinge, Sweden

Hassan Kanj, M.D. Endocrinology Fellow, Department of Medicine, UMDNJ-Robert Wood Johnson Medical School, One Robert Wood Johnson Place-CN19, New Brunswick, N.J. 08903-0019

Zebulon V. Kendrick, Ph.D. Associate Professor of Physical Education, Department of Physical Education, Temple University, Philadelphia, PA 19122

Joseph M. Krisanda, Ph.D. Assistant Research Professor, Department of Medicine, Boston University School of Medicine, 75 East Newton Street, Boston, MA 02118

Martin J. Kushmerick, M.D., Ph.D. Associate Professor of Physiology and Biophysics, Department of Radiology, Harvard Medical School, Brigham and Women's Hospital, 25 Shattuck Street, Boston, MA 02115

David T. Lowenthal, M.D., Ph.D. Professor of Geriatrics, Medicine and Pharmacology, Mount Sinai Medical Center, 1 Gustave L. Levy Place, New York, NY 10029

Timothy S. Moreland, Ph.D. Research Fellow, Department of Radiology, Harvard Medical School, Brigham and Women's Hospital, 25 Shattuck Street, Boston, MA 02115

Daphne A. Roe, M.D. Professor of Nutrition, Division of Nutritional Sciences, Cornell University, Ithaca, NY 14853

Neil B. Ruderman, M.D. Professor of Medicine and Physiology, Boston University School of Medicine, University Hospital, Section of Diabetes and Metabolism, 75 East Newton Street, Boston, MA 02118

Bengt Saltin, M.D. Professor of Physiology, August Krogh Institute, University of Copenhagen, 13, Universitetsparken, DK-2100 Copenhagen 0, Denmark

Steven H. Schneider, M.D. Associate Professor of Clinical Medicine, UMDNJ-Robert Wood Johnson Medical School, One Robert Wood Johnson Place-CN 19, New Brunswick, NJ 08903-0019

Ethan A.H. Sims, M.D. Professor of Medicine,

Emeritus, Department of Medicine, University of Vermont, School of Medicine, Given Building C-352, Burlington, VT 05405

Lawrence L. Spriet, Ph.D. Assistant Professor of Human Biology, School of Human Biology, University of Guelph, Guelph, Ontario N1G 2W1, Canada

Marcia L. Stefanick, Ph.D. Research Associate, Stanford Center for Research in Disease Prevention, Stanford Medical School, 730 Welch Road, Palo Alto, CA 94303

Robert Superko, M.D. Clinical Assistant Professor of Medicine, Stanford Center for Research in Disease Prevention, Stanford Medical School, 730 Welch Road, Palo Alto, CA 94303

John Wahren, M.D. Professor of Clinical Physiology, Department of Clinical Physiology, Huddinge University Hospital, Huddinge, Sweden

CONTENTS

Preface   v
Contributors   vii

1. Whole-Body Metabolism
   Per-Olof Åstrand, M.D.   1

2. Muscle Fiber Recruitment Patterns and Their Metabolic Correlates
   Robert B. Armstrong, Ph.D.   9

3. ATP Supply and Demand During Exercise
   Joseph M. Krisanda, Ph.D., Timothy S. Moreland, Ph.D., and Martin J. Kushmerick, M.D.   27

4. Fuel for Muscular Exercise: Role of Carbohydrate
   Bengt Saltin, M.D., and Philip D. Gollnick, Ph.D.   45

5. Fuel for Muscular Exercise: Role of Fat
   Philip D. Gollnick, Ph.D., and Bengt Saltin, M.D.   72

6. Amino Acid and Protein Metabolism
   Michael N. Goodman, Ph.D.   89

7. Glucose Homeostasis During and After Exercise
   Ola Björkman, Ph.D., and John Wahren, M.D.   100

8. Metabolic Consequences of Endurance Exercise Training
   John O. Holloszy, M.D.   116

9. Dietary Intake Prior to and During Exercise
   Eric Hultman, M.D., and Lawrence L. Spriet, Ph.D.   132

10. Fluid and Electrolyte Balance During Prolonged Exercise
    Bengt Saltin, M.D., and David Costill, Ph.D.   150

11. Influence of Exercise on Gastrointestinal Function
    Alexander Bortoff, Ph.D.   159

12. Vitamin Requirements for Increased Physical Activity
    Daphne A. Roe, M.D.   172

13. Trace Minerals and Exercise
    Richard A. Anderson, Ph.D., and Helene N. Guttman, Ph. D.   180

14. Drug-Nutrient Interactions
    Zebulon V. Kendrick, Ph.D., and David T. Lowenthal, M.D., Ph.D.   196

15. Influence of Exercise on Plasma Lipids and Lipoproteins
William L. Haskell, Ph.D., Marcia L. Stefanick, Ph.D., and Robert Superko, M.D.   213

16. Exercise and Diabetes Mellitus
Hassan Kanj, M.D., Steven H. Schneider, M.D., and Neil B. Ruderman, M.D.   228

17. Exercise and Energy Balance in the Control of Obesity and Hypertension
Ethan A. H. Sims, M.D.   242

Index   259

Exercise, Nutrition, and Energy Metabolism

Chapter 1

WHOLE-BODY METABOLISM

Per-Olof Åstrand, M.D.

The two main processes responsible for energy provision in the resynthesis of adenosin triphosphate (ATP) are the anaerobic breakdown of glucose and glycogen to pyruvate and lactate and the aerobic oxidation of lipid, protein, and carbohydrates (CHO). The importance of each substrate as an energy source during exercise has been the topic of much research over the years. At the turn of this century, it was assumed that contracting skeletal muscle used carbohydrate exclusively as a fuel. This conclusion was based on studies of isolated muscles that were poorly oxygenated. Therefore, the anaerobic breakdown of glycogen was probably the sole energy source available. The contribution of fat toward energy metabolism in muscle was convincingly documented by Christensen and Hansen [5], who in 1939 published a series of papers demonstrating that both carbohydrate and fat could be oxidized during exercise. In this classic work, the respiratory quotient (RQ; the ratio of the CO_2 production rate to the O_2 consumption rate) was used to study how various factors could modify the choice of substrates in muscle. Then in the 1950s, a new technique made it possible to insert catheters in blood vessels and to determine regional blood flow and arteriovenous differences of substances (e.g., across skeletal muscles). These measurements revealed a substantial uptake of free fatty acids (FFA) by exercising muscle. Many authors concluded that utilization of FFA was the dominant source for muscle

energy metabolism. The fact that muscle normally has a large quantity of glycogen stored within its cells was overlooked. Oxidation of this carbohydrate source could not be traced just by studying the exchange of substrates between the arterial blood and the active muscle.

In the 1960s, Bergström and coworkers [3] made use of the biopsy needle to obtain samples of the working muscle to study events going on within the muscle during exercise. They actually repeated and confirmed Christensen and Hansen's experiments and added information about endogenous substrates and enzymatic processes within the muscle itself. Thus, over time the interpretation of energy metabolism in exercising skeletal muscle has changed—the pendulum has swung back and forth. The forthcoming chapters will fully develop the various factors that influence muscle metabolism and the balance between the different energy substrates utilized by working muscle.

TOTAL ENERGY OUTPUT

During 24 hours, the basal metabolic rate for a nonobese 75-kg man may be about 7 MJ (1700 kcal). Is this a high or a low energy output? As a comparison, the extra energy demand for this person for walking 35 to 40 km above the resting level would be on the same magnitude. In other words, staying in bed during 24 hours is as energy demanding as walking those many kilometers (obviously the training effects of the two lifestyles are *not* similar!)

This example makes clear that it is not relevant always to express the energy content of beer, Danish pastry, chocolate, and so on in terms of how many kilometers the consumer must walk to spend the energy taken in. Our relatively high resting metabolic rate is, to a great degree, the price we pay for our relatively warm (~37°C) internal environment. The high efficiency of walking at a modest speed (4–5 km·hr⁻¹) must have provided an essential benefit for early humans. At times, the food needed for an adequate energy intake was sparse, and the hunters and gatherers were forced to walk many kilometers a day to find enough food. If walking were an expensive physical activity, the food energy collected might scarcely cover the energy demand of the walking, let alone the energy demand of the rest of the day. Anyone who has devoted time to walking in an attempt to lose weight has experienced lack of significant weight loss in the short term. For a 75-kg person, the extra energy output of a daily 2-km walk over a month will be equivalent to the energy content of approximately 350 g of fatty tissue. Since body weight observed in the morning can vary up to 1 kg from that of the previous day due to variations in water content, it is easy to understand that an actual loss of 350 g of fatty tissue is difficult to measure. However (still from a mathematical point of view), a 2-km walk taken daily for 10 years increases the energy output of a 75-kg person by approximately 1200 MJ (300,000 kcal). This is equivalent to the energy content in approximately 45 kg of fatty tissue, which is quite significant! One cannot, however, apply strict mathematical principles to all biological systems. Actual weight loss achieved by habitual walking is probably still less than the amount calculated from the extra energy output. Further, weight gain if regular walking is stopped is less than predicted [6, 10]. In this context it is interesting to note that jogging at a low speed costs approximately twice as much energy per kilometer as walking at the same speed (Figure 1). At higher speeds, walking becomes more inefficient in comparison with jogging or running, which costs approximately the same units of energy per kilometer and per kilogram of body weight irrespective of speed.

There is great interest in data on the energy output of, say, walking, running, swimming, or skiing a given distance or playing tennis, golf, or basketball for a given

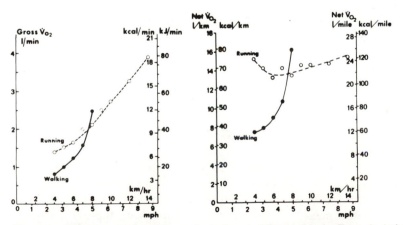

Figure 1. Energy cost of walking and running at different speeds. For calculation of the net energy output (right panel), oxygen uptake during sitting was subtracted from oxygen uptake during walking and running, respectively. The body weight of the subject was 75 kg. (From Åstrand, P.-O., and K. Rodahl. *Textbook of Work Physiology*. 3rd ed. New York: McGraw-Hill, 1986.)

time. Such data must, however, be considered very approximate and sometimes even misleading. Figure 1 illustrates how the velocity of walking affects energy demand. Figure 2 takes into account additional factors. In Figure 2, with walking speed constant, oxygen uptake varied from 0.8 to 2.1 L·min^{-1} depending on the slope of the road and the velocity of a head wind. It should be emphasized that the classic and most accurate estimation of whole-body aerobic metabolism derives from measurement of the rate of oxygen uptake. Namely, consumption of 1 L of oxygen in the mitochondria yields approximately 20 kJ (or 5 kcal) (Range 19.7–21.2 kJ [4.7–5.05 kcal] depending on the combination of free fatty acids and carbohydrates utilized as substrates).

Another example of individual variations in energy output at given tasks is evident from swimming. When swimming freestyle at 0.8 m·s^{-1}, a relatively good swimmer's oxygen uptake was 3.6 L·min^{-1}, but an elite swimmer consumed only 1.8 L·min^{-1}, that is, this swimmer's efficiency was much higher [7]. The energy demand of swimming butter-fly or breaststroke at a given speed is significantly higher than that of freestyle or backstroke [cf. 7]. Thus, in physical activities in which skill and technique can be much improved (e.g., in swimming, cross-country skiing), the distance or time spent in the activity is poor information about the person's energy output.

Actually, a person's maximal oxygen uptake (maximal aerobic power, $\dot{V}o_2$max) is quite decisive for that person's potential to spend energy aerobically. Recommended levels of oxygen uptake in a training program aiming at improvement of the oxygen transport system vary between 50 and 80% of the individual's $\dot{V}o_2$max, depending on the initial fitness level (athletes excluded). Table 1 illustrates how critical this maximum is for the power tolerated during physical activity. Exercising at 50% of her $\dot{V}o_2$max for 60 minutes, a 25-year-old woman's energy expenditure may be 1.4 MJ (335 kcal). Her exercising mother's energy output during these 60 minutes may be 1.2 MJ (290 kcal), and her exercising grandmother's, 0.8 MJ (200 kcal). The perceived exertion will be approximately the same for the three women. In contrast, with less effort a top male athlete will go through the 60-minute exercise bout at 50% of his $\dot{V}o_2$max, spending 4.5 MJ (1100 kcal), that is, more than three times as much energy as the young woman. Interestingly, in such activities as submaximal walking and bicycling, the mechanical efficiency for adults is similar irrespective of sex and age.

Figure 3 presents some extremes in energy expenditure for individuals involved in various activities. The highest 24-hour energy output reported is 78 MJ (18,600 kcal) in an athlete running 250 km in a 24-hour race. This extremely high energy expenditure would necessitate an inordinately large volume of food for return to caloric balance. Obviously, this extreme in energy output cannot be attempted on a daily basis. Further, it is apparent that nutritional supplementation (e.g., fluid and carbohydrate) is required for optimal performance.

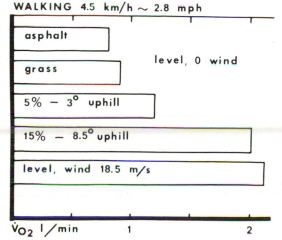

WALKING 4.5 km/h ~ 2.8 mph

asphalt	
grass	level, 0 wind
5% — 3° uphill	
15% — 8.5° uphill	
level, wind 18.5 m/s	

$\dot{V}o_2$ l/min   1   2

Figure 2. Energy expenditure of walking under different conditions. (From Åstrand, P.-O. and K. Rodahl. *Textbook of Work Physiology.* 3rd ed. New York: McGraw-Hill, 1986.)

Table 1.   AEROBIC POWER DURING DIFFERENT RATES OF EXERCISE FOR AVERAGE INDIVIDUALS COMPARED WITH TOP ATHLETES.

SUBJECT	EXERCISE AT 100% $\dot{V}O_2MAX$		EXERCISE AT 80% $\dot{V}O_2MAX$		EXERCISE AT 50% $\dot{V}O_2MAX$		EXERCISE (1 HR) AT 50% $\dot{V}O_2MAX$
	L/min	kJ	L/min	kJ	L/min	kJ	MJ
Average Male							
Age 25	3.3	70	2.6	55	1.65	34	2.0
Age 50	2.7	55	2.2	45	1.35	28	1.7
Age 75	2.0	40	1.6	33	1.0	20	1.2
Athlete							
Age 25	7.4*	155	5.9	120	3.7	75	4.5
Average Female							
Age 25	2.3	50	1.8	38	1.5	24	1.4
Age 50	1.9	40	1.5	30	0.95	20	1.2
Age 75	1.4	30	1.1	24	0.7	14	0.8
Athlete							
Age 25	4.5*	95	3.6	75	2.25	45	2.7

*Highest figures reported.

DIET AND EXERCISE

Under normal conditions, most of the energy demand in exercising muscles is derived from free fatty acids and carbohydrate, especially glycogen. The higher the work rate in relation to the individual's maximal aerobic power, the higher is the share from carbohydrate. The relative contribution of each substrate oxidized during prolonged exercise requiring not more than approximately 70% $\dot{V}O_2max$ will be affected by the

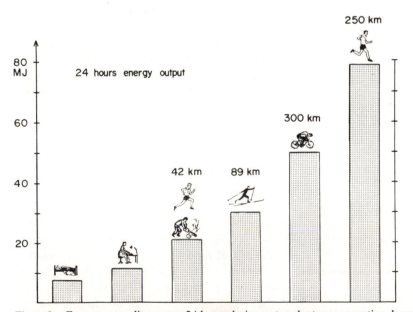

Figure 3.   Energy expenditure over 24 hours during rest, sedentary occupation, heavy manual work/running the marathon, 89-km cross-country skiing ("Vasaloppet"), 300-km bicycle race, and 250-km running (24-hour race). Energy output was partly measured, in some cases predicted from the heart rate in "calibrated" subjects or taken from standard tables.

composition of the diet. For example CHO utilization will dominate muscle metabolism if a CHO-rich diet is consumed. In contrast, lipid oxidation is favored when a high-fat diet is consumed. Endurance training will also enhance fatty acid utilization as a substrate. Increasing the energy contribution from lipid oxidation is important, since this reduces the rate of glycogen utilization. This can significantly improve endurance performance.

Table 2 illustrates how a given glycogen store (2 mol or 360 g of 6-carbon units) can be emptied after 150 minutes if the individual, exercising at 80% of $\dot{V}o_2$max, is untrained. Another person, who by training has increased $\dot{V}o_2$max from 2.5 to $3.0 \cdot min^{-1}$, could exercise approximately 40 more minutes at the same oxygen uptake before the glycogen store became exhausted (the lower RQ for the trained person indicates a relatively higher combustion of FFAs, compared with the untrained person).

A popular belief is that low-intensity exercise should be more effective in reducing an unwanted mass of fatty tissue, because FFA oxidation dominates as the fuel. However, the important factor is overall energy output in relation to energy intake, not the actual combustion of FFAs during exercise. If during exercise glycogen is oxidized, the depot will be restored after exercise. This process demands energy. If FFA is the preferred substrate during exercise, the glycogen stores are better maintained. However,

excess energy intake, for example in the form of carbohydrate, will then be stored in the fatty tissue.

From this short review it should be evident that for most habitually active people, the extra energy output should be balanced with an increased intake of carbohydrate and fat. Under normal conditions, protein is not the preferred substrate for activated skeletal muscles. These aspects of substrate utilization will be considered in detail in subsequent chapters.

LIMITING FACTORS FOR WHOLE BODY METABOLISM

There is general agreement that the potential of the skeletal muscles to consume oxygen far exceeds the potential of the central circulation to deliver oxygen [2, 9]. In other words, normally more than enough mitochondria, enzymes, and substrates are available to back up the individual's maximal oxygen uptake, for example, when running or skiing at maximal speed, but not enough oxygen is offered to the mitochondria.

Some observations will illustrate this statement. During exercise at a maximal rate, the highest oxygen uptake attained in one-leg cycling is 65 to 70% of the peak value observed in two-leg cycling. When use of the second leg is "superimposed" on the one-leg activity, vasoconstriction and re-

Table 2. ENDURANCE OF TWO SUBJECTS WITH SAME MAXIMAL OXYGEN UPTAKE ($\dot{V}o_2$max) BUT DIFFERENT TRAINING, EXERCISING AT 80% OF THEIR $\dot{V}o_2$max UNTIL EXHAUSTION.*

SUBJECT	OXYGEN UPTAKE (L/MIN)		RESPIRATORY QUOTIENT	CARBOHYDRATE METABOLISM			EXERCISE TIME ON 2.0 MOL† GLYCOGEN/MIN
	Maximum	80%		kJ/min	%	mmol/min	
Untrained	3.0	2.4	0.95	50.1	83	13.3	150
Trained	3.0	2.4	0.90	49.5	66	10.6	189

*For calculations, an eventual protein metabolism was not considered.
†glycosyl units

Source: Åstrand, P.-O. Diet, performance, and their interaction. In Barker, L. M. (ed.). *The Psychology of Human Food Selection.* Westport, Conn. AVI Publishing, 1982, p. 17.

duced blood flow occur in the first leg [9]. During swimming with arm strokes only, the legs kept passive, the highest oxygen uptake attained by a trained swimmer was 2.7 $L \cdot min^{-1}$ [8]. During swimming with leg kicks only, the arms kept passive, the swimmer's highest oxygen uptake was 3.4 $L \cdot min^{-1}$. During normal swimming with both arm and leg strokes, the maximum was certainly not 6.1 $L \cdot min^{-1}$ but rather 3.6 $L \cdot min^{-1}$, only 60% of the potential combined maximum. A similar discrepancy was obtained with an untrained swimmer [8]. Most likely some muscle groups are engaged in both one-leg and two-leg exercise as well as in arm and leg strokes in swimming, but the difference in the theoretical maximal oxygen uptake and the actually measured one in the different types of exercise is quite dramatic. So, again, the dimensions and functional potential of the central circulation to provide oxygen are not analogous to the capacity of the total mitochondrial mass in the skeletal muscles to consume oxygen during metabolism.

However, it seems as if peripheral factors limit endurance performance during exercise lasting 1 hour or longer. It has already been illustrated that in heavy exercise the size of the glycogen store in the muscles may be crucial (Table 2). During very prolonged but milder exercise, the effectiveness of the liver to maintain an optimal blood glucose concentration may become reduced. As discussed in Chapter 9, the resultant hypoglycemia can cause cessation of exercise. However, adaptive changes induced within working muscles by endurance training serve to greatly enhance exercise performance. Probably fundamental are metabolic changes related to the enhanced mitochondrial content of the trained muscle. (cf. Chapter 8). The extreme is evident with elite endurance athletes whose muscle fibers exhibit a uniform and extremely high capacity for aerobic metabolism. In contrast, in normal sedentary individuals muscle fibers generally show much lower metabolism and wider extremes in mitochondrial content (cf. Chapter 2).

ADEQUACY OF DIETARY INTAKE

By definition, when energy intake equals energy output there is an energy balance and the energy content of the body is maintained constant. An imbalance in the equation during a few weeks is not normally catastrophic: A well-fed person has enough energy stored in fatty tissue to cover a minimum of a few weeks' energy output. An excess of energy intake is readily stored as fatty tissue. In contrast, the body's store of oxygen is very limited and is sufficient for approximately 1 minute's oxygen demand before negative symptoms develop (e.g., dysfunction of the central nervous system). However, this limited store is normally not a problem since we live in an ocean of oxygen.

Lack of fluid intake for 1 day will induce negative effects on the circulation and on physical performance, particularly in a hot environment and during exercise with profuse sweating (cf. Chapter 10). Total elimination of vitamins in the diet gradually causes a malfunction. The time course varies with the vitamin. A deficiency in vitamin B_1 (thiamine) is evident after a few weeks, whereas a deficiency in vitamin B_{12} is apparent only after a year or so. As mentioned, protein is normally not an important substrate quantitatively for active muscles. There are no real extraneous stores of protein in the body. A diet deficient in protein does, however, lead to transfer of amino acids from some tissues, such as skeletal muscles, to other tissues with apparently higher priority for survival.

The conclusion is that except for oxygen and fluid, humans can function relatively well physiologically for a number of days without food. However, it is clear that optimal performance of certain exercise tasks requires an adequate dietary intake of appropriate foods.

Blix [4] studied intake of some essential nutrients in individuals with different occupations and in retired people. He found a high correlation between intake of many nutrients (protein, calcium, vitamin A, thiamine, iron) and daily energy intake (Figure

4). This energy intake varied from approximately 5 MJ (1200 kcal) for elderly women to 19 MJ (4500 kcal) for lumberjacks. It is important to note that the demand for these nutrients is relatively independent of physical activity (with the exception of the vitamin B complex). Through the centuries humans have chosen a food intake sufficient to provide an energy intake of 12 MJ (about 3000 kcal) or more. This dietary intake also provides all the needed nutrients. A potential problem could occur with physically inactive individuals who reduce their nutrition intake by calorie restriction in an attempt to limit body weight gains. This could cause malnutrition and produce related disturbances in well-being. The dilemma may be particularly evident for elderly individuals, because the basal metabolic rate declines with aging and in addition older individuals tend to become less active physically. With a reduction in energy output, it is normally recommended that energy intake be proportionately decreased. The inevitable risk in the older person is reduced intake of many essential nutrients (see data presented in Figure 4). Since the older person apparently needs approximately the same intake of essential nutrients as he or she did when younger, the nutritional situation may become critical.

Again it should be emphasized that activation of skeletal muscles is the only factor that markedly increases the body's total metabolic rate and therefore the demand for more energy. The extra energy requirement can easily be covered by increased dietary intake, with the advantage of an increase in the intake of essential nutrients. This is significant, since the demand for essential nutrients increases with physical activity far less than the elevation in energy output would seem to warrant. Therefore, physically active individuals can better secure an adequate intake of essential nutrients with a well-balanced mixed diet than can sedentary individuals who have a relatively smaller caloric balance. From this point of view, it is particularly important for elderly persons to include at a minimum 1 hour of physical activity in their daily routine. The same argument can be applied to obese individuals attempting to lose weight by a combination of caloric restriction and increased physical activity.

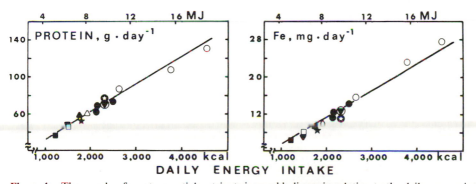

Figure 4. The supply of most essential nutrients is roughly linear in relation to the daily energy intake. The demand for such nutrients remains constant. ○ Lumberjacks (18.9 MJ); metal workers (15.7 MJ); clerks (11.0 MJ); △ elderly men, two cooked meals daily; ▲ elderly women, two cooked meals daily; ◑ female clerks, 16-20 years, two cooked meals daily; ▲ female clerks, 21–34 years, two cooked meals daily; ● wives of lumberjacks (10.5 MJ), of metal workers (9.0 MJ), of clerks (9.0 MJ); □ elderly men, one cooked meal daily; ■ elderly women, one cooked meal daily; ★ female clerks, 16–20 years, one cooked meal daily; ▼ female clerks, 21–34 years, one cooked meal daily. The risk for malnutrition is minimal among high-energy consumers, i.e., the physically active person. (Modified from Blix, G. A study on the relation between total calories and single nutrients in Swedish food. *Acta Soc. Med. Upsal.* 70:117–129, 1965.)

This chapter might well conclude with a quotation about activity versus inactivity from an earlier edition of ref. 2:

The question is frequently raised whether a medical examination is advisable before commencing a training program. Certainly anyone who is doubtful about his state of health should consult a physician. In principle, however, there is less risk in activity than in continuous inactivity. In a nutshell, our opinion is that it is more advisable to pass a careful medical examination if one intends to be sedentary in order to establish whether one's state of health is good enough to stand the inactivity!. (Åstrand and Rodahl [2], 1st ed. 1970, p. 608.

REFERENCES

1. Åstrand, P.-O. Diet, performance, and their interaction. In Barker, L.M. (ed.). *The Psychobiology of Human Food Selection.* Westport, Conn.: AVI Publishing, 1982, p. 17.
2. Åstrand, P.-O., and K. Rodahl. *Textbook of Work Physiology.* 3rd ed. New York: McGraw-Hill, 1986.
3. Bergström, J., L. Hermansen, E. Hultman, and B. Saltin. Diet, muscle glycogen and physical performance. *Acta Physiol. Scand.* 71:140–150, 1967.
4. Blix, G. A Study on the relation between total calories and single nutrients in Swedish food. *Acta Soc. Med. Upsal.* 70:117–129, 1965.
5. Christensen, E.H., and O. Hansen. Arbeitsfhäigkeit und Ehrnärung. *Skand. Arch. Physiol.* 81:160–171, 1939.
6. Garrow, J.S. *Energy Balance and Obesity in Man,* New York: Elsevier, 1978.
7. Holmér, I. Physiology of swimming man, *Acta Physiol. Scand.* (Suppl.) 407:1–55, 1974.
8. Holmér, I., and P.-O. Åstrand. Swimming training and maximal oxygen uptake. *J. Appl. Physiol.* 33:510–513, 1972.
9. Saltin, B. Hemodynamic adaptations to exercise. *Am. J. Cardiol.* 55:42D–47D, 1985.
10. Widdowson, E.M. The response to unlimited food. In *Studies in Undernutrition.* Wuppertal 1946–1949. Spec. Rep. No. 375. London: Medical Research Council, 1951.

Chapter 2

MUSCLE FIBER RECRUITMENT PATTERNS AND THEIR METABOLIC CORRELATES

Robert B. Armstrong, Ph.D.

Skeletal muscles perform a broad range of contractile activities on a daily basis. Contrast, for example, the precise control of the extrinsic flexor muscles of the fingers in playing a Chopin polonaise with the performance of the same muscles in grasping a barbell in a dead lift. These radical alterations in muscle function in the performance of various motor tasks are dependent both on central nervous system control of contraction and on intrinsic differences among the fibers in the muscles. Change in the force that the muscle produces or in the velocity of shortening or lengthening of the muscle is primarily dependent upon the patterns and magnitude of neural activation of the muscle cells. The neural activation patterns, however, are superimposed on a population of muscle fibers that display a spectrum of contractile properties. Activation of the appropriate muscle fibers with the appropriate patterns of neural input leads to the desired movement.

Performance of any given activity in turn depends on metabolic processes in the muscle fibers, since adenosine triphosphate (ATP), which provides the energy for contractions, is consumed at high rates when active tension is produced. It is therefore not surprising that the specific fibers activated to produce force in a muscle undergo acute metabolic changes designed to maintain ATP levels in the cells adequate to support the

particular level of contractile activity. Just as fibers within a muscle have differing contractile properties suited for particular types of activity, the fibers have different metabolic capacities designed to meet their energy needs when they are recruited. Thus, within a given skeletal muscle the physiological and metabolic properties of the individual fibers reflect the particular functions of the fibers, and the central nervous system has a variety of fiber types available for accomplishing various motor tasks.

The purpose of this chapter is to discuss (a) the properties of the different types of fibers in the skeletal muscles, (b) the patterns of distribution of the fiber types within and among the muscles, (c) the patterns of recruitment of the fibers during exercise, and (d) the patterns of metabolic changes that occur in the active muscles. Recent references, particularly reviews, that will give the reader detailed coverage of the topic, are listed at the end of the chapter.

PROPERTIES OF THE SKELETAL MUSCLE FIBER TYPES

The basic functional contractile unit in skeletal muscle in a conscious human or animal is the motor unit, which consists of one alpha-motoneuron and the group of muscle fibers it innervates and controls. The cell body of the alpha-motoneuron resides in the ventral horn of the spinal cord (or in the nucleus of one of the cranial nerves), and the axon projects out to the muscle through a spinal (or cranial) nerve (Figure 1). In the muscle the axon diverges to innervate its constituent muscle fibers. The number of muscle fibers innervated by each alpha-motoneuron varies from several to more than 1000 [9]. In mammalian skeletal muscles, each muscle fiber is innervated by only one alpha-motoneuron, so each motor unit consists exclusively of one neuron and its constituent muscle cells.

It is generally assumed that all of the muscle fibers of a given motor unit have the same contractile and metabolic characteristics, that is, that the constituent fibers are of the same type [9, 34]. In fact, the fiber type of the muscle cells in a given motor unit is primarily dictated by the innervating alpha-motoneuron; alteration of the normal neural stimulation pattern to a motor unit results in a change in the fiber composition [30]. Each skeletal muscle then consists of a population of motor units with varying physiological and biochemical properties suited to the functional requirements of the particular muscle.

The fibers of a given motor unit are not clustered together in the muscle, but are distributed so that adjacent fibers in cross section normally belong to different motor units. This gives the muscle a typical "checkerboard" appearance when transverse sections of the muscle are cut and treated histochemically to identify the different fiber types (Figure 2). On the other hand, the constituent fibers of a particular motor unit are normally not distributed homogeneously throughout the entire muscle, but congregate within general geographical regions (e.g., anterior, posterior, medial, etc.) in the muscle [9].

For most skeletal muscles in mammals, the constituent motor units exhibit a quantitative spectrum for any given physiological or metabolic characteristic (Table 1). For example, in medial gastrocnemius muscle of the cat, the twitch contraction times for the total population of motor units vary in a continuous spectrum from about 20 to about 100 ms, a five fold difference [11]. Similarly, the metabolic capacities of the fibers in a particular muscle vary over a spectrum from relatively low to relatively high. The oxidative enzymes of individual fibers in rabbit muscles, for example, cover about a 13-fold range in activities [40]. For both the physiological and metabolic characteristics, the values among the population of motor units in the muscle are continuous, with no clear lines of demarcation. Nonetheless, by means of histochemistry, the fibers in a muscle can be divided into different populations and classified as different fiber types (Figure 2). Whereas this classification of the fibers into several types is convenient for the study of muscle function, the divisions are to a certain extent arbitrary, since the various physiological and biochemical properties do not always fall into distinct categories.

In most muscle fiber type classification systems based on histochemistry, the primary assay is for myofibrillar adenosine triphosphatase (ATPase) activity. When the

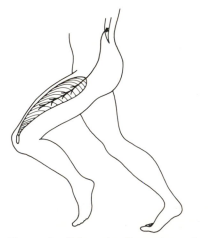

Figure 1. Schematic illustration of an alpha-motoneuron projecting from the spinal cord through a peripheral nerve to innervate a population of fibers in the muscle. The neuron and muscle fibers constitute a motor unit.

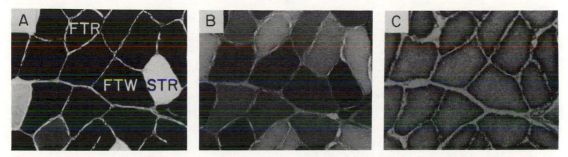

Figure 2. Serial sections of rat plantaris muscle histochemically assayed for myofibrillar adenosine triphosphatase (ATPase) activity after alkaline preincubation (A), myofibrillar ATPase activity after acid preincubation (B), and nicotinamide adenine dinucleotide (NADH)-tetrazolium reductase activity (C). Three fibers are identified on the section for ATPase after alkaline preincubation: slow-twitch red (STR); fast-twitch red (FTR); and fast-twitch white (FTW). See Table 1 for other nomenclature.

Table 1. PROPERTIES OF SKELETAL MUSCLE FIBER TYPES IN RODENT AND CAT MUSCLES.*

CHARACTERISTIC	FIBER TYPE		
	Slow-Twitch Red	Fast-Twitch Red	Fast-Twitch White
Histochemistry (rodent)			
Reaction to Myofibrillar ATPase assay, alkaline preincubation	Low	High	High
Reaction to Myofibrillar ATPase assay, acid preincubation	High	Low	Medium
Reaction to oxidative enzyme assay (NADH tetrazolium reductase)	High	High	Low
Reaction to glycolytic enzyme assay (Phosphorylase)	Low	High	High
Morphology (rodent)			
Fiber diameter	Small	Small-medium	Large
Capillary supply	Large	Large	Small
Biochemistry (rodent)			
Succinate dehydrogenase activity (μmol/min/g)	3.36	5.04	1.71
Phosphofructokinase activity (μmol/min/g)	17.20	49.80	57.60
Myoglobin (mg/g)	1.39	1.44	0.31
Physiology (cat)			
Twitch contraction time (ms)	58–130	30–55	20–47
Maximum tetanic tension (g/motor unit)	1.2–35	4.5–55	30–130
Fatigue index	>0.75	>0.75	<0.25

ATPase, adenosine triphosphatase; NADH, nicotinamide adenine dinucleotide, reduced form.

*Near-equivalent fiber type nomenclature:

Slow-twitch red: slow-twitch oxidative (SO) [29]
type I [8]
slow (S) [11]

Fast-twitch red: fast-twitch oxidative glycolytic (FOG) [29]
type IIa [8]
fast-twitch fatigue resistant (FK) [11]

Fast-twitch white: fast-twitch glycolytic (FG) [29]
type IIb (8)
fast-twitch fatigable (FF) [11].

myofibrillar ATPase assay is performed on mammalian muscle tissue preincubated in an alkaline medium (pH 10.3), the fibers generally exhibit either an intense reaction or no reaction for the enzyme (Figure 2). Fibers with an intense reaction (fast-twitch) have a relatively high myofibrillar ATPase activity as determined biochemically, and those with no reaction (slow-twitch) have a relatively low ATPase activity (Table 1) [9, 34]. The fibers with high ATPase activity have relatively fast contraction times, while those with low reactivity are relatively slow. Because of these relationships, we have a general classification scheme that identifies fast-twitch (high myosin ATPase) and slow-twitch (low myosin ATPase) fibers [9, 34]. When the muscle fibers are histochemically assayed for myofibrillar ATPase following an acid preincubation (pH 4.3–4.7), a reverse staining pattern is generally evident and the fast-twitch fibers can be subdivided into subtypes (Figure 2).*

Histochemical fiber type classification systems also may include an assay for a mitochondrial enzyme, which provides an indication of the oxidative capacity of the fibers (Table 1 and Figure 2). As already pointed out, a spectrum of oxidative capacities exists among the fibers within a given muscle, but the fibers can arbitrarily be divided into populations with relatively high and relatively low oxidative capacities. In most mammals, slow-twitch fibers have a relatively high capacity and are red in appearance; on the other hand, the fast-twitch fibers typically have a broader range of oxidative enzyme capacities [2, 34]. Thus, it is common to divide the fast-twitch fibers into high and low oxidative capacity subpopulations. Fast-twitch red fibers (high oxidative) identified with an assay for an oxidative enzyme tend to be the same fibers as those classed as type IIa fibers (cf. Table 1) using the myofibrillar ATPase assay after acid preincubation, but the relationship is not constant and cannot be depended upon [28].

The fiber types can also be classed according to their glycolytic enzyme capacities. This analysis is usually based upon an assay for one or more of the primary enzymes in the glycogenolytic (e.g., phosphorylase) or glycolytic (e.g., phosphofructokinase or lactate dehydrogenase) pathways in the fibers. In most mammals, the slow-twitch fibers have a relatively low glycolytic capacity, and the fast-twitch fibers have a relatively high capacity (Table 1 and Figure 3) [10, 23, 29, 34].

From the foregoing, it is clear that skeletal muscle fiber types have been classified in different ways [cf. 10, 12, 34]. It is important to recognize that, for any classification scheme, relative differences between fiber types of a given species may not be directly applicable

*This histochemical procedure is the basis for a classification scheme in which fibers are identified as type I (slow-twitch) and type II (fast-twitch) fibers [8]. There is a general correspondence with the nomenclature used throughout this volume. All slow-twitch red fibers would be classified as type I. Most fast-twitch red fibers would be identified as type IIa, and most fast-twitch white fibers would be identified as type IIb. It is in the fast-twitch fiber population that some discrepancies exist between the two systems. Also, with the acid preincubation ATPase method there is a fourth fiber type, identified as type IIc. This fiber type exists in relatively small numbers in most muscles and may represent a transitional form of myosin.

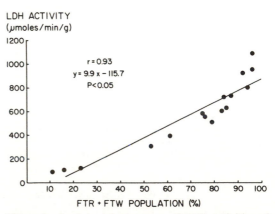

Figure 3. Lactate dehydrogenase (LDH) activities of various skeletal muscles of miniature swine plotted as a function of total fast-twitch (red & white) fiber populations of the muscle samples. LDH activity was assayed with pyruvate as the substrate (unpublished results).

to the fiber types of another species (e.g., humans). In the present volume, we have chosen to use a descriptive nomenclature that refers to both the contractile and the metabolic properties of the fibers. The fibers will be classed into three types: fast-twitch red (FTR), fast-twitch white (FTW), and slow-twitch red. These three fiber types appear to be present in most locomotory muscles in most mammalian species [1, 2]. As is obvious from the nomenclature, this system of classification incorporates both physiological (i.e., fast/slow twitch) and metabolic (i.e., oxidative capacity) characteristics in the identification scheme. The advantage of this system is that even those not familiar with the nuances of fiber type classification can quickly grasp the salient properties of the fibers. The primary disadvantages of the system are that (a) the determination of whether a fast fiber is designated oxidative or not is arbitrary because of the spectrum of oxidative capacities represented in the fibers in a muscle (Figure 2) and (b) the oxidative capacity of a given fiber is very plastic, so that fiber classification is dependent upon the contractile history of the fiber. The general correspondence between this fiber type nomenclature and three other commonly used classification schemes is provided in Table 1.

Finally, it should be stressed again that although the fibers within a given motor unit are homogeneous regarding their physiological and metabolic properties, the different motor units within a muscle present a quantitative spectrum for any given variable. Thus, the designation of fiber types is somewhat arbitrary, and simply provides a convenient means of grouping muscle fibers into general functional categories for study.

DISTRIBUTION OF MUSCLE FIBER TYPES

The function(s) of a skeletal muscle is (are) reflected in its fiber composition. For example, the flight muscles of small bats that fly for extended periods with high wing-beat frequencies are composed entirely of fast-twitch red fibers, and the flexor muscles of slow arboreal mammals like the sloth and the slow loris contain high populations of slow-twitch red fibers. Also, different muscles within a given animal differ markedly in their fiber compositions, which permits the animal to perform a variety of motor tasks.

If a particular muscle is required to perform contractions that produce high shortening velocities, then it must possess fibers with high myosin ATPase activity, since shortening speed is proportional to ATPase activity of the myosin in the fiber. However, high ATPase activity results in rapid ATP hydrolysis by the muscle fiber, so recruitment of these fibers is energetically costly. For postural maintenance or contractions requiring relatively slow shortening velocities, it is more economical to recruit fibers with low myosin ATPase activities, that is, slow-twitch red fibers. These fibers are resistant to fatigue because their rate of ATP hydrolysis is relatively low and because they possess a relatively high aerobic capacity [9, 34] and blood flow [25]. Thus, for prolonged periods of contraction they are able to provide adequately for their energy needs.

On the other hand, fast-twitch fibers, when recruited for high power or rapid shortening contractions, have a much higher ATP utilization rate and are less resistant to fatigue than are slow-twitch red ribers [9]. Fast-twitch red fibers have a high oxidative capacity (in rodents, higher than slow-twitch red fibers, Table), so they are more fatigue resistant than fast-twitch white fibers, but less resistant than slow-twitch red fibers, because of the higher rate of ATP use.

In terrestrial quadrupedal and bipedal mammals, distinguishable patterns of fiber type distribution occur in the extensor and flexor muscle groups [1, 2, 25]. Normally the most deeply located muscle in an antigravity extensor group is composed primarily of slow-twitch red fibers, and the more superficially situated muscles in the group contain higher populations of fast-twitch fibers (Figure 4). For example, soleus

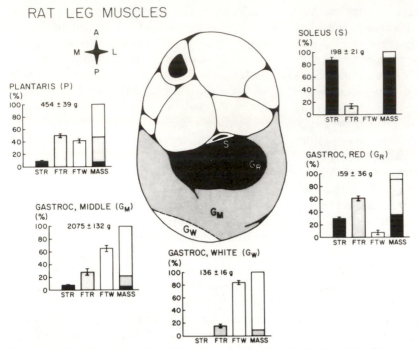

Figure 4. Cross-sectional view of the rat leg showing the distribution of the fiber types (STR, slow-twitch red; FTR, fast-twitch red; FTW, fast-twitch white) in the ankle extensor muscles. Included in the histograms are the muscle masses (g), the populations (%) of the fiber types in the muscles, and the proportion of the muscle mass composed of three fiber types. (From Armstrong, R.B., and M.H. Laughlin. Muscle function during locomotion in mammals. In Gilles, R. [ed.]. *Circulation, Respiration, and Metabolism, Current Comparative Approaches.* Berlin: Springer-Verlag, 1985, pp. 56–63).

muscle in most mammals (including man) has a high percentage of slow-twitch red fibers, whereas gastrocnemius muscle contains more fast-twitch fibers. In flexor muscle groups, the deep muscle is not composed of slow-twitch red fibers.

Characteristic patterns of fiber type distribution can also be found within individual muscles [2, 25]. In most mammals including humans, the deepest portions of locomotory muscles have the highest proportion of the slow-twitch red fibers that are present in the muscle (Figure 4). Also, the fast-twtich red fibers in the muscle tend to concentrate in the deeper portions of the muscle. The most superficial parts of the muscle, then, have the highest percentage of fast-twitch white fibers in the muscle. The degree of stratification of the fiber types within muscles varies among different mammals; human muscles generally show a lesser degree of stratification of fibers

than do those of other animals that have been studied [25]. However, the general pattern of fiber distribution in locomotory muscles from deep to superficial regions is slow-twitch red to fast-twitch red to fast-twitch white.

RECRUITMENT OF THE MUSCLE FIBER TYPES

Muscle function is a result of change in the relationship between the external load or resistance and the internal force of the muscle. For the velocity of a concentric (shortening) contraction to increase, the active tension produced by the contractile elements of the muscle must increase; for the velocity of an eccentric (lengthening) contraction to increase, the active tension must decrease. The amount of active tension produced by a muscle at any given time during a motor task is the critical controlled variable in the performance of the task.

The central nervous system changes the amount of tension actively produced by a muscle at any given moment by two primary means: (a) by varying the number of motor units (and hence, muscle mass) that are active and (b) by varying the force generated by a given active motor unit by altering the discharge frequency of the innervating alpha-motoneuron (which alters the amount of force produced by the crossbridges that is transmitted to the bone of insertion through the series elastic element) [9, 18]. These two phenomena may be referred to as "spatial recruitment" and "rate coding," respectively (Figure 5).

Spatial recruitment and rate coding are dependent upon both control of the motor units by the central nervous system and direct afferent feedback from the muscles themselves. Control is exerted at the level of the motoneuron pool, which is composed of the cell bodies of the alpha-motoneurons innervating a particular muscle (or, more globally, those innervating the muscles of a

synergistic muscle group [9, 18, 19]. The cell bodies of the alpha-motoneurons are spatially localized in the ventral horn of the spinal cord or in the nucleus of a cranial nerve, and are all influenced by excitatory and inhibitory presynaptic neural influences impinging on the pool from central and peripheral pathways. Although the synaptic input into the alpha-motoneuron pool for a particular muscle is similar for all the neurons in the pool, the responses of the neurons to the input differ because of variation in the functional thresholds of the constituent alpha-motoneurons [9]. For a given level of excitation (or comparable decrease in inhibition) of the pool of neurons from presynaptic pathways, only a fraction of the motoneurons in the pool reach threshold and generate action potentials. The remainder of the neurons in the pool are facilitated but fail to reach threshold and discharge. An increase in the excitatory input into the pool allows more alpha-motoneurons to reach threshold and begin to discharge, which in turn increases the number of active motor units and the force produced by the muscle [19]. This progression accounts for changes

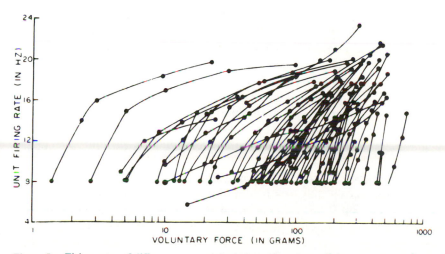

Figure 5. Firing rates of different motor units in human extensor digitorum communis muscle as a function of voluntary isometric force. Note that the muscle increases voluntary force both by increasing the firing rate of individual motor units and by progressively recruiting new motor units. Motor units begin discharging at about the same frequency and increase their rate of discharge twofold to threefold. (From Monster, A.W., and H. Chan. Isometric force production by motor units of extensor digitorum communis muscle in man. *J. Neurophysiol.* 40:1432–1443, 1977.)

in spatial recruitment. In addition, a greater excitation of the pool by presynaptic pathways increases the rate of discharge of the active motor units, which increases the force the motor units produce through the process of rate coding. When an action potential is produced in a given alpha-motoneuron, it is transmitted to the constituent muscle fibers under most circumstances. The final integration of motor control thus occurs at the level of the motoneuron pool.

Although the factors that influence the functional thresholds of the motoneurons in a motoneuron pool are complex, one property of the neurons that is related to threshold is size [19]. The smallest alpha-motoneurons have the lowest functional thresholds. These are the first motor units to be recruited during low-force contractile efforts. With increasing muscular forces, successively larger alpha-motoneurons attain threshold and begin to discharge. This relationship between motoneuron size and excitability is known as the "size principle" [19]. For many motor tasks that have been studied, variations in muscular force are achieved through successive recruitment or derecruitment of motoneurons (and the accompanying changes in rate coding in the active motor units) according to the size principle (Figure 6). There is also a relationship between the size of the alpha-motoneurons in the pool (and hence, the order of recruitment) and the types of muscle fibers they innervate [19]. The smaller motoneurons in the pool innervate slow-twitch red fibers; successively larger motoneurons innervate fast-twitch red fibers, and the largest neurons innervate fast-twitch white fibers. According to the size principle, the fibers that would be recruited for low-force contractions would be slow-teitch red. With progressive increases in muscular force, the central nervous system would successively and fast-twitch red and then fast-twitch white fibers to the population of active fibers.

It is not the purpose of this chapter to discuss neural recruitment mechanisms in detail. It should be mentioned, however, that

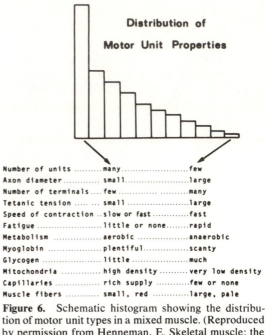

Figure 6. Schematic histogram showing the distribution of motor unit types in a mixed muscle. (Reproduced by permission from Henneman, E. Skeletal muscle: the servant of the nervous system. In Mountcastle, V.B. [ed.]. *Medical Physiology*, 14th ed. St. Louis: C. V. Mosby Co., 1980).

the recruitment order is not just a function of size of the alpha-motoneurons but may be changed under some circumstances. For example, group Ia afferent fibers from the muscle spindles preferentially synapse to a greater extent with alpha-motoneurons to slow-twitch red motor units than with those to fast-twitch motor units [9]. Hence, preferential recruitment of slow-twitch red units during periods of group Ia discharge (for example, during muscle stretch) is not entirely due to their relative size. Second, the apparent order of recruitment among the motor units may be altered during performance of some motor tasks. During high-frequency oscillating limb movements in cats, for example, fast-twitch fibers may be recruited without activation of slow-twitch red units [38].Nonetheless, the normal sequential recruitment, that is, slow-twitch red to fast-twitch red to fast-twitch white, can be observed when animals progress from standing to high-speed locomotion. While standing, the motor units that produce force to maintain posture are principally of the slow-twitch red type [9, 39, 43]. When the animal begins to walk, fast-twitch red fibers are recruited in addition to the active slow-twitch red fibers to provide the necessary increases in force [5]. With increasing locomotory speed, additional motor units are activated, until during high speed running, fibers of all three types may be involved [5, 9, 43]. During contractions requiring maximal strength, it is probable that all motor units in at least some muscles are recruited to contribute to the force production, although this has not been demonstrated with any certainty.

The fibers in motor units are able to adapt to altered usage. For example, when the alpha-motoneurons of fast-twitch motor units are chronically stimulated over several weeks with electrical stimulation patterns and frequencies similar to those found in slow-twitch red motor units, the fibers show increased oxidative capacities (i.e., increased mitochondrial, myoglobin, and capillary density), decreased glycolytic enzyme activities, and decreased myosin ATPase activities [30]. In other words, the fast-twitch fibers transform to resemble slow-twitch red fibers. These chronic stimulation experiments have shown unequivocally that the basic properties of the muscle fibers can be changed with altered usage.

Changes in physiological use patterns, such as occur during prolonged endurance training, also can cause alterations in the fibers. It has been known for some time that endurance exercise training results in elevated oxidative capacities of the fibers recruited during the exercise [20]. Thus, relatively high-intensity endurance exercise stimulates increases in aerobic potential of all of the fiber types in the active muscles [20, 34]. Recently, convincing evidence has also been obtained that myosin can be transformed with prolonged moderate-intensity endurance training, so that active muscles demonstrate increases in the proportions of slow-twitch red fibers [30]. The decrease in myosin ATPase in fibers with endurance training presumably increases the economy (i.e., force produced per energy utilized) of force production during contraction.

Many earlier studies did not demonstrate changes of fast-twitch to slow-twitch fibers with training [34]. Apparently the intensity and duration of the training required to induce changes in myosin are quite high. However, the tendency for competitive endurance athletes to have more slow-twitch red (type I) fibers in the muscles that are primarily used in their events than do sedentary persons (or athletes who are not involved in high-endurance events) [34] may be explained by training-induced transformation of the myosin. Alternatively, higher populations of slow-twitch red fibers in endurance athletes may represent genetic differences among groups. Hence, world-class athletes may have more slow-twitch red fibers because they have selected events for which they are already well endowed with high economy muscle fibers (slow-twitch red). Whether selection or fiber transformation is the explanation for the observed group differences among world-class athletes remains to be determined, but it seems possible that both could contribute.

METABOLIC CORRELATES TO RECRUITMENT PATTERNS

Muscle Oxidative Capacity

Given the selectivity and reproducibility in recruitment order of motor units during exercise, it could be predicted that the metabolic capacities of the fibers in the motor units would be matched to the particular functions of the units. As pointed out earlier, this matching is evident in the relative oxidative capacities of the fibers. Slow-twitch red fibers, which are normally recruited during most muscle contractions, have relatively high aerobic potentials and a high resistance to fatigue (Table 1) [9, 34]. The fatigue resistance presumably accrues both from the high oxidative capacity and from a low rate of ATP utilization. Thus, the slow-twitch red motor units may be successfully recruited for prolonged periods. At the other extreme, fast-twitch white motor units are recruited only during forceful contractions (or when the units with greater oxidative capacity have fatigued after prolonged use). How often these fast-twitch white fibers are recruited depends on the behavior of the person or animal. Sedentary, cage-confined laboratory rats have a high population (about 70%) of fast-twitch white fibers in their total hind limb musculature [6]. On the other hand, active foraging animals such as dogs have no fast-twitch white fibers [7]. All of the fibers in the dog hind limb muscles have high-oxidative capacities (i.e., fast-twitch red or slow-twitch red). Similarly, sedentary humans have a relatively high population of low-oxidative capacity fast-twitch white fibers, whereas all of the fast-twitch (and slow-twitch) fibers in the conditioned muscles of highly trained endurance athletes may be highly oxidative [15].

These observations, and those demonstrating that the oxidative capacity of the muscles rapidly decreases during detraining [34], suggest that the muscle maintains the oxidative capacity at the lowest level consistent with the fibers' daily energy requirements. When daily use of the fibers increases, the oxidative capacity increases. These increases in oxidative capacity in working muscles are disproportionately larger than the elevations in maximal oxygen consumption ($\dot{V}O_2$max) induced by the training program [34, 35].

Muscle Blood Flow

When an athlete changes from rest to intense exercise requiring $\dot{V}O_2$max, there may be a 20 to 25-fold increase in the rate of oxygen use by the body [31, 36]. More specifically, resting oxygen, consumption of a 70-kg man is about 0.20 L/min, of which ap-

proximately 20% is due to needs of the skeletal muscles (which constitute about 40% of the body mass). With these values, the $\dot{V}O_2$ of the total skeletal musculature at rest would be about 0.04 L/min. During exercise at $\dot{V}O_2$max, whole body $\dot{V}O_2$ may increase to 5 L/min. During this intense exercise, at least 80% of the oxygen may be used by the skeletal muscles [31]. These simple calculations demonstrate that total muscle $\dot{V}O_2$ may increase from 0.04 to 4 L/min, a 100-fold increase in aerobic metabolism. Similar alterations in distribution occur for the cardiac output (Figure 7).

Although measurements of how much of the muscle mass is active during exercise at maximal oxygen consumption have not been made, it is probable that a relatively small percentage of the muscle fibers in the body are simultaneously recruited. If it is assumed that half of the muscle fibers are active during exercise at $\dot{V}O_2$max (which prob-

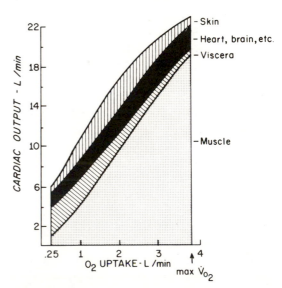

Figure 7. Schematic representation of the changes in magnitude and distribution of cardiac output in human subjects during exercise as a function of exercise intensity (expressed as oxygen uptake). (From Rowell, L.B. Circulation to skeletal muscle. In Ruch, T.C., and H. D. Patton [eds.]. *Physiology and Biophysics II*. Philadelphia: W. B. Saunders, 1974, pp. 200–214.)

ably is an overestimate), that 40% of the body mass is skeletal muscle, and that 80% of the oxygen used is consumed by the active muscle fibers (which may be an underestimate), it can be calculated that the active muscle fibers in a 70-kg man with a $\dot{V}O_2$max of 5 L/min would consume oxygen at a rate of close to 300 ml/min/kg of active muscle fiber mass. This is similar to the oxygen consumption of the quadriceps muscle group (250-450 ml/min/kg) during one-legged maximal bicycle exercise [33]. The oxygen consumption by the specific muscle fibers that are active is considerably higher than the calculated whole body $\dot{V}O_2$max of 71 ml/min/kg.

In terms of pure biological economy, it is logical that the metabolic apparatus in the skeletal muscles and the metabolic delivery system (i.e., the circulation) be designed so that the specific muscle fibers that are recruited over the normal range of activities, up to $\dot{V}O_2$max, have adequate enzymatic capacity for oxidative phosphorylation and adequate extracellular and intracellular capacities for O_2 and substrate delivery. Recall that the slow-twitch red and fast-twitch red fibers have the highest oxidative capacities (Table 1) and are the fibers recruited most often according to the size principle. Fast-twitch white fibers, which are recruited less frequently, have lower oxidative capacities and are more dependent upon anaerobic processes when they are active.

The question may be asked why animals (or humans) do not all have 100% high oxidative motor units in their muscles and high maximal aerobic powers to support the muscles. Some animals do have very high aerobic capacities and completely oxidative muscles [2, 7]—many breeds of dogs fit this description. The best answer to the question appears to be that it is energetically costly to maintain high oxidative capacities in the muscles and the associated respiratory and cardiovascular structure. It is well known that during detraining there is rapid loss of muscle aerobic capacity [34]. Further, animal species (and humans) that are relatively

inactive have low aerobic capacities. Thus, it appears to be a law of nature that the muscle oxidative system and the supporting cardiovascular system be maintained at as low a level as possible to support some "average" daily activity level. A reasonable assumption is that this represents energy economy on the part of the organism.

Delivery of O_2 at a rate of 30 ml/min/100 g of active muscle fibers (see preceding calculations) would require a minimum blood flow of 200 ml/min/100 g of muscle if it is assumed that O_2 extraction is 15 ml/100 ml of blood. Since cardiac output for the 70-kg subject would be about 25 L/min, average blood flow in all tissues would be about 36 ml/min/100 g. Thus, delivery of the required blood flow of 200 ml/min/100 g of muscle to the active high-oxidative capacity muscle fibers requires that the circulatory system shunt blood from inactive muscle and nonmuscular organs to the active fibers. Blood flow in some of the visceral organs and inactive skeletal muscles (e.g., facial muscles) decreases considerably during brief bouts of high-intensity locomotory exercise [24, 25].

Because exercise at $\dot{V}O_2$max taxes the cardiovascular system to its limit to provide adequate oxygen to the active muscle fibers, it is clear that the system must be designed to deliver the oxygenated blood preferentially to the specific muscle fibers that are active during the bout of exercise. Moreover, the system should ideally be designed so that the blood flow is made available specifically to the muscle fibers that have the metabolic apparatus to oxidize substrates for ATP synthesis aerobically.

Distribution of cardiac output among and within muscles has been studied extensively in exercising rats, and most of the predictions suggested in the preceding paragraph appear to be true [24]. When the animals are simply standing on the treadmill, the highest blood flow among muscles is in those with relatively high proportions of slow-twitch red fibers, which are known to be active during postural maintenance [24, 25]. For example, preexercise (PE) blood flow in rat soleus muscle is two to six times higher than in the other ankle plantar flexor muscles (Figure 8). When the animal begins to walk on the treadmill, blood flow in the slow-twitch red regions remains relatively high, but there is also rapid elevation in perfusion of fast-twitch red fibers (red gastrocnemius muscle, walking at 15 m/min, Figure 8). During slow locomotion, blood flow in muscles predominantly composed of fast-twitch white fibers actually decreases below the preexercise level (white gastrocnemius muscle, walking at 15 m/min, Figure 8). Hence, blood flow is specifically distributed to the oxidative mus-cle fibers that are recruited for the exercise according to the size principle.

The mechanisms that control blood flow in muscles during exercise have been studied in detail, particularly in isolated muscle experiments [14, 21, 22, 25, 37, 41, 42]. Much is still not known, but the primary mechanisms for blood flow redistribution appear to be the two opposing influences of sympathetic nervous system vasoconstriction mediated through alpha-adrenergic receptors, and local metabolic factor vasodilation. With exercise there is a general elevation in the activity of the sympathetic nervous system,

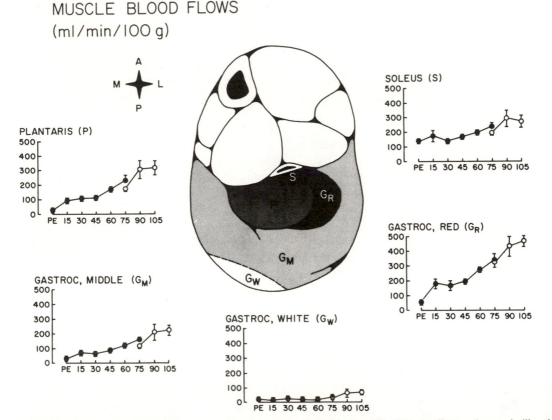

Figure 8. Muscle blood flows in rat ankle extensor muscles during preexercise (PE) standing on the treadmill and at 1 minute of exercise from fast walking (15 m/min) through high-speed galloping (105 m/min). The intensity of shading of the muscles in cross section is proportional to the population of high oxidative capacity (slow-twitch red & fast-twitch red) fibers. (From Armstrong, R.B., and M.H. Laughlin. Muscle function during locomotion in mammals. In Gilles, R. [ed.]. *Circulation, Respiration, and Metabolism. Current Comparative Approaches.* Berlin: Springer-Verlag, 1985, pp. 56–63).

resulting in increases in circulating cat-echolamines and norepinephrine release from sympathetic postganglionic neurons. When these adrenergic humoral and trans-mitter substances bind to alpha-adrenergic receptors in the vascular smooth muscle, they stimulate constriction of the arteriolar resistance vessels, which in turn increases the resistance to blood flow in the tissues. Under these conditions, blood flow de-creases in the inactive skeletal muscle regions and in other tissues. However, in the active muscles, a variety of local metabolic factors (e.g., low PO_2 or elevated K^+, phos-phate, lactate, adenosine, or osmolarity) can cause smooth muscle to relax so the resis-tance vessels dilate. In this way flow may be elevated specifically to the muscle fibers that are recruited during the exercise. Unfortu-nately, as indicated previously, the details of these mechanisms are still not known.

With increasing locomotory speeds, as the animal progressively recruits more motor units in the muscles, there is a corresponding elevation of blood flow to the regions of the activated fibers [24]. For example, flow does not significantly increase in the regions of fast-twitch white fibers until the animal at-tains relatively high running speeds and these fibers are recruited (white gastroc-nemius muscle, running at 75 m/min, Figure 8). Thus, in the rat there is a close rela-tionship between the patterns of recruitment in the muscles and the patterns of blood flow for oxygen delivery [24].

There is also a close correspondence be-tween the maximal blood flows that are achieved in the muscles and the oxidative capacities of the constituent muscle fibers [25]. In terms of biological economy, this is the sensible way to structure the system. The fibers with the greatest density of mi-tochondria and myoglobin [20] have the highest blood flows during exercise. In the rat, the fast-twitch red fibers fit this descrip-tion. There also are differences in the number of capillaries adjacent to the different types of fibers. The high-oxidative capacity fibers have more surrounding capillaries than do the fast-twitch white fibers [3]. Thus, in the rat there is a relationship between the capil-larity and the maximal blood flow capacities. In some animals, including humans, it is probable that the slow-twitch red fibers dem-onstrate this relationship, since these fibers have higher oxidative capacities in these species.

At the present time no methods are avail-able for measuring the distribution of blood flow within human muscles during locomo-tory exercise, so whether the distinctive dis-tribution patterns observed in rats also occur in humans is not known. Since the fiber types are distributed more homogeneously within human muscles than in those of most mam-mals, and since the oxidative capacities and capillarities of the fiber types are more simi-lar in human muscles [34], the distinctive patterns of blood flow distribution described for the rat may be less evident in humans. Nonetheless, the same principle that blood flow is specifically directed to recruited muscle fibers during exercise, undoubtedly pertains.

Glycogen Loss Patterns

Another metabolic factor that has been shown to follow recruitment patterns in muscles is glycogen loss. In fact, the map-ping of patterns of glycogen loss in fibers provides a convenient method of obtaining rough estimates of which fibers in the mus-cles have been active during a bout of exer-cise.

When human subjects perform submax-imal prolonged exercise, the first fibers to lose glycogen in the active muscles are the slow-twitch red fibers (Figure 9) [16, 34]. Because these fibers would be the least likely to lose glycogen if all fibers in the muscles were active (because of their low ATPase activities, high oxidative capacities, and sub-strate preferences), this finding provides evi-dence that the slow-twitch red fibers are recruited to a greater extent than the fast-twitch fibers during low-intensity exercise.

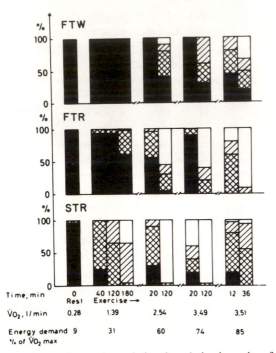

Figure 9. Schematic depicting the relative intensity of the periodic acid Schiff (PAS) stain for glycogen in the different fiber types in human subjects at rest and after exercise at varying intensities and durations. Intensity ratings: dark, high glycogen; cross hatched, moderate glycogen; hatched, low glycogen; open, no glycogen. (From Saltin, B., and P.D. Gollnick. Skeletal muscle adaptability: Significance for metabolism and performance. In Peachey, L.D., R.H. Adrian, and S.R. Geiger [eds.]. *Handbook of Physiology. Sec 10: Skeletal Muscle*. Bethesda, Md.: American Physiological Society, 1983, pp. 555–631.)

high intensities [17, 34], slow-twitch red and fast-twitch fibers initially lose glycogen, indicating that all fiber types have been recruited, The extent of slow-twitch red fiber recruitment in high-intensity exercise will usually be underestimated from glycogen loss because of the fibers' high oxidative capacity and reliance on fatty acids as a metabolic substrate.

In animal studies it has been shown that during treadmill walking, both slow-twitch red and fast-twitch red fibers lose glycogen [5, 9]. These same fibers continue to lose glycogen during slow to moderate trotting speeds, but during fast trotting, fast-twitch white fibers may also be involved. During galloping, fibers of all three types lose glycogen.

Enzymatic Adaptation to Training

One of the primary changes that takes place in the skeletal muscles with exercise training is elevation in the mitochondrial volume and in the activities of enzymes of the Krebs cycle and components of the respiratory chain [20, 34]. The molecular mechanisms that regulate these changes in the muscle cells are not known, but the changes are related to the intensity and duration of the exercise bouts and occur in the specific muscles utilized in the exercise. It is reasonable to assume that the increase in mitochondrial components is therefore stimulated by factors associated with the increased metabolic fluxes in the active muscle fibers. From foregoing discussion, it would be predicted that elevation in oxidative capacity should occur specifically in the motor units that are recruited at the training intensity used. This relationship has in fact been demonstrated in rats trained at different intensities [13]. When the animals train at slow treadmill speeds, the increase in oxidative capacity occurs exclusively in the deep red muscles. These findings are in keeping with the fact that at slow treadmill speeds the animals recruit slow-twitch red and fast-

This is consistent with the general concept of the size principle [19]. With continued exercise, the slow-twitch red fibers eventually lose their glycogen stores and the fast-twitch fibers begin to lose their glycogen as well [16]. This progression of loss of glycogen continues until the subject cannot continue the exercise. These observations have been interpreted to indicate that the slow-twitch red fibers are initially recruited to support the submaximal exercise, but as their glycogen stores are depleted and they are not metabolically able to continue to produce the required forces, fast-twitch fibers are progressively activated to maintain the muscle output. When human subjects exercise at

twitch red motor units in the locomotory muscles. However, with increasing training speeds, oxidative capacity progressively increases in the more peripheral white motor units.

Similar conclusions are reached if the oxidative capacity of individual fiber types is determined in human subjects following different intensities of training or life-style [34] (Figure 10). In deconditioned subjects, oxidative enzyme capacity is uniformly low regardless of muscle fiber type. In normal sedentary subjects, enzyme activity is highest in slow-twitch red fibers and relatively low in the two fast-twitch fiber populations. In active subjects involved in recreational sports, enzyme activity is increased in slow-twitch red and fast-twitch red fibers but there is little change in fast-twitch white fibers. However, in highly trained endurance athletes, oxidative capacity is uniformly high in all three fiber types. These observations may be interpreted to indicate that in inactive muscles none of the fiber types are recruited to a significant extent, and therefore they all have relatively low oxidative enzyme capacities. In active subjects there is recruitment of both slow-twitch red and fast-twitch red fibers, so both types show elevated enzyme activities. In highly trained athletes, all fibers are recruited during training and all show increased enzyme activity. Thus, fibers that are recruited on a regular basis during training have elevated enzyme activity proportional to their use.

Other Considerations

All metabolic processes in muscles are unquestionably influenced by the patterns of fiber recruitment and the types of fibers activated for the particular exercise. However, unlike alterations in glycogen loss, blood flow, and enzymatic adaptation, it is not technically possible to measure alterations in many of the other metabolic processes within muscles as a function of spatial fiber-type recruitment patterns. For example, lactate content of plasma or muscle serves as an important indicator of glycolysis in active muscles and has been studied in considerable detail. However, to the present time it has not been possible to measure with any degree of certainty the rate of lactate production by a muscle fiber (or for that matter, by a whole muscle) during locomotion. The difficulty stems from the fact that lactate produced by a given fiber may be reconverted to pyruvate for complete oxidation or for glycogen resynthesis (or for conversion to other amphibolic intermediates) either in the same fiber or in adjacent fibers with greater oxidative capacity. In other words, since muscle fibers produce and release lactic acid, as well as take it up and oxidize it, measurement of the amount of lactate in the muscle fibers at a given time during exercise does not provide definitive information about the source or rate of production of the lactate. Nonetheless, after intense locomotory exercise, lactate concentrations are significantly

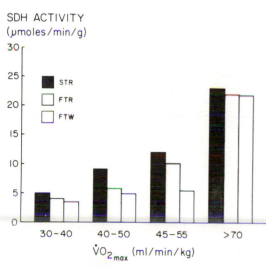

SDH ACTIVITY
(μmoles/min/g)

Figure 10. Succinate dehydrogenase (SDH) activity in the three fiber types of human subjects categorized by their maximal oxygen consumption ($\dot{V}O_2$max). (Drawn from data tabulated by Saltin, B., and P.D. Gollnick. Skeletal muscle adaptability: Significance for metabolism and performance. In Peachy, L.D., R.H. Adrian, and S.R. Geiger [eds.]. *Handbook of Physiology. Sec. 10: Skeletal Muscle.* Bethesda, Md.: American Physiological Society, 1983, pp. 555–631).

higher in fast-twitch white fibers than in slow-twitch red or fast-twitch red fibers [26]. This difference probably results from the greater reliance of fast-twitch white fibers on anaerobic glycogenolysis for ATP resynthesis and from the lower blood flows to fast-twitch white fiber regions, which would reduce efflux of lactate from the fibers into the circulation.

When blood lactate concentration during "steady state" exercise is plotted as a function of exercise intensity, the well-known lactate threshold can be identified at a relative intensity between 50 and 80% of $\dot{V}_{O_2}$max, depending on the individual studied. Below this break point, little lactate accumulates in the blood; above this point, lactate concentration increases disproportionately with exercise intensity. The mechanism(s) underlying the lactate threshold is currently a topic of debate, but one hypothesis holds that it represents the exercise intensity at which fast-twitch white fibers begin to be recruited during progressive exercise. There are compelling arguments against this concept [34], and for the technical reasons outlined in the previous paragraph, the question remains unanswered. However, the relationships between the spatial recruitment patterns of the different fiber types in the active muscles and the overall metabolic response to exercise remain interesting topics for further experimentation.

CONCLUSIONS

It is clear that muscle fiber recruitment patterns and associated metabolic support systems (i.e., intrinsic fiber metabolic potentials and the circulatory delivery system) are closely matched. Biological economy requires that excessive development of the metabolic support systems be avoided. However, when motor units are used on a regular basis, oxidative capacity and the cardiovascular delivery system adapt to meet the requirements. This matching of functional use to structural, biochemical, and

physiological capacity generally fits the principle of "Symmorphosis" as described by E. Weibel [44]. According to this principle, "the formation of structural elements (morphogenesis) that occurs during growth, and during maintenance of structures in the grown-up organism, should be regulated to satisfy but not exceed the requirements of the functional system" [44]. In general terms, this principle appears to describe the relationship between muscle fiber activity level and the magnitude of the metabolic response.

REFERENCES

1. Ariano, M.A., R.B. Armstrong, and V.R. Edgerton. Hindlimb muscle fiber populations of five mammals. *J. Histochem. Cytochem.* 21:51–55, 1973.
2. Armstrong, R.B. Properties and distributions of the fiber types in the locomotory muscles of mammals. In Schmidt-Neilsen, K., and C.R. Taylor (eds.). *Comparative Physiology: Primitive Mammals.* Cambridge: Cambridge University Press, 1980, pp. 243–254.
3. Armstrong, R.B., P.D. Gollnick, and C.D. Ianuzzo. Histochemical properties of skeletal muscle fibers in streptozotocindiabetic rats. *Cell Tiss. Res.* 162:387–394, 1975.
4. Armstrong, R.B., and M.H. Laughlin. Muscle function during locomotion in mammals. In Gilles, R. (ed.), *Proceedings of the First Congress on Comparative Physiology and Biochemstry.* Berlin: Springer-Verlag, 1985, pp. 56–63.
5. Armstrong, R.B., P. Marum, C.W. Saubert, IV, H.W. Seeherman, and C.R. Taylor. Muscle fiber activity as a function of speed and gait. *J. Appl. Physiol.* 43:672–677, 1977.
6. Armstrong, R.B., and R.O. Phelps. Muscle fiber type composition of the rat hindlimb. *Am. J. Anat.* 171:259–272, 1984.
7. Armstrong, R.B., C.W. Saubert IV, H.J. Seeherman, and C.R. Taylor. Distribution of fiber types in locomotory muscles of dogs. *Am. J. Anat.* 163:87–98, 1982.
8. Brooke, M.H., and K.K. Kaiser. Three "myosin adenosine triphosphatase" systems: The nature of their pH lability and sulfhydryl dependence. *J. Histochem. Cytochem.* 18:670–672, 1970.
9. Burke, R.E. Motor units: Anatomy, physiology and functional organization. In Brooks, V.B. (ed.). *Handbook of Physiology. Sec. 1: The Nervous System.* Vol. II, Bethesda, Md.: American Physiology Society, 1981, pp. 345–422.
10. Burke, R.W., and V.R. Edgerton. Motor unit properties and selective involvement in movement. *Exerc. Sport Sci. Rev.* 3:31–81, 1975.

11. Burke, R.E., D.N. Levine, F.E. Zajac III, P. Tsaairis, and W.K. Engel. Mammalian motor units: Physiological-histochemical correlations of three types in cat gastrocnemius. *Science* 174:709–712, 1971.

12. Close, R.I. Dynamic properties of mammalian skeletal muscles. *Physiol. Rev.* 52:129–197, 1972.

13. Dudley, G.A., W.A. Abraham, and R.L. Terjung. Influence of exercise intensity duration on biochemical adaptations in skeletal muscle. *J. Appl. Physiol.* 53:844–850, 1982.

14. Duling, B.R., and B. Klitzman. Local control of microvascular function: Role in tissue oxygen supply. *Annu. Rev. Physiol.* 42:373–382, 1980.

15. Gollnick, P.D., R.B. Armstrong, C.W. Saubert IV, K. Piehl, and B. Saltin. Enzyme activity and fiber composition in skeletal muscle of untrained and trained men. *J. Appl. Physiol.* 33:312–319, 1972.

16. Gollnick, P., R.B. Armstrong, C.W. Saubert IV, W.L. Sembrowich, and R.E. Shepherd. Glycogen depletion patterns in human skeletal muscle fibers during prolonged work. *Pflügers Arch.* 244:1–12, 1973.

17. Gollnick, P.D., R.B. Armstrong, W.L. Sembrowich, R.W. Shepherd, and B. Saltin. Glycogen depletion pattern in human muscle fibers after heavy exercise. *J. Appl. Physiol.* 34:615–618, 1973.

18. Hasan, Z., R.M. Enoka, and D.G. Stuart. The interface between biomechanics and neurophysiology in the study of movement: Some recent approaches. *Exerc. Sport Sci. Rev.* 13:169–234, 1985.

19. Henneman, E., and L.M. Mendell. Functional organization of motoneuron pool and its inputs. In Brooks, V.B. (ed.).*Handbook of Physiology. Sec. 1. The Nervous System.* Vol. II. Bethesda, Md.: American Phyiological Society, 1981, pp. 423–507.

20. Holloszy, J.O., and F.W. Booth. Biochemical adaptations to endurance exercise in muscle. *Annu. Rev. Physiol.* 38:273–291, 1976.

21. Honig, C.R. Contributions of nerves and metabolites to exercise vasodilation: A unifying hypothesis. *Am. J. Physiol.* 236:H705–H719, 1979.

22. Hudlicka, O. *Muscle Blood Flow: Its Relationship to Muscle Metabolism and Function.* Amsterdam: Swets and Zeitlinger, 1973.

23. Ianuzzo, C.D., and R.B. Armstrong. Phosphofructokinase and succinate dehydrogenase activities of normal and diabetic rat skeletal muscle. *Hor. Metab. Res.* 8:244–245, 1976.

24. Laughlin, M.H., and R.B. Armstrong. Muscular blood flow patterns during exercise in the rat. *Am. J. Physiol.* 243:H296–H306, 1982.

25. Laughlin, M.H., and R.B. Armstrong. Muscle blood flow during exercise. *Exerc. Sports Sci. Rev.* 13:95–136, 1985.

26. Meyer, R.A., G.A. Dudley, and R.L. Terjung. Ammonia and IMP in different skeletal muscle fibers after exercise in rats. *J. Appl. Physiol.* 49:1037–1041, 1980.

27. Monster, A.W., and H. Chan. Isometric force production by motor units of extensor digitorum communis muscle in man. *J. Neurophysiol.* 40:1432–1443, 1977.

28. Nemeth, P., H.W. Hofer, and D.Pette. Metabolism heterogeneity of muscle fibers classified by myosin ATPase. *Histochemistry* 63:191–201, 1979.

29. Peter, J.B., R.J. Barnard, V.R. Edgerton, C.A. Gillespie, and K.E. Stemel. Metabolic profiles of three types of skeletal muscle in guinea pigs and rabbits. *Biochemistry* 11:2627–2633, 1972.

30. Pette, D., and G. Vrbova. Invited review: Neural control of phenotypic expression in mammalian muscle fibers. *Musc. Nerv.* 8:676–689, 1985.

31. Rowell, L.B. Human cardiovascular adjustments to exercise and thermal stress. *Physiol. Rev.* 54:75–159, 1974.

32. Rowell, L.B. Circulation to skeletal muscle. In Ruch, T.C., and H.D. Patton (eds.). *Physiology and Biophysics* (II). Philadelphia: W.B. Saunders, 1974, pp. 200–214.

33. Saltin, B. Malleability of the system in overcoming limitations: Functional elements. *J. Exp. Biol.* 115:345–354, 1985.

34. Saltin, B., and P.D. Gollnick. Skeletal muscle adaptability: Significance for metabolism and performance. In Peachey, l.D., R.H. Adrian, and S.R. Geiger (eds.). *Handbook of Physiology. Sec. 10: Skeletal Muscle.* Bethesda, Md.: American Physiological Society, 1983, pp. 555–631.

35. Saltin, B., J. Henriksson, E. Nygaard, E. Jansson, and P. Andersen. Fiber types and metabolic potentials of skeletal muscles in sedentary man and endurance runners. *Ann. NY Acad. Sci.* 301:3–29, 1977.

36. Saltin, B., and L.B. Rowell. Functional adaptations to physical activity and inactivity. *Fed. Proc.* 39:1506–1513, 1980.

37. Shepherd, J.T. Circulation to skeletal muscle. In J.T Shepherd and F.M. Abboud (eds.), *Handbook of Physiology. The Cardiovascular System. Sec. 2, Peripheral Circulation.* Bethesda, Md.: American Physiological Society, 1983, pp. 319–370.

38. Smith, J.L., B. Betts, V.R. Edgerton, and R.F. Zernicke. Rapid ankle extension during paw shakes: Selective recruitment of fast ankle extensors. *J. Neurophysiol.* 40:612–620, 1980.

39. Smith, J.L., V.R. Edgerton, B. Betts, and T.C. Collatos. EMG of slow and fast ankle extensors of cat during posture, locomotion, and jumping. *J. Neurophysiol.* 40:503–513, 1977.

40. Spamer, C., and D. Pette. Activities of malate dehydrogenase, 3-hydroxyacyl-CoA dehydrogenase and fructose-1,6-diphosphatase with regard to metabolic subpopulations of fast- and slow-twitch fibers in rabbit muscles. *Histochemistry* 60:9–19, 1979.

41. Sparks, H.V. Effect of local metabolic factors on vascular smooth muscle. In D.F. Bohr, A.P. Somlyo, and H.V. Sparks, Jr. (eds.). *Handbook of Physiology. Sec. 2: The Cardiovascular System. Vol II: Vascular Smooth Muscle.* Bethesda, Md.: American Physiological Society, 1980, pp. 475–514.

42. Vanhoutte, P.M. Physical factors of regulation. In *Handbook of Physiology. Sec. 2: The Cardiovascular System. Vol II: Vascular Smooth Muscle.* Bethesda, Md.: American Physiological Society, 1980, pp. 443–474.

43. Walmsley, B., J.A. Hodgson, and R.E. Burke. Forces produced by medial gastrocnemius and soleus muscles during locomotion in freely moving cats. *J. Neurophysiol.* 41:1103–1216, 1978.

44. Weibel, E.R. *The Pathway for Oxygen.* Cambridge, Mass.: Harvard University Press, 1984.

Chapter 3

ATP SUPPLY AND DEMAND DURING EXERCISE

Joseph M. Krisanda, Ph.D., Timothy S. Moreland, Ph.D., and Martin J. Kushmerick, M.D., Ph.D.

INTRODUCTION

Skeletal muscle cells are organized as motor units, that is, one nerve cell body located in the spinal cord and all the muscle cells with which that nerve forms synapses. These neural connections control all muscle activity. Anatomical connections to the skeleton allow active force to be developed for useful movement. The energy for this muscular activity is ultimately derived from metabolic oxidation of substrates, which typically are stored within the muscle cells (e.g., glycogen and triglyceride) and in "storage depots" (e.g., adipose tissue) in the animal. Skeletal muscles have the secondary function of providing heat to the animal via shivering and nonshivering mechanisms of thermogenesis, and also supply gluconeogenic precursors in the starved state by net protein degradation.

Muscle is therefore a chemomechanical converter that can be studied from two vantage points. The first tends to focus on the chemical energy demands of the actomyosin interaction, the nature and regulation of the actomyosin chemomechanical transduction, and the mechanisms of electrical and osmotic work, which accompany contractile activity. The second considers the first group of mechanisms as an energy sink. The focus here is the integrated operation of metabolic pathways, the flux through which provides the necessary chemical potential energy for energy-supplying reactions, both in steady-state and non-steady-state contractile activities. Thus, considerations of muscle energetics and metabolism offer a broad scope and a wonderfully quantitative and integrative exercise in molecular and cellular physiology.

The conceptual organization of the metabolism and energetics of all cells is that originally outlined by Lipmann [31]. Oxidative metabolism supplies effective concentrations of relatively few intermediates, which in turn supply chemical potential energy for cellular function. Lipmann coined the phrase "energy-rich phosphate compounds" to focus attention on their role as readily convertible forms of chemical potential energy necessary to provide the driving forces for all cellular processes that do not otherwise proceed spontaneously. We now recognize adenosine triphosphate (ATP) and phosphocreatine (PCr) as the most ubiquitous examples of energy-rich phosphate compounds, and together they are referred to as "high-energy phosphate" compounds; in this chapter we use the term "~P" to denote these high-energy phosphate compounds, and refer to ATP or PCr only when we need to specify the more detailed chemistry. Cells have evolved a set of metabolic reactions, the net result of which is the production of a store of chemical potential energy. They also have evolved a wide variety of mechanisms by which this free energy is mechanistically coupled to spontaneous processes useful for the cell. Examples of these mechanisms include formation of solute and electrical potential gradients, macromolecular biosynthesis, and cell movements. Specifically, in muscle we are concerned with the coupled adenosine triphosphatase (ATPase) of actomyosin, the sarcoplasmic reticulum Ca^{2+} pump, sarcolemmal sodium/potassium transport, and other active ion pumps. We can thus distinguish stored substrates and products (glycogen, triglyceride) and other forms of metabolic substrate from $\sim P$, which is the coin of that realm with regard to the transactions of cellular energetics.

BASIC ENERGETIC MODEL

One distinguishing characteristic of muscle cells compared with other cells is that the metabolic rate may increase many times on transition from the resting to the contracting state. The most striking known example is the frog sartorius muscle. The basal oxygen consumption at 0°C accounts for more than 90% of the total energy requirements of the muscle, and is approximately 7nmol O_2/g wet weight/min. This corresponds to a steady-state turnover of approximately 0.8 nmol $\sim P$/g wet weight of muscle/s. However, in the first few seconds of an isometric tetanus, it has been demonstrated that the rate of energy turnover is nearly 1000-fold higher. Moreover, the transition from the basal to the high ATPase state occurs in tens of milliseconds. The reverse transition from an elevated rate of aerobic metabolism to the basal state takes considerably longer, and is measured with a time scale of minutes.

The basic paradigm of muscle energetics incorporates concepts developed from studies of isolated muscles and exercising animals [29]. The paradigm has two aspects: (a) There is a net decrease in chemical potential energy content during muscle activity (for brief contractions the major reaction is the utilization of PCr) and (b) there exists a recovery period after mechanical relaxation in which oxidative metabolism utilizes substrate to regenerate the initial precontraction steady state of $\sim P$ compounds, and so restores the initial chemical potential energy content. Under certain experimental conditions at least, it is thought possible to completely separate the processes occurring in the contraction phase (e.g., PCr splitting) from those occurring in the recovery phase (e.g., oxygen consumption). The basis for the separability into two phases lies in the greatly differing rate constants of the relevant chemical processes. For the example given in the preceding paragraph of amphibian skeletal muscle at 0°C, the rate constant for utilization of PCr is approximately $0.1 \cdot s^{-1}$ during tetanic contractions, whereas for aerobic resynthesis the rate constant is on the order of $0.01 \cdot s^{-1}$. For mammalian skeletal and cardiac muscles at body temperature, the rates are each about 10-fold higher and, because of differences in mitochondrial content and intrinsic actomyosin ATPase activity, there is a wide variation in the relative rates of $\sim P$ resynthesis compared with $\sim P$ utilization.

This energetic paradigm is schematically illustrated in Figure 1. The contractile phase is on the left; progression from left to right indicates a contraction-recovery cycle. Figure 1A shows the development of isometric force upon stimulation. During the recovery period (on the right) there is no mechanical activity. In Figure 1B the ATPase rate is plotted as the most direct and explicit measure of energy utilization. Before stimulation there is a small positive value equivalent to the basal rate of energy metabolism (dashed line). With the onset of stimulation the ATPase rate rapidly rises. Current evidence suggests that the rate may not be steady [12], at least in some types of muscles. During the maintained tetanus, the steady rate is much higher than the basal rate. As a consequence of the increased rate of utilization, and on the assumption that PCr and ATP are near equi-

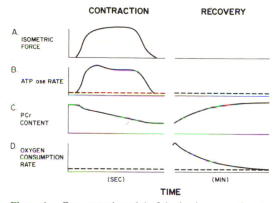

CONTRACTION   RECOVERY

A. ISOMETRIC FORCE

B. ATP ase RATE

C. PCr CONTENT

D. OXYGEN CONSUMPTION RATE

(SEC)   (MIN)

TIME

Figure 1. Conceptual model of the basic energetic relationships for fast-twitch skeletal muscle during and following a single tetanus. Left side of figure indicates mechanical and chemical events during contraction, and right side illustrates events during recovery period. See text for detailed explanation. (Modified from Kushmerick, M.J. Energetics of muscle contraction. In Peachey, L., R. Adrian, and S.R. Geiger [eds.]. *Handbook of Physiology. Skeletal Muscle*. Bethesda, Md.: American Physiological Society, 1983, pp. 189–236.)

librium with each other via the creatine phosphokinase (CK) reaction (see below), the PCr levels follow the time course indicated in Figure 1C, that is, a rapid decrease during the tetanus in proportion to the ATP turnover rate. Figure 1D indicates that oxygen consumption remains at basal levels during brief contractions (dashed line).

An obvious feature of the model in Figure 1 is that the contractile events are much more rapid than the rate of oxidative metabolism during contraction. During a long contraction, or at some time after a brief contraction, the oxygen consumption rate increases to a rate less than the maximal (Figure 1D, right). Thereafter, the rate of oxygen consumption declines exponentially to basal values as PCr levels are restored. The return of oxygen consumption to basal values marks the end of the recovery period. The increased rate of oxygen consumption above basal values during recovery and the (assumed) very low basal ATPase rate during the recovery period (Figure 1B, right) allow the PCr levels to return to precontractile levels (Figure 1C, right). The rate of PCr

resynthesis is directly proportional to the oxygen consumption rate in this simple model.

The schematic model in Figure 1 considers a maximal tetanus, which is not a physiological state of contractile activity. A second energetic scheme, one that is probably the most physiologically common, can be considered. This scheme represents steady states of mechanical activity at levels that are sustainable. Steady-state running or swimming is one example; similar steady-state activities have been studied in animal experiments. Here the ~P demand, integrated over time, is much lower than what the maximal tetanic rate would be and is within the range of the steady-state ~P-generating potential of the muscle.

The pattern of chemical changes under a third scheme is illustrated in Figure 2. Panel A of that figure shows schematically the steady-state oxygen consumption rate as a function of stimulation rate for a slow-twitch, highly oxidative muscle and for a fast-twitch muscle with smaller aerobic ~P-generating capacity. An example of the former might be the soleus muscle and of the latter the gastrocnemius or biceps muscle. At lower rates of stimulation, both kinds of muscle can sustain steady-state contractile activities so long as the supply of substrate and removal of product are intact. The fast-twitch muscle, per contraction, uses more ~P and subsequently has a greater rate of steady-state oxygen consumption, because the actomyosin and other ATPase activities are greater than in the slow-twitch muscle. The fast-twitch muscle reaches its maximal oxygen consumption at a lower twitch rate than the slow-twitch muscle. The reason is that the fast-twitch muscle has a greater ~P "cost" per contraction than the slow-twitch muscle, and because it has a lower ~P-generating capacity. Thus, on the schematic diagram, the slope of the curve of oxygen consumption rate versus stimulation frequency for the slow-twitch muscle is less than for the fast-twitch, but the absolute rate of oxygen consumption is greater in the

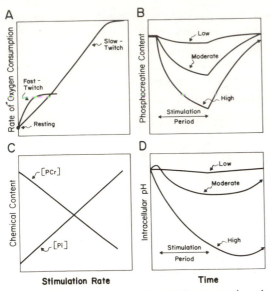

Figure 2. Conceptual model of the energetic relationships for skeletal muscle during steady-state contractile activity. Panel A shows that steady-state rate of oxygen consumption rises above the basal rate as a function of steady-state twitch rate. For fast-twitch muscle, the maximal O_2 consumption rate is reached before the tetanic fusion frequency is reached, whereas for slow-twitch muscle, high rates of stimulation above the mechanical fusion frequency are needed to reach the maximum. The slope is greater for fast-twitch muscles, but the maximal level achieved at plateau is greater for slow-twitch muscles. Panel B diagrams temporal events during the onset and the recovery period of steady-state stimulation at increasing twitch rates or equivalently increasing "wash" load. Panel C indicates a stoichiometric relationship between phosphocreatine (PCr) decrease and inorganic phosphate (Pi) increase measured during the steady-state period of contractile activity. Note that the abscissa coordinate is now in relative terms, i.e., a schematic decrease in PCr and even in ~Pi occurs over a range of stimulation frequencies whose absolute values differ for fast-twitch and slow-twitch muscle; the maxima diagrammed in Panel A would be on the right of panel C. Panel D diagrams the change in intracellular pH during and following a period of steady-state twitch activity. (Modified from Kushmerick, M.J., and R.A. Meyer. Chemical changes in rat leg muscle by phosphorus nuclear magnetic resonance. *Am. J. Physiol.* 249 [*Cell Physiol.* 18]:C362–C365, 1985.)

slow-twitch muscle and occurs at stimulus frequencies above the maximal for fast-twitch muscles.

Panel B illustrates several features. For steady-state stimulation rates, where ~P utilization is less than the maximal ~P-

generating ability, the PCr content declines from the resting value [30] after the stimulation begins. After a short time, PCr content levels off. The concentration of PCr at which this leveling off occurs is a function of the balance between ~P utilization and ~P-generating capacity. The greater the stimulation rate, the greater the net ~P utilization rate, and therefore the lower the steady-state plateau reached. When the stimulation stops, the PCr concentration rises to the original resting level at the end of the recovery period.

Panel C shows that the relationship between the decrease in PCr content and the increase in inorganic phosphate (Pi) content is stoichiometric, and of course opposite in sign. Panel D illustrates that changes in the intracellular pH are more complex than the patterns seen among ~P compounds. In general, the results obtained so far are the following. (a) For relatively small rates of stimulation (i.e., mild exercise), there is relatively little change in the intracellular pH from the resting value of 7.0. (b) There is evidence, especially in muscles with a low glycolytic capacity, that there is a transient alkalinization [37] during the period when PCr is decreasing most rapidly. This of course occurs during the early part of steady-state stimulation. (c) With exercise that is intense enough to cause large decreases in PCr, even in muscles with low glycolytic capacity, the intracellular pH declines slowly and reversibly through each value as lactate accumulates, even in the range of pH 6.0. Such low pH values have been measured both in isolated animal muscles *in vitro* and during human voluntary exercise. After the end of the stimulation, the pH tends to decrease further during the early part of the recovery period, and finally returns to control values. Thus, the time course of recovery of intracellular pH is considerably slower than that of ~P.

The metabolic events explaining these descriptive results are briefly discussed later. For our present purposes, it is sufficient to point out that despite a very large amount of data derived from isolated mitochondria [8, 27] and from reconstituted glycolytic systems, the details of physiological regulation are not quantitatively settled [17, 27, 55].

CHEMICAL REACTIONS AND METABOLIC PRINCIPLES

All cells extract the energy necessary for their internal functions from substrates available in their environment. By highly integrated sequences of chemical reactions, metabolic pathways convert these substrates into cellular components, chemical and osmotic gradients, and storage of chemical potential energy. In aerobic cells, the net metabolic strategy is the controlled oxidation of substrates. Oxygen is the ultimate electron acceptor. Energy made available by metabolic sequences is stored by accumulation of ATP, PCr, and a few other so-called "energy-rich" phosphate compounds to provide the driving force for most cellular processes; of other compounds such as reduced nicotinamide adenine dinucleotide phosphate (NADPH), which provides reducing power for biosynthesis; and of acetyl coenzyme (CoA), which is the carrier of "activated" acyl groups. The strategy is a simple one. Many processes necessary for cell and organism survival do not proceed spontaneously. This type of process is called "endergonic," and examples are maintenance of intracellular ionic gradients, protein synthesis, and muscle mechanical work. In order for an endergonic process to proceed efficiently, three conditions must be met: (a) Chemical potential energy must be available, (b) a coupling mechanism must exist for conversion, and (c) the spontaneous uncoupled chemical reaction should not proceed in the absence of coupling. What is controlled in governing the rate of the endergonic process is usually not the chemical potential, but rather the rate of the energetic processes. Hydrolysis of ATP to adenosine diphosphate (ADP) and Pi is thermodynamically spontaneous, or "exergonic"; in the cell, the

concentration ratio of products to substrates is such that the free energy is very favorable, that is, there is a very negative value for the Gibbs–Helmholtz free energy. Nature has evolved a large variety of endergonic processes, which are necessary for cellular survival, and a limited number of exergonic metabolic reactions that can provide the required energy. A specific chemical mechanism must also have evolved that enables coupling between the exergonic and endergonic reactions, such that there is a net extent of reaction for both. If the coupling mechanism did not exist, only the exergonic reaction would occur, because it is spontaneous. The net result of such an uncoupling would be dissipation of the chemical potential into heat, but no advance of the endergonic reaction. It is important to realize that the chemical nature of these compounds, the energetics of their interconversions, and the stoichiometry of the coupled metabolic processes are not predictable from chemical and thermodynamic principles. Obviously, the magnitude of the potential energy in the coupled exergonic reaction must exceed that of the coupled endergonic reaction for both to proceed at some finite rate.

The central role of ATP in cellular energetics as discussed above is embodied by Lipmann in his phrase "energy-rich phosphate compounds" [31]. The term does not refer to any physical-chemical characteristic of the phosphorus atomic bonds per se, but to three biological facts: (a) The ubiquity of ATP and related compounds in cellular energy interconversions, (b) the arrangement of metabolic reactions that act to maintain the concentration ratio, $[ATP]/([ADP] \cdot [Pi])$, sufficiently large so that the hydrolysis of ATP is very favorable; and (c) the specific coupling requirement of many cellular processes for ATP and related compounds. Therefore the experimental focus of chemical energetics of muscle is on ~P consumption and generation during the contraction-recovery cycle.

One might be tempted to extrapolate to the hypothesis that all interconversions of energy are linked to energy-rich phosphate compounds, but this view is not valid. Most transformations are, but the example of respiration-dependent Ca^{2+} uptake by mitochondria is one well-documented exception. However, with respect to actomyosin interactions and Ca^{2+}, Na^+, and K^+ movements across the cell and sarcoplasmic reticulum membranes, ATP is certainly the primary physiological source of energy. PCr is not a direct substrate for any of these processes.

CHEMOMECHANICAL ENERGY TRANSDUCTION SETS THE METABOLIC DEMAND

Three functions are driven by utilization of ATP during a cycle of contraction and relaxation. The first and quantitatively the most important of these is the action of actomyosin ATPase. Demand for ATP by actomyosin varies among muscle types, as discussed below. The second function coupled to hydrolysis of ATP is calcium transport. Relaxation from the contractile state is achieved through uptake of calcium by the sarcoplasmic reticulum, which lowers the cytoplasmic free calcium level from approximately 10^{-5} M to 10^{-7} M. Uptake is an active process mediated by a membrane-bound $Ca^{2+}Mg^{2+}$ATPase. Calcium transport follows Michaelis–Menten kinetics (apparent K_m [substrate concentration at which enzymatic reaction proceeds at one-half maximal velocity] of 1–4 μM) and occurs with a stoichiometry of two Ca^{2+} ions translocated per ATP molecule hydrolyzed. An excellent review of relaxation in vertebrate skeletal muscle has recently been published [22]. The third function during the contraction-relaxation cycle that requires ATP is maintenance of the cellular membrane potential. Contraction is triggered by an action potential that results in a net efflux of potassium ions and an influx of sodium ions. The initial ionic distribution, which is altered only slightly, is restored by the action of a Na/K ATPase pump during the recovery period.

The relative importance of these three ATP-utilizing processes has been estimated earlier in this chapter for frog muscle at 0°C; about two-thirds of the total energy cost is due to actomyosin interactions [29]. Demand by actomyosin under conditions of maximal contractile activity is approximately 1.4 μmol ~P/g muscle/s and 0.3 to 0.4 μmol ATP/g muscle/s during a sustained tetanus. Roughly 0.2 to 0.6 μmol/g Ca^{2+} is released during a twitch, and its uptake during relaxation would therefore require 0.1 to 0.3 μmol ATP/g muscle/s. The degree to which calcium is simultaneously taken up and released during a tetanus is not certain, but the energy demand of sarcoplasmic reticulum (SR) ATPase is estimated to be 0.1 μmol/g muscle/s. A single action potential causes a relatively small disturbance in the distribution of sodium and potassium across the sarcolemma, and the energy cost to restore the resting condition is probably on the order of 2 nmol ATP/g muscle/s. As a first approximation, the energy needed to maintain membrane potential during a tetanus can be taken as the product of this value and the stimulation frequency, for example, 0.04 μmol ATP/g muscle/s at 20 Hz stimulation frequency.

The onset of contraction is accompanied by a rapid and dramatic increase in the rate of actomyosin ATP demand. Energy utilization of a typical mammalian muscle in the active contractile state may exceed the resting rate by a factor of 100, somewhat less than in the example given earlier for frog muscle. This difference is due to the higher rate of resting metabolism in the mammal compared with the amphibian, even at the same temperature [29]. Ultimately this increased demand for chemical energy is met by an increased flux through the catabolic pathways of energy provision, notably glycolysis and oxidative phosphorylation (discussed below). Although it is useful to consider the active contractile phase as being separate from the recovery phase, as illustrated in Figure 1, it should be noted that the temporal relationship between the two is quite variable. Nearly complete separation of the contractile and recovery phases can be experimentally achieved, and such separation is observed to a varying extent in different skeletal muscles, giving rise to the phenomenon of oxygen debt. In other muscle tissues, notably heart, the two processes can occur nearly simultaneously, thereby permitting the attainment of a steady-state relationship between contractile activity and metabolic energy supply, averaged over a single contraction-relaxation cycle.

For muscles in which the active contractile phase can be separated from the processes of recovery metabolism (Figure 1), it is typically observed that ATP concentration in working muscle does not decrease in proportion to demand for ATP. The reason is that ATP and the products of hydrolysis —ADP, Pi, and H+—participate in a second reaction with creatine (Cr) and PCr, catalyzed by the enzyme CK:

$$MgADP + \alpha\, H^+ + PCr \leftrightarrow MgATP + Cr$$

The fractional proton, denoted by α, reflects the fact that the participants of the reaction possess differing values of pKa (negative logarithm of dissociation constant of an acid); the value for α is close to 1 under cellular conditions [21, 29]. A corollary to this fact is that the equilibrium concentrations of ATP, ADP, PCr, and Cr are a function of pH and of intracellular Mg^{2+}. The consequence of the CK reaction is that contractile activity (prior to any subsequent recovery processes) is observed to result in the stoichiometric breakdown of PCr to Cr and Pi, while ATP concentration remains relatively constant, as diagrammed in the model (Figures 1 and 2). The CK reaction therefore acts as a buffer of $\sim$P, and this process forms the basis of what might be termed the "classical" view of the function of the CK reaction. An alternative view of PCr function has been proposed, the "PCr shuttle," which focuses on the principal function of the CK reaction as one of transport of $\sim$P. It holds that most flux of $\sim$P between mitochondria and myofibril

occurs not as ATP/ADP, but as PCr/Cr [2], because there are compartments or poorly exchanging pools of adenine nucleotides localized at the myofibril and mitochondrion, and CK isoforms are located on the myofibril, cytosol, and mitochondrion. However, measurements of unidirectional flux through CK by ^{31}P nuclear magnetic resonance (NMR) suggest that the reaction is in a near-equilibrium steady state in skeletal muscle [19, 35, 51], and that the apparent lack of near equilibrium in the myocardium [26, 42] is now known to be the result of an incorrect biochemical model for the interpretation of the ^{31}P NMR data. The biochemical model was initially thought to be an exchange between PCr and ATP; however, it is now recognized that exchange also occurs between ATP and Pi in the beating heart, due to a significant activity of actomyosin ATPase. This three-site exchange model can fully account for the observed NMR spin transfer data. We believe that the classical and shuttle interpretations of PCr/Cr function, which emphasize temporal and spatial buffering of adenine nucleotides, respectively, can both be defined by considering the CK reaction as an example of facilitated diffusion similar to the role of myoglobin in oxygen transport [38]. Given that the CK reaction is close to equilibrium averaged over the entire cell, and that [PCr] > [ATP] and [Cr] $\gg$ [ADP], it follows that PCr and Cr have an important transport role in the steady state and transient state, and there is no need to postulate poorly mixed microenvironments.

Another important reaction is that catalyzed by the enzyme adenylate kinase (myokinase):

$$2\, ADP \leftrightarrow ATP + AMP$$

This reaction is thought to be near-equilibrium in skeletal muscle [4, 6, 14, 45], and ATP can thus be regenerated from two molecules of ADP with the stoichiometric production of adenosine monophosphate (AMP). However, this reaction is ADP-limited due to the buffering action of CK until the available concentration of PCr is substantially reduced and cytosolic ADP levels rise above the tens of of micromolar concentration. For example, in mammalian skeletal muscle at rest, the metabolically active concentration of ADP has been estimated to be on the order of 10 to 20 μM [51]. The concentration rises to 100 to 200 μM as PCr is depleted to about 10% of initial values. Assuming an equilibrium constant of 1 for the adenylate kinase reaction at pH 7.0 and an MgATP concentration of 8 mM, one can easily calculate the AMP concentration to be on the order of 15 nM at rest when ADP is 10 μM; 3μM when ADP is 150μM. Thus, until PCr is completely depleted and the ATP concentration declines significantly, there will be insufficient AMP for a large flux through the adenylate kinase reaction. Because over this normal range of changes in $\sim$P the AMP concentration varies 200-fold, enzymes sensitive to AMP concentration in the nanomolar range will be affected.

METABOLIC PATHWAYS SUPPLYING METABOLIC DEMAND

Glycolysis

The basic mechanisms and a description of the intermediates and enzymes in the glycolytic pathway are given in Chapter 4 of this volume. This section will be devoted to defining those parameters that are important in the regulation of flux through the glycolytic pathway. Previous evidence concerning regulation of key enzymes was based on the integration of studies of the behavior of enzymes in dilute solutions. Information gained in this manner has been useful in defining the metabolic pathways and directing attention to possible sites of regulation. More recent evidence collected using nuclear magnetic resonance spectroscopy to study "*in vivo*" enzyme kinetics, and a revision of our understanding of the characteristics of enzymes in the cytosol, are beginning to revolutionize

our concepts of regulatory control of metabolism. A suitable example of our advance can be seen from a brief review of research concerning the regulation of glycolysis. The glucose transport enzymes, glycogen phosphorylase and synthase, phosphofructokinase and pyruvate dehydrogenase, will be considered.

Glucose is transported into the muscle cell by a facilitated transport mechanism. The carrier for the glucose molecule is a protein inserted in the plasma membrane. Evidence in favor of a carrier-mediated process comes from observations that the rate of glucose transport can be saturated, suggesting the presence of a limited number of carriers and a finite capacity, and that the rate of transport can be increased by the action of hormones such as insulin and by muscle contractile activity [39]. The significance of the action of insulin is that in the fed state an enhanced rate of glucose transport into the muscle cell facilitates both removal of excess glucose from the bloodstream and stimulation of the replenishment of glycogen stores required for future muscle activity. This transport process does not require energy because the glucose molecule is transported down a concentration gradient. The intracellular concentration of glucose is maintained at a very low level by the enzyme hexokinase, which phosphorylates glucose to glucose-6-phosphate (Glu-6-P) and traps the charged molecule inside the cell.

The hexokinase reaction is regulated by the cellular concentration of Glu-6-P. The Glu-6-P concentration depends on the activities of phosphofructokinase (PFK) and glycogen synthase. The rate of glycogen synthesis is determined by the relative activities of the enzymes glycogen synthase, responsible for synthesis of glycogen from glucose, and glycogen phosphorylase, responsible for glycogen degradation and subsequent metabolism. Both the phosphorylase and synthase enzymes are regulated by a phosphorylation-dephosphorylation mechanism, whereby the covalent attachment of a phosphate molecule to the enzyme molecule modifies enzyme activity [43]. Phosphorylation of the synthase and phosphorylase enzymes is achieved by the action of a Ca^{2+}-sensitive kinase that results in the inhibition of the synthase and activation of the phosphorylase. Contractile activity of muscle due to increased intracellular levels of Ca^{2+} results in the concomitant degradation of glycogen to Glu-1-P and subsequent metabolism by the glycolytic pathway.

Investigators studying human skeletal muscle have observed increases in phosphorylase activity during exercise [10]. These increases can be attributed to changes in the intracellular calcium concentration during stimulation, but this mechanism cannot totally account for the observed enzyme activity. It has been suggested that increases in Pi must accompany phosphorylation of the phosphorylase enzyme for glycogen breakdown to proceed at physiological rates. The Pi is derived from the net hydrolysis of PCr. By the argument presented above, AMP levels are too low to activate phosphorylase. The initial increase in phosphorylase activity declines during fatigue. The drop in intracellular pH is thought to inactivate the enzyme.

PFK is a key regulatory enzyme of carbohydrate metabolism. This allosterically regulated enzyme catalyzes the conversion of fructose-1-phosphate to fructose-1,6-diphosphate. The interaction of the sites is such that binding of a molecule to the regulatory site effects a conformational change in the enzyme that alters catalytic activity. It has been proposed that flux through this enzyme may be increased by the effectors Pi, AMP, and NH_4^+, and flux may be inhibited by ATP, protons, and citrate. The efficacy of these regulators and the activity of the enzyme itself appear to depend on the concentration of the enzyme. Recent studies that have attempted to simulate cellular concentrations of PFK have clarified the control characteristics of PFK [3]. In the presence of inhibiting concentrations of ATP, the proposed effectors listed above show the classical response observed from the study of the enzyme in dilute solutions. If the ATP concentration is reduced, however, regulation is essentially absent. The conclusion is that inhibition by ATP is the primary allosteric mechanism, and this inhibition is further modulated by the other effectors. Since, under most physiological degrees of exercise, ATP levels do not change substantially, PFK is under constant inhibition by ATP. An additional and important consequence of this work is that enzyme concentration itself can modulate activity, so that cells with high concentrations of enzyme will exhibit elevated activities in excess of that expected from a simple linear relationship between enzyme concentration and activity.

Glucose is metabolized to pyruvate by the enzymes of the glycolytic pathway. Glucose can be further metabolized either to lactate, by lactate dehydrogenase with the net synthesis of 2 mol ATP, or oxidized completely to $CO_2 + H_2O$, by the mitochondria with a net synthesis of 36 mol ATP. If the glycosyl unit is derived from glycogen, an additional mole of ATP is synthesized because the phosphorylation of blood-derived glucose by hexokinase is bypassed.

Pyruvate dehydrogenase is a multienzyme complex that catalyzes the conversion of pyruvate into acetyl CoA [52]. The pyruvate dehydrogenase complex is located on the inner membrane-matrix of the mitochondrion. It is composed of three major enzymes: Pyruvate dehydrogenase, lipoate acetyltransferase, and lipoamide dehydrogenase. The observation has been made in isolated perfused rat heart and isolated diaphragm muscle that pyruvate oxidation is inhibited by fatty acid and ketone body oxidation [20]. The pyruvate dehydrogenase reaction can be regulated by the acetyl CoA concentration, possibly the energy state of the tissue (the chemical potential of ATP), and a phosphorylation-dephosphorylation mechanism. The latter mechanism is most likely operational during long-term exercise such as marathon running, where a metabolic steady state has been achieved and the athlete is dependent on triglyceride metabolism for energy supply.

Oxidative Phosphorylation

Quantitatively the most important process supplying ATP for muscle function is mitochondrial oxidative phosphorylation. A complex of enzymes that are intimately associated with the inner mitochondrial membrane catalyzes the transfer of electrons from reduced cofactors (NADH, flavin adenine dinucleotide [$FADH_2$]) to molecular oxygen, forming water. Electron transfer is coupled to translocation of protons from the matrix across the inner mitochondrial membrane. The resulting electrochemical proton gradient subsequently drives ATP synthesis, thereby capturing a significant fraction of the free energy of cofactor oxidation as ~P. Reduced cofactors are generated by dehydrogenation reactions in catabolic pathways, such as the tricarboxylic acid cycle and fatty acid oxidation. These pathways are fueled in turn by metabolites derived from degradation of lipids, carbohydrates, and amino acids. Oxidative phosphorylation, the electron transport chain, and control of respiration have been the subject of several recent reviews [17, 24, 36], and the reader may wish to consult these for a more comprehensive account.

The original studies of Chance and Williams [9] provide a means to understand the metabolic status of isolated mitochondria and control of mitochondrial oxidative phosphorylation (Table 1.). In this scheme, respiratory activity of a suspension of mitochondria provided with saturating levels of reduced substrate and oxygen is limited by availability of ADP, an acceptor for synthesis of ATP (state 4). Oxygen consumption is enhanced by addition of ADP, and is limited by the intrinsic catalytic capacity of the respiratory chain (state 3). The apparent K_m for ADP for this increase is on the order of 10 μM. These in vitro results have long been viewed as a paradigm for control of respiratory activity in vivo. Mitochondria of well-perfused aerobic muscle are thought to be saturated with reduced substrate and oxygen, and therefore might be considered to be in a condition analogous to state 4 of isolated mitochondria. Similarly, contractile activity generates ADP, which could relieve the rate-limiting condition of substrate availability and induce a transition to state 3 respiration. The question is, how can this model explain the graded steady-state rate of oxidative phosphorylation observed in submaximal exercise?

The scheme of respiratory control outlined in Table 1 is almost certainly valid for suspensions of isolated mitochondria. However, extrapolation of this model to the situation in

Table 1.   RESPIRATORY STATES OF ISOLATED MITOCHONDRIA.

STATE	CHARACTERISTICS					PERCENT REDUCTION IN STEADY STATE	
	Respiration Rate	ADP Concentration	Oxidizable Substrate	O_2 Concentration	Rate-limiting Substance	NADH	Cytochrome a
1	Slow	Low	Low	>0	ADP	90	0
2	Slow	High	Low	>0	Substrate	0	0
3	Maximal	High	High	>0	Respiratory chain	53	<4
4	Slow	Low	High	>0	ADP	>99	0
5	0	High	High	0	O_2	100	100

ADP, adenosine diphosphate; NADH, reduced form of nicotinamide adenine dinucleotide phosphate.

vivo is not straightforward, since it does not address the mechanisms linking cytosolic processes of ATP utilization with mitochondrial ATP synthesis. Two hypotheses are being evaluated as models of regulation of oxidative metabolism in the intact cell. The first has been referred to as the "near-equilibrium steady-state hypothesis," and has as its basic tenet that a network of reactions near thermodynamic equilibrium link cytosolic and mitochondrial reactions of energy metabolism [55]. The second class of hypotheses denies that such an equilibrium exists between cytosol and mitochondria, and instead proposes that exchange of ADP from cytosol to mitochondria is the rate-limiting step in respiration. The latter is conceptually similar to the scheme of Table 1, and can be considered to include proposals that a PCr shuttle exerts a regulatory role in the integration of cellular energy metabolism [27, 33].

The near-equilibrium steady-state hypothesis of control of mitochondrial function is based upon evidence from both isolated mitochondria [16] and intact cellular preparations [23, 54, 55] that the reactions of the electron transport chain corresponding to sites one and two of ATP synthesis are at or close to equilibrium with the cytosolic phosphorylation potential

$$\frac{[ATP]}{[ADP] \cdot [Pi]}$$

(excluding for the moment the role of H^+). The probable rate-limiting step of respiration is the reaction catalyzed by cytochrome c oxidase (cytochrome aa_3 [17]). The rate of the cytochrome oxidase reaction (and therefore of mitochondrial respiration) is a function of the concentration of its participating substrates, molecular oxygen and reduced cytochrome c. The concentration of reduced cytochrome c is linked in turn by the near-equilibrium condition to the intramitochondrial [NAD]/[NADH] redox couple and to the cytosolic phosphorylation potential. The rate of mitochondrial respiration

therefore reflects the following four interrelated factors [17]:

1. Intramitochondrial [NAD]/[NADH], which in turn is governed by substrate availability and the status of intermediary metabolism
2. The net catalytic capacity of the respiratory chain, which is a function of the concentration of the respiratory chain proteins
3. Cytosolic [ATP]/([ADP] · [Pi]), which is determined by the rate of cellular ATP demand
4. The concentration of available molecular oxygen

Control by the four factors is analogous to the conditions described by states 2 through 5 in Table 1, respectively, for isolated mitochondria. The distinction is that the original proposal of Chance and Williams [9] emphasizes kinetic control by availability of acceptor (e.g., ADP), whereas control in the near-equilibrium model is a function of the mass-action ratio of participating substrates and products (e.g., the phosphorylation potential at pH 7, [ATP]/([ADP] · [Pi]).

In contrast to the near-equilibrium model, the second hypothesis being considered holds that exchange of adenine nucleotides between cytosol and mitochondria is the rate-limiting step in oxidative phosphorylation. Current debate centers on the role of adenine nucleotide translocase, which exchanges ADP^{3-} for ATP^{4-} (antiport) across the inner mitochondrial membrane. An implicit assumption of the near-equilibrium hypothesis is that this exhange is near equilibrium; in effect, cytosol and mitochondrial matrix approximate one compartment with regard to adenine nucleotides. If, however, the exchange reaction is indeed far removed from equilibrium, mitochondrial respiration (given adequate levels of oxidizable substrate and oxygen) could be regulated by the rate at which ADP is delivered to the matrix via adenine translocase. This view is therefore similar to the original proposal of respiratory control by Chance and Williams [9], depicted in Table 1.

A complete description of the mechanisms linking cytosolic ATP utilization with mitochondrial ATP supply must include a consideration of the creatine kinase reaction. As stated above, the result of both the proposed PCr shuttle model and the steady-state-facilitated diffusion model is that transport of most high-energy phosphate between myofibril and mitochondria does not occur as ATP/ADP, but instead as PCr/Cr. It has been suggested that the mitochondrial isoform of CK is "functionally coupled" to adenine translocase by virtue of physical proximity; in other words, the translocase provides mitochondrially produced ATP to CK which, in turn, generates ADP for the translocase (see reference 27 for review). A corollary is that, if flux of ADP per se from myofibril to mitochondrion is sufficiently small, the rate-limiting step in mitochondrial respiration in muscle could be the generation of ADP by the mitochondrial CK reaction [27].

To summarize, the near-equilibrium model of mitochondrial respiration describes a network of cytosolic and mitochondrial reactions that are held close to equilibrium in a steady-state preparation. In this context, contractile activity can be viewed as altering concentration ratios of particpating compounds (e.g., adenine nucleotides, Pi, and PCr), thus inducing a perturbation in the near-equilibrium condition. The rate of oxidative phosphorylation initially increases in response to the perturbation, and subsequently returns to a basal level as the system relaxes to the resting steady state. Under physiologically normal situations, mitochondria are supplied with saturating concentrations of oxygen and reduced substrate, so that the relevant parameter for control of respiration is the cytosolic phosphorylation state ratio (the mass-action ratio of ATP hydrolysis), $[ATP]/([ADP] \cdot [Pi])$. The alternative view postulates that mitochondrial respiration is controlled by availability of ADP, with the rate-limiting step being exchange of adenine nucleotides across the inner mitochondrial membrane. Here the relevant parameter describing the rate of translocation, and therefore oxidative phosphorylation, is the ratio $[ATP]/[ADP]$. Distinguishing between the two models is conceptually simple, requiring only knowledge of the status of the adenine nucleotide translocase reaction. This information is difficult to obtain experimentally, however, and available data are equivocal [17, 53]. An interesting approach has been developed by Wilson, Erecinska, and Schramm [53], in which intramitochondrial concentrations of free ADP and ATP are determined by means of a linked phosphoenolpyruvate carboxykinase assay system. Their data indicate that the intramitochondrial $[ATP]/[ADP]$ ratio is as great as or greater than the extramitochondrial $[ATP]/[ADP]$ ratio, and that the adenine nucleotide translocase reaction is therefore not a rate-limiting step in respiration.

An assumption was made at several points in the preceding discussion that mitochondrial respiration is not limited by availability of oxidizable substrate or oxygen. While this is generally true in the case of well-perfused aerobic tissues, clearly it may not always be so. Availability of reduced substrates at the cellular level can be influenced by the nutritional and endocrine status of the individual, and oxygen supply can be limiting in pathological conditions or as a result of intense physical activity. The rate of cellular respiration is zero order with respect to ambient oxygen tension above a "critical Po_2," typically several torr [8]. It is important to note, however, that oxygen concentration may be a limiting commodity for respiratory metabolism even at a Po_2 above this critical level. The rate of cellular respiration can remain relatively constant at subsaturating concentrations of oxygen by means of compensatory adjustments in other portions of the mitochondrial near-equilibrium network. For example, a lowered $[NAD]/[NADH]$ or a more reduced state for the near-equilibrium concentration of cytochrome c could maintain the respiratory rate even though oxygen concentration is not saturating [17, 29].

SUPPLY-DEMAND STRATEGIES

The metabolic variables important in defining performance limitations involve the storage and type of fuels utilized by the muscle as well as the metabolic capacity of the system. Metabolic capacity can be loosely defined as the maximum rate at which the muscle can resynthesize ATP; it entails the consideration of enzyme activity (differing catalytic rate of enzyme isoforms); the actual quantity of metabolic enzymes present; and the effective concentrations of substrate, products, activators, and inhibitors. The muscles that are capable of a wide performance range are the skeletal and cardiac muscles. Skeletal muscle performs physical work against the environment, and cardiac muscle pumps the blood required to maintain adequate tissue perfusion. Adaptive changes in vascular smooth muscle have not been investigated and appear to be less likely than in skeletal muscle, since the former serves the more passive function of regulating the flow and distribution of the blood in the cardiovascular system.

The specific adaptations that occur during training depend on the particular type of exercise that is being performed. It is obvious that skeletal muscles adapt in different ways to the short-term burst activity of the sprinter and the long-term continuous activity of the marathon runner. The leg muscles of sprinters and the arm muscles of weightlifters recruit a greater fraction of their fast-twitch white fibers, whereas the legs of the long-distance runner primarily use high-oxidative capacity slow-twitch red and fast-twitch red fibers [47]. Changes in muscle fibers during force overload training consist primarily of an increase in muscle size, which serves to place a greater proportion of the myofibrils in parallel. This is reflected in the greater forces that can be developed dur-

ing contraction. There is some evidence that a slight increase in the concentration of key glycolytic enzymes, such as PFK, also occurs [50]. This increase is small, however, and suggests that the capacity of the cell to supply ATP through anaerobic glycolysis is optimal for the demands of the contractile apparatus during short-term burst activity. The parameters that lead to fatigue in these muscles may reside in the ability of the cell to tolerate changes in intracellular pH. Factors involved are cellular buffering capacity, proton pumps and translocases, and blood flow to the working muscle determining the rate of washout of metabolites.

Metabolic changes in muscle during endurance training provide a different situation. Studies on enzyme changes in mammalian skeletal muscle have revealed a pattern of changes during endurance training programs [25]. The predominant observation has been a general increase in the quantity of oxidative enzymes in all muscle fiber types that are exercised [18]. This increase is accompanied by an increase in concentration of the enzymes responsible for fatty acid oxidation. The latter change concurs with a general increase in fatty acid metabolism and conservation of glycogen. The conservation of glycogen appears to be an important determinant of performance for endurance athletes. It has been shown that performance declines dramatically when glycogen reserves are depleted [1]. Consequently, one result of endurance training is to conserve glycogen and increase the overall reserves of this compound. The reason for the dependence of performance of endurance exercise on glycogen content is not clear.

The total increase in concentration of mitochondrial enzymes of trained muscle does not reflect a major change in enzyme content per mitochondrion, but rather results from an increase in the mitochondrial fractional content of the cell. The significance of an increased mitochondrial content may be grasped by a look at cardiac muscle, where a large mitochondrial volume decreases the diffusion distance between the ATP-synthesizing sites and the contractile apparatus, thus allowing the muscle to supply ATP adequately from the oxidation of fatty acids [38]. This view is consistent with the observation that changes in total enzyme activity are not induced by exercise in cardiac muscle. This muscle already contains sufficient mitochondria to meet metabolic demands. The basic changes are directed toward hypertrophy of the muscle in the ventricular wall in order to increase stroke volume and, consequently, cardiac output.

Changes in vascular smooth muscle metabolism have not been documented. As with the case of cardiac muscle, a dramatic alteration of smooth muscle metabolism resulting from endurance training is not expected. Vascular smooth muscle performs essentially the same task as the heart, maintaining blood pressure and distribution through slow cyclic and tonic contractions. Experimental work on this tissue has involved the use of isolated strips of muscle studied in organ baths in the presence of glucose. Data suggest that the metabolic profile of this tissue is complex and the simple oxidation of glucose does not provide a complete picture. As with cardiac muscle, smooth muscle appears to be able to metabolize endogenous stores of fatty acids [7]. Endurance training-induced changes in blood concentration of fatty acids and hormones may alter smooth

muscle metabolism in important ways that relate to the overall health of the tissue. This area has not been adequately studied and may provide insights into the physiology and pathophysiology of this muscle type.

SPECIAL MUSCLE TYPES

The special muscle types, cardiac and smooth muscle, are defined relative to skeletal muscle (Table 2). The metabolic pattern that distinguishes these muscles from skeletal muscle is that both smooth and cardiac muscle rely explicitly on the close temporal matching of oxidative metabolism to changes in the metabolic demand. The incursion of an oxygen debt is not observed, and the glycolytic pathway may serve functions other than primarily maintaining the supply of ATP to the contractile apparatus in times of insufficient rates of oxidative metabolism. Consequently, these tissues have developed mechanisms (a) to ensure an adequate supply of oxygen, by increased vascularization, and (b) to prevent the occurrence of an oxygen debt, by decreasing the lag time between increase in energy demands of the contractile apparatus and onset of oxidative metabolism.

Cardiac muscle is not characterized by periods of activity followed by long periods

Table 2. SPECIAL MUSCLE TYPES

MUSCLE TYPE	MITOCHONDRIAL VOLUME FRACTION*	TENSION COST†	MYOSIN CONTENT‡	CELL DIAMETER§
Fast-twitch white	Low	High	High	Large
Fast-twitch red	Medium	High	High	Large
Slow-twitch red	Medium	Medium	High	Large
Cardiac	High	Medium	High	Medium
Smooth	Low	Low	Low	Small

*Represents the fraction of the total cellular volume that is composed of mitochondria. Data for skeletal and cardiac muscle from [11] and [15], for smooth muscle from [48].

†Represents energy cost of developed tension. Data for skeletal muscle from [46], for cardiac and smooth muscle from [34].

‡ See [40].

§ See [11] for skeletal muscle, [49] for cardiac muscle, and [5] for smooth muscle.

of inactivity: The heart beats continuously, throughout the lifetime of the body. Adjustments to the activity of the cardiac muscle are accomplished by increasing or decreasing the strength and rate of contraction. The maintained beating of the heart requires a steady supply of ATP to the contractile apparatus. Unlike the situation in skeletal muscle, in the heart during normal function the supply of ATP is not met by a large breakdown in PCr [23, 27a]. It is possible that small changes in PCr concentration occur during contraction. This is a source of controversy, however, and must be resolved by the refinement of current techniques to detect very small changes in tissue phosphagen content. It is sufficient to say that the magnitude of the proposed hydrolysis of PCr during contraction of cardiac muscle is small enough for the PCr to be completely resynthesized during the relaxation phase of the cardiac cycle.

The cardiac cell is small compared with the cell of skeletal muscle. This characteristic of cardiac muscle is important for enhancing the spread of excitation and the synchronous contraction of the heart. It also serves a key role in preventing the occurrance of an oxygen debt in this tissue. In muscle, the site of ATP synthesis in the mitochondria is spatially separated from the site of ATP hydrolysis in the contractile apparatus. In skeletal muscle, large cell diameter and low mitochondrial density result in a large diffusion distance between ATP-synthesizing reactions and ATP-utilizing reactions. Consequently, the ATP concentration in the contractile apparatus is maintained constant during brief bursts of activity by hydrolysis of PCr. The relatively small diameter of cardiac muscle, coupled with a lower actomyosin ATPase activity and large mitochondrial volume, serves to drastically reduce the diffusion distance between the mitochondria and the contractile proteins. It is observed that the metabolic demands of the heart are met exclusively by mitochondrial oxidative phosphorylation, and that the oxygen supply to the healthy heart is more than adequate. Anaerobic glycolysis is not stimulated except in extreme cases of cardiac dysfunction, for example, when stress is imposed on individuals with coronary artery disease.

Vascular smooth muscle surrounds the arteries and veins of the vasculature. During exercise, vascular smooth muscle directs blood to the working muscle and reduces blood flow to other areas of the body, such as the stomach and intestine. The unique feature of vascular smooth muscle that allows it to serve this function well is the high economy of tension maintenance of this tissue. The economy of tension maintenance is the rate of ATP utilization that is required to support a given level of force. In comparison with skeletal muscle, smooth muscle can support the same level of isometric force with an ATPase rate that is 1/500th that of fast skeletal muscle. It has been estimated that vascular smooth muscle can support the tone of the total vasculature while using only 1% of the basal rate of ATP hydrolysis of a 70-kg person [44].

Vascular smooth muscle is considered to be an oxidative muscle. Measurements of tissue oxygen consumption correlate well with the level of maintained isometric force. The rate of anaerobic glycolysis, unlike in cardiac and skeletal muscles, is high in the resting tissue. Data suggest that ATP derived from the metabolism of glucose, and the subsequent production of lactate, is used to supply energy to membrane processes such as the Na-K ATPase and ultimately to calcium transport mechanisms [32]. This separation of the oxidative and glycolytic metabolic pathways has been termed "functional compartmentalization" to suggest a functional separation rather than a separation due to a physical barrier. Although this hypothesis is of interest, it requires further experimentation concerning the use of substrates other than glucose in the reaction medium. It is important to realize that smooth muscle does not appear to derive all of the energy required to sustain contraction and maintain ion gradients from glucose and glycogen. A large fraction of the energy may be derived from endogenous and exogenous supplies of fatty acids [7].

Similar to cardiac muscle, smooth muscle has a relatively small cellular diameter. The medial layer of smooth muscle that surrounds the blood vessels is composed of a large number of cells that are serially connected to form a continuous network [13]. Smooth muscle is a tonic muscle capable of maintaining tension for long periods of time. This is accomplished without the incurrence of an oxygen debt. Tissue measurements of PCr do not reveal a significant decrease in PCr ($\pm$ 20%) from basal levels to full activation (28). This means that the ATP used by the contractile apparatus is resupplied by ATP synthesis employing oxidative metabolism. The small diameter of the smooth-muscle cell again is useful for reducing diffusion distances between the mitochondria and the contractile apparatus. Although smooth muscle relies on oxidative metabolism to supply ATP for tension development, the mitochondrial volume is similar to, if not less than, that of skeletal muscles. This tissue has a low actomyosin ATPase activity and a low myosin content relative to that of skeletal and cardiac muscle [41]. The net result is the low rate of ATP utilization required to support tension. Because of this low rate combined with the reduced diffusion distances due to the small cell diameter, the existing oxidative capacity is sufficient to supply ATP for tension maintenance in the steady state.

Maximum stimulation of vascular smooth muscle results in a twofold increase in tissue oxygen consumption, while PCr does not change more than 20%. If a simple Michaelis–Menten control theory is applied to the regulation of oxidative phosphorylation, the calculated change in ADP is not sufficient to account for the change in oxygen consumption. If the outcome is coupled with calculations that suggest that the cellular free ADP concentration in smooth muscle is approximately 100 μM, a concentration sufficient to saturate oxidative phosphorylation,

then regulation by this mechanism seems unlikely. It is important to realize that these calculations are based on cytosolic metabolite concentrations and may not reflect the concentrations actually in the mitochondrion. It is apparent, however, that a simple correlation between free ADP concentrations and the rate of tissue oxygen consumption is not obvious, and that other factors may have a regulatory function. A possible regulator may be the availability of substrates for oxidation or changes in intracellular calcium concentrations. This is an area of active research that is challenging the notion of sole ADP regulation in favor of multiple sites of regulation and the consequent greater flexibility that is derived from such a system.

REFERENCES

1. Åstrand, P.-O., and K. Rodahl. *Textbook of Work Physiology.* New York: McGraw-Hill, 1970, p. 466.
2. Bessman, S.P., and P.J. Geiger. Transport of energy in muscle: The phosphorylcreatine shuttle. *Science* 211:448–452, 1981.
3. Boscá, L., J.J. Aragon, and A. Sols. Modulation of muscle phosphofructokinase at physiological concentration of enzyme. *J. Biol. Chem.* 260:2100–2107, 1985.
4. Bowen, W.J., and T.D. Kerwin. The kinetics of myokinase. II. Studies of heat denaturation, the effects of salts and the state of equilibrium. *Arch. Biochem. Biophys.* 64:278–284, 1956.
5. Burnstock, G. Structure of smooth muscle and its innervation. In Bulbring, E., et al (eds.). *Smooth Muscle.* London: Arnold, 1970, pp. 1–69.
6. Carlson, F.D., and A. Siger. The mechanochemistry of muscular contraction. I. The isometric twitch. *J. Gen. Physiol.* 44:33–60, 1960.
7. Chace, K.V., and R. Odessey. The utilization by rabbit aorta of carbohydrates, fatty acids, ketone bodies, and amino acids as substrates for energy production. *Circ. Res.* 48:850–858, 1981.
8. Chance, B. Reaction of oxygen with the respiratory chain in cells and tissues. *J. Gen. Physiol.* 49(Suppl.):163–188, 1965.
9. Chance, B., and G.R. Williams. The respiratory chain and oxidative phosphorylation. *Adv. Enzymol.* 17:65–134, 1956.
10. Chasiotis, D. The regulation of glycogen phosphorylase and glycogen breakdown in human skeletal muscle. *Acta Physiol. Scand.* (Suppl.) 518:1–68, 1983.

11. Close, R.I. Dynamic properties of mammalian skeletal muscles. *Physiol. Rev.* 52:129–197, 1972.

12. Crow, M.T., and M.J. Kushmerick. Chemical energetics of slow- and fast-twitch muscles of the mouse. *J. Gen. Physiol.* 79:147–166, 1982.

13. Driska, S.P., D.N. Damon, and R.A. Murphy. Estimates of cellular mechanics in an arterial smooth muscle. *Biophys. J.* 24:525–540, 1978.

14. Egglton, G.P., and P. Eggleton. A method of estimating phosphagen and some other phosphorus compounds in muscle tissue. *J. Physiol. London* 68:193–211, 1929–1930.

15. Eisenberg, B.R. Quantitative ultrastructure of mammalian skeletal muscle. In Peachy, L.D., et al. (eds.). *Handbook of Physiology. Sec 10: Skeletal Muscle.* Bethesda, Md.: American Physiological Society, 1980, pp. 73–112.

16. Erecínska, M., R.L. Veech, and D.F. Wilson. Thermodynamic relationships between the oxidation-reduction reactions and the ATP synthesis in suspensions of isolated pigeon heart mitochondria. *Arch. Biochem. Biophys.* 160:412–421, 1974.

17. Erecínska, M., and D.F. Wilson. Regulation of cellular energy metabolism. *J. Membrane Biol.* 70:1–14, 1982.

18. Essén-Gustavsson, B., and J. Henriksson. Enzyme levels in pools of microdissected human muscle fibres of identified type: Adaptive response to exercise. *Acta Physiol. Scand.* 120:505–515, 1984.

19. Gadian, D.G., G.K. Radda, T.R. Brown, E.M. Chance, M.J. Dawson, and D.R. Wilkie. The activity of creatine kinase in frog skeletal muscle studied by saturation-transfer nuclear magnetic resonance. *Biochem. J.* 194:215–228, 1981.

20. Garland, P.B., E.A. Newsholme, and P.J. Randle. Regulation of glucose uptake by muscle. *Biochem. J.* 93:665–678, 1964.

21. George, P., and R.J. Rutman. The "high energy phosphate bone" concept. *Prog. Biophys. Chem.* 10:2–53, 1960.

22. Gillis, J.M. Relaxation of vertebrate skeletal muscle. A synthesis of the biochemical and physiological approaches. *Biochim. Biophys. Acta* 811:97–145, 1985.

23. Hassinen, I.E., and K. Hiltunen. Respiratory control in isolated perfused rat heart: Role of the equilibrium relations between the mitochondrial electron carriers and the adenylate system. *Biochim. Biophys. Acta* 408:319–330, 1975.

24. Hatefi, Y. The mitochondrial electron transport and oxidative phosphorylation system. *Annu. Rev. Biochem.* 54:1015–1069, 1985.

25. Holloszy, J.O., and F.W. Booth. Biochemical adaptations to endurance exercise in muscle. *Annu. Rev. Physiol.* 38:273–291, 1976.

26. Ingwall, J.S., and E.T. Fossel. Measurement of unidirectional phosphate fluxes in the creatine kinase reaction in normal and spontaneously hypertensive rat hearts using 31-P saturation transfer NMR. (Abstract) *Circulation* 62:III–19, 1980.

27. Jacobus, W.E. Respiratory control and the integration of heart high-energy phosphate metabolism by mitochondrial creatine kinase. *Annu. Rev. Physiol.* 47:707–725, 1985.

27a. Koretsky, A.P., S. Wang, J. Murphy-Boesch, M.P. Klein, T.L. James, and M.W. Weiner. 31P NMR spectroscopy of rat organs, in situ, using chronically implanted radiofrequency coils. *Proc. Natl. Acad. Sci. USA* 80:7491–7495, 1983.

28. Krisanda, J.M., and R.J. Paul. Phosphagen and metabolite content during contraction in porcine carotid artery. *Am. J. Physiol.* 244 (*Cell Physiol.* 13):C385–C390, 1983.

29. Kushmerick, M.J. Energetics of muscle contraction. In Peachey, L., R. Adrian, and S.R. Geiger (eds.). *Handbook of Physiology. Sec. 10: Skeletal Muscle.* Bethesda, Md.: American Physiological Society, 1983, pp. 189–236.

30. Kushmerick, M.J., and R.A. Meyer. Chemical changes in rat leg muscle by phosphorus nuclear magnetic resonance. *Am. J. Physiol.* 249 (*Cell Physiol.* 18):C362–365, 1985.

31. Lipmann, F. Metabolic generation and utilization of phosphate bond energy. *Adv. Enzymol.* 1:99–162, 1941.

32. Lynch, R.M., and R.J. Paul. Glucose uptake in porcine carotid artery: Relation to alterations in active Na$^+$-K$^+$ transport. *Am. J. Physiol.* 247 (*Cell Physiol.* 16):C433–C440, 1984.

33. Mahler, M. First-order kinetics of muscle oxygen consumption, and an equivalent proportionality between Q_{O2} and phosphorylcreatine level: Implications for the control of respiration. *J. Gen. Physiol.* 86:135–165, 1985.

34. Marston, S.B., and E.W. Taylor. Comparison of the myosin and actomyosin ATPase mechanisms of the four types of vertebrate muscles. *J. Molec. Biol.* 139:573–600, 1980.

35. McGilvery, R.W., and T.W. Murray. Calculated equilibria of phosphocreatine and adenosine phosphates during utilization of high energy phosphate by muscle. *J. Biol. Chem.* 249:5845–5850, 1974.

36. Mela-Riker, L.M., and R.D. Bukoski. Regulation of mitochondrial activity in cardiac cells. *Annu. Rev. Physiol.* 47:645–663, 1985.

37. Meyer, R.A., T.R. Brown, B.L. Krilowicz, and M.J. Kushmerick. Phosphagen and intracellular pH changes during contraction of creatine-depleted rat muscle. *Am. J. Physiol.* 250 (*Cell Physiol.* 19):C264–C274, 1986.

38. Meyer, R.A., H.L. Sweeney, and M.J. Kushmerick. A simple analysis of the "phosphocreatine shuttle." *Am. J. Physiol.* 246 (*Cell Physiol* 5):C365–C377, 1984.

39. Morgan, H.E., D.M. Regen, and C.R. Park. Identification of a mobile carrier-mediated sugar transport system in muscle. *J. Biol. Chem.* 239:369–374, 1964.

40. Murphy, R.A. Mechanics of vascular smooth muscle. In Bohr, D.F., A.P. Somblyo, and H.V. Sparks (eds.). *Handbook of Physiology. Sec. 2: The Cardiovascular System.* Bethesda, Md.: American Physiological Society, 1980, pp. 325–351.

41. Murphy, R.A., J.T. Herlihy, and J. Megerman. Force-generating capacity and contractile protein content of arterial smooth muscle. *J. Gen. Physiol.* 64:691–705, 1974.

42. Nunnally, R.L., and D.P. Hollis. Adenosine tri-

phosphate compartmentation in living hearts: A phosphorus nuclear magnetic resonance saturation transfer study. *Biochemistry* 18:3642–3646, 1079.

43. Palm, D.R., R. Goerl, and K.J. Burger. Evolution of catalytic and regulatory sites in phosphorylases. *Nature (London)* 313:500–502, 1985.

44. Paul, R.J. Chemical energetics of vascular smooth muscle. In Bohr, D.F., A.P. Samlyo, and H.V. Sparks (eds.). *Handbook of Physiology. Sec. 2: The Cardiovascular System*, Bethesda, Md.: American Physiological Society, 1980, pp. 201–236.

45. Rose, I.A. The state of magnesium in cells as estimated from the adenylate kinase equilibrium. *Proc. Natl. Acad. Sci. USA* 61:1079–1086, 1968.

46. Saltin, B., and P.D. Gollnick. Skeletal muscle adaptability: Significance for metabolism and performance. In Peachy, L.A., R.M. Adrian, and S.R. Geiger (eds.). *Handbook of Physiology. Sec. 10: Skeletal Muscle*. Bethesda, Md.: American Physiological Society, 1983, pp. 555–631.

47. Shephard, R.J. *Physiology and Biochemistry of Exercise*. New York: Praeger, 1982, p. 111.

48. Somlyo, A.V. Ultrastructure of vascular smooth muscle. In Bohr, D.F., A.P. Somlyo, and H.V. Sparks (eds.). *Handbook of Physiology. Sec. 2: The Cardiovascular System*, Bethesda, Md.: American Physiological Society, 1980, pp. 33–67.

49. Sommer, J.R., and E.A. Johnson. Ultrastructure of cardiac muscle. In Berne, R.M., et al. (eds.). *Hand-book of Physiology. The Cardiovascular System.* Bethesda, Md.: American Physiological Society, 1979, pp. 113–186.

50. Thorstensson, A., B. Hulten, W. von Dobeln, et al. Effect of strength training on enzyme activities and fibre characteristics in human skeletal muscle. *Acta Physiol. Scand.* 96:392–398, 1976.

51. Veech, R.L., J.W.R. Lawson, N.W. Cornell, and H.A. Krebs. Cytosolic phosphorylation potential. *J. Biol. Chem.* 254:6538–6547, 1979.

52. Wieland, O.H. The mammalian pyruvate dehydrogenase complex: Structure and regulation. *Rev. Physiol. Biochem. Pharmacol.* 96:123–170, 1983.

53. Wilson, D.F., M. Erecinska, and V.L. Schramm. Evaluation of the relationship between the intra- and extramitochondrial ATP]/[ADP] ratios using phosphoenolpyruvate carboxykinase. *J. Biol. Chem.* 258:10464–10473, 1983.

54. Wilson, D.F., M. Stubbs, N. Oshino, and M. Erecinska. Thermodynamic relationships between the mitochondrial oxidation-reduction reactions and cellular ATP levels in ascites tumor cells and perfused rat liver. *Biochemistry* 13:5305–5311, 1974.

55. Wilson, D.F., M. Stubbs, R.L. Veech, M. Erecinska, and H.A. Krebs. Equilibrium relations between the oxidation-reduction reactions and the adenosine triphosphate synthesis in suspensions of isolated liver cells. *Biochem. J.* 140:57–64, 1974.

Chapter 4

FUEL FOR MUSCULAR EXERCISE: ROLE OF CARBOHYDRATE

Bengt Saltin, M.D., and Philip D. Gollnick, Ph.D.

Speculations about how food is used by the body, and specifically about how food is utilized as substrate in the muscles to produce mechanical work, date far back in history [109]. During the seventeenth and eighteenth centuries these speculations began to be based on observations and measurements from experiments performed on muscles from various species or on intact animals, including humans (for references, see Needham [88]). It was soon learned that protein did not play a major role as a substrate for the energy turnover of contracting skeletal muscles, but that carbohydrate and fat did [96]. The respiratory exchange ratio (RER or R-value, also RQ in older literature) was found to become elevated with increasing exercise intensities [11], but with more prolonged exercise the R-value fell slightly [76, 85]. Thus, some very basic facts concerning the role of carbohydrate for muscular work, such as its greater role at higher exercise intensities and its lesser role in prolonged light efforts, have long been known. The effects of diet on the relative utilization of substrate at rest and during exercise, as well as the effects of endurance training on the metabolic response to exercise, have also been known for a long time. Thus, R-values were found to be lower at rest and during a given submaximal work level after a fat-protein diet than after a carbohydrate-protein diet [23]. With the latter diet, the time to fatigue was

increased and the time to exhaustion was markedly prolonged. The physically well-trained person could exercise at a given submaximal intensity with a lower R-value, indicating that muscle can adapt and reduce its dependence upon carbohydrate as a fuel [22]. In separate experiments performed in part on the same subjects, Bang [9] demonstrated that lactate concentrations in the blood were lower in trained subjects during submaximal exercise. This effect of training on the accumulation of lactate in blood is illustrated schematically in Figure 1.

In this and the following chapter, these findings will be discussed in some depth, the focus being on what regulates the rate by which the demands of the substrate turnover are met. First, however, some basic facts will be presented about carbohydrate use by humans.

CHARACTERISTICS AND DIETARY SOURCES OF CARBOHYDRATE

Carbohydrate (CHO) is a major energy source for muscle during exercise. This class of energy compounds is composed of repeating units of CH_2O. The name "carbohydrate" comes from the fact that within the molecular structure, each carbon is present in a ratio to hydrogen and oxygen the same as that found in water. The simplest CHOs

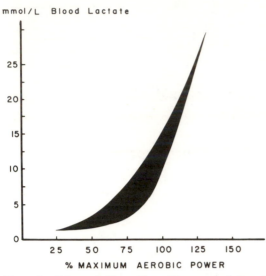

mmol/L   Blood Lactate

% MAXIMUM AEROBIC POWER

Figure 1. Schematic illustration of the accumulation of lactate in blood as a function of exercise intensity. Endurance training is associated with a delayed accumulation of lactate, as indicated by the lower portion of the curve. At high-intensity exercise, trained individuals generate as high or higher values than sedentary individuals.

that are metabolically important, sugars, have the general structure $C_6H_{12}O_6$. This formula encompasses a group of sugars that are collectively referred to as "monosaccharides," some of which are not metabolically important. Glucose and fructose, the most important of the monosaccharides for metabolism, are found in nature and are present in some foods. Their single greatest dietary source is sucrose, which is formed by the condensation of glucose and fructose. This disaccharide is derived in large amounts from sugar cane or sugar beets and is present in the diet as refined sugar. In the digestive process, sucrose is converted into equal portions of glucose and fructose. An important consideration in the comparative value of monosaccharides in metabolism, particularly the metabolism of exercise, is the fact that the rate of glucose absorption via the gut is more than twice that of fructose [25]. A large part of the fructose is used by the liver, where it is phosphorylated by fructokinase. Both glucose and fructose can be phosphory-

lated by hexokinase; however, the affinities of muscle and liver hexokinases for glucose are 10 and 1000 times greater, respectively, than for fructose [31, 48]. Thus, of the monosaccharides, glucose is the most important to the exercising muscle, as it can be taken up and utilized by the metabolic machinery of the muscle.

The greatest source of CHO in the average diet is starch, found in such foods as cereal grains and potatoes. Starches are large polymers of glucose that are degraded to glucose in the stomach and gut. The glucose is then absorbed into the blood, where it is transported to tissues for metabolism or storage. Glycogen, a polymer of glucose that differs from plant starch, is the method used by animals to store glucose. If more glucose is available in the body than can be stored as glycogen, the glucose is converted to fat and stored as triacylglycerol in adipocytes.

STORAGE OF CARBOHYDRATE IN THE HUMAN BODY

The overall storage of CHO in the body as glycogen is rather small. The priniciple sites of storage and the amount of glycogen stored in each are summarized in Table 1. Although the highest concentration of glycogen is found in the liver, this organ is not the largest site of glycogen storage. The large mass of skeletal muscle, and its relatively high glycogen concentration, results in skeletal muscle having the most stored glycogen. Glycogen in animal tissue differs from plant starch in that in addition to the normal α-1,4 bonds that produce the single straight chain of glucose, it possesses branch points produced by α-1,6 bonds (Figure 2). These branch points represent about 8% of the total glucose stored in glycogen. There are several important aspects of the α-1,6 bonds and the branch points of glycogen: (a) These points increase the availability of α-1,4 bonds for phosphorolysis by the enzyme phosphorylase, compared with what would be available in a single straight chain of the same molecu-

Table 1. PRINCIPAL SITES OF GLYCOGEN CARBOHYDRATE [CHO] STORES IN THE BODY AND STORAGE RATE (70-kg, NONOBESE MAN).

STORAGE SITE	GLYCOGEN WEIGHT OR VOLUME	MIXED DIET	HIGH CHO DIET	LOW CHO DIET
Liver	1.2 kg	40–50 g	70–90 g	0–20 g
Extracellular fluid	12 L	9–10 g(90 mg%)	10–11 g(100 mg%)	8–9 g(70 mg%)
Muscle	32 kg	350 g	600 g	300g

lar weight. (b) The points provide more sites for the addition of glucose units to the molecule during synthesis. (c) The points increase the solubility of the molecule. (d) During glycogen degradation, the debranching process releases free glucose into the cell. The role of the glycogen stored in liver and in skeletal muscle in total body metabolism are also different. Liver is the sole contributor of glucose to maintain glucose homeostasis, except in periods of prolonged starvation, when the kidney also contributes. The priority for storage of glucose that exceeds the needs of the body is in the skeletal muscle rather than the liver [40, 82, 83, 112]. In the postexercise period when the muscle is glycogen depleted, the liver does not take up significant amounts of glucose until the stores of the muscles are reasonably well filled. In periods of low CHO intake, such as during starvation or during days when only a small amount of CHO is present in the diet, glucose may be stored in muscle but not in the liver [12, 58]. The mechanisms responsible for the preferential refilling of the glycogen stores of muscle are unknown, and the signal to transfer storage to the liver after the muscles are adequately filled is equally unknown.

In the resting state, the uptake of glucose by muscle is controlled by insulin, as is the conversion of glycogen synthase from the D

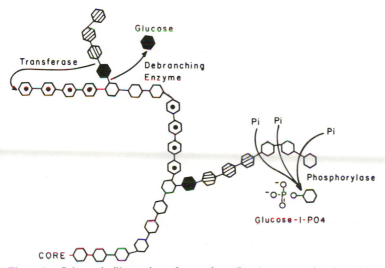

Figure 2. Schematic illustration of a portion of a glycogen molecule and its degradation. The glucosyl units with block dots represent the "limit dextran" beyond which phosphorylase cannot function, those with crosshatching represent the units transferred from the branch point to extend the straight chain to enable further degradation, and those of solid black are cleaved by the debranching enzyme to release free glucose.

form to the I form (glucose-6-phosphate [Glu-6-P]-dependent to Glu-6-P-independent forms), which probably is mediated via a reduction in cyclic adenosine monophosphate (cAMP). This "second messenger" is influenced by the catecholamines, and it is also known that glycogen concentration influences glycogen synthase I activity. Thus, in addition to high blood insulin concentration, a low glycogen concentration and minimum sympathetic activity are essential for a high rate of glycogen synthesis. Muscle may also use lactate, in addition to glucose, as a precursor for glycogen formation [56, 86]. This may be of practical significance only after intense exercise, when there are high concentrations of lactate in skeletal muscle. Glycogen synthesis in muscle appears to occur in spite of low or almost nonexistent concentrations of the enzymes malic enzyme, phosphenolpyruvate carboxykinase, and fructose-1,6-bisphosphatase in human skeletal muscle.

In the liver, gluconeogenesis plays a major role for glucose production from precursors such as glycerol, lactate, and some amino acids. However, storage of glycogen in the liver is unlikely to be influenced by this function, because the peak rate of gluconeogenesis coincides with shortage of glucose in the extracellular space, as in prolonged exercise or starvation.

Although the magnitude of the glucose taken up by the liver is independent of insulin concentration [73], there is uncertainty as to whether insulin has an effect on the conversion of glycogen synthase from the D to the I form similar to its effect in muscle. Even if it does affect conversion, other controls of the rate at which glucose is stored as glycogen in the liver must be present, sincle plasma insulin concentrations are higher in the portal vein than in the systemic blood. The liver is innervated by the parasympathetic and sympathetic nervous systems, and both systems affect the enzymes controlling the synthesis and degradation of glycogen. It is not known, however, whether they play a role in glucose homeo-stasis at rest. If they do, they provide a mechanism for precise control. The possibility has also been discussed that gastrointestinal peptides (peptides produced in the intestine) interact with insulin to control glycogen storage in the liver.

The content of CHO in the diet markedly influences the storage of glycogen in the body. This is true for both the rate at which storage occurs and the magnitude of storage in the liver [89, 90] and in muscle [29]. When a CHO rich diet is consumed over a couple of days preceded by a prolonged exercise period and some days of no significant CHO intake or of starvation, a doubling or tripling of the CHO stores of the body is observed [12]. For muscle, this effect is local, that is, it occurs only in the muscle or muscle fibers that have become glycogen depleted during the exercise bout [14]. This is sometimes called "supercompensation." This phenomenon has been extensively studied but the mechanisms by which it is regulated are not understood. Glycogen content of the cell is a potent inhibitor of glycogen synthase, but even if it brings down the percentage of the I form of synthase below 10 to 15% of total glycogen synthase activity, glycogen storage still occurs, as evidenced by increasing concentrations of muscle glycogen. The absolute amount of the enzyme appears to play a role in both the magnitude and the rate by which restorage of glycogen can take place. Endurance-trained muscle contains more glycogen synthase (both D and I forms) [93, 110], and these muscles can store an above-normal glycogen content in 10 to 15 hours if adequately supplied with CHO. This compares with a requirement of 24 to 48 hours for similar storage to occur in untrained muscle. It has been proposed that the enzyme glycogen synthase has a given number of sites for glycogen synthesis and that during synthesis these sites become covered. When all are covered, synthesis stops. Trained muscle has more glycogen synthase, and thus more glycogen can be stored. The glycogen stored in the human skeletal muscle appears to be evenly distributed within the muscle fiber, but fast-twitch fibers* contain slightly more glycogen than do slow-twitch fibers (see Saltin and Gollnick [105]). It is noteworthy that glycogen storage is associated with the binding of water. In the liver, 1 g of glycogen has been found to bind to 3 g of water, and there is indirect evidence for the same binding in muscle [92].

CARBOHYDRATE DEGRADATION

In all tissues, glycogen is degraded to glucose-1-phosphate (Glu-1-P) by action of the enzyme phosphorylase (PHOS) (Figure 2), after which it is converted to Glu-6-P by the enzyme Glu-6-P isomerase. The uniqueness of phosphorylated glucose molecules is that they do not diffuse out of tissues, such as skeletal muscle, and therefore, in a sense, they are captive metabolites. However, liver possesses a specific phosphatase, Glu-6-P phosphatase, which degrades Glu-6-P to glucose and inorganic phosphate (Pi). By this process, glucose can be produced from glycogen and released into the blood for transport to tissues that have limited storage capacities for glycogen, such as the central nervous system.

The complete oxidation of CHO proceeds through two distinct phases. The first series of reactions in this process occurs without consumption of oxygen through a series of reactions that are known collectively as the "Embden–Meyerhof pathway." It is also referred to as "anaerobic glycolysis" or sometimes simply as "glycolysis." However, since glycolysis means a breakdown of sugar and does not specifically identify whether breakdown occurs with or without oxygen, the initial (without oxygen) aspects of this process will henceforth be referred to as the Embden–Meyerhof pathway. When the source of CHO is glycogen, initial degradation is to Glu-1-P, which is converted to Glu-6-P. A unique role of Glu-6-P is that it is

also produced by the action of hexokinase on free glucose. Thus, it represents a merge point between the entry of glucose units derived from glycogen and the glucose taken up from the blood into a common pathway for CHO metabolism. The enzyme PHOS is specific for hydrolysis of the α-1,4 bonds of glycogen (Figure 2). This hydrolysis of glycogen by PHOS occurs only on the straight chain portion of the glycogen molecule and only until hydrolysis proceeds to within 4 glucose units of a α-1,6 branch point. At this point a specific transferase transfers the 3 glucose units to the α-1,4 part of the glycogen chain to form a straight chain, leaving behind the α-1,6-linked glucose unit. Exposure of the α-1,6 bond leads to its cleavage by a debranching enzyme. Degradation of glycogen then proceeds to the next sequence around an α-1,6 branch point, where the process is repeated. Thus, the transferase and debranching enzymes operate in concert to maintain the α-1,4 bonds that are susceptible to the action of PHOS and to produce free glucose.

The degradation of the glucose units provided to the Embden–Meyerhof pathway proceeds, through a series of reactions that occur in the cytosol, to the production of pyruvate. Under normal conditions, in which the cell is adequately oxygenated, the majority of the pyruvate formed is transported into the mitochondria for terminal oxidation to carbon dioxide and water. However, pyruvate can be reduced to lactate under conditions of both adequate and inadequate oxygen supply during high rates of glycogenolysis (Figure 3). Some energy is captured as adenosine triphosphate (ATP) in the cytosolic (Embden–Meyerhof) phase of this CHO degradation. The total energy released in the complete oxidation of 1 mol of glucose to CO_2 and H_2O is 686 kcal (1 kcal = 4.19J). When the initial glucose unit is derived from glycogen, there is a net ATP production of 3 mol of ATP for every 1 mol of glucose flux through the Embden–Meyerhof pathway. This is an energy recovery of 21 kcal. However, the energy in

---

*See chapter 2, Table 1 for fiber type nomenclature.

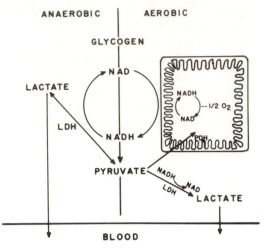

Figure 3. Schematic illustration of the production of pyruvate from glycogen. The prime purpose of the pyruvate is its delivery to mitochondria for terminal oxidation. However, any excess pyruvate produced under conditions of adequate oxygenation can be reduced to lactate via a mass action reaction of the lactate dehyrogenase reaction. Under conditions of very heavy exercise, the production of lactate may be associated with oxygen lack or the need to produce more energy than is being derived from the terminal oxidative processes associated with mitochondria.

pyruvate or lactate is still 634 kcal. There is thus a drop in total energy of 52 kcal in the degradation of 1 mol of glucose to 2 mol of lactate or pyruvate. The net energy recovery of the process is about 40%. When the initial source of glucose is blood glucose or glucose from the debranching step, the energy yield is only 2 mol per mol of glucose and the net efficiency of energy recovery as ATP falls to about 27%. This demonstrates that metabolically it is more efficient to use glycogen than to take up glucose from the blood. In the complete degradation of glycogen to CO_2 and H_2O, 36 mol of ATP is generated per mol of glucose units oxidized. The net energy capture is 252 kcal, which is an efficiency of about 37%. The important point here is that both aspects of the degradation, the "anaerobic" and the "aerobic" phases, are about equally efficient when considered from the standpoint of net energy captured as ATP, compared with the fall in free energy from the initial compound to the end

products. The oxidation of CHO gives 5.05 kcal of energy per liter of oxygen taken up.

REGULATION OF THE EMBDEN–MEYERHOF PATHWAY

All metabolic pathways and reactions within pathways require regulation to match the flux of substrate through the pathway (or step) to the need for the product of that pathway. In the case of exercise, the need is for ATP, and this can be derived from the degradation of glucose units. The breakdown of glycogen within muscle and acceleration of metabolism must be linked in some manner to the hydrolysis of ATP to adenosine diphosphate (ADP) during the contractile cycle.

Of the enzymes of the Embden-Meyerhof pathway, PHOS and phosphofructokinase (PFK) have perhaps been the most extensively studied, because they have properties that can be altered to regulate the rate of glucose flux through the pathway [52]. The study of these enzymes has identified many factors as either stimulating or inhibiting their activities. A full discussion of all factors is beyond the scope of this chapter, and therefore only a few points will be made. As indicated previously, PHOS occupies the key role in initiating the degradation of glycogen into Glu-1-P units. The enzyme exists in two forms. One, PHOS *b*, predominates at rest and does not catalyze the phosphorolysis of glycogen in the absence of rise in the AMP concentration. PHOS *b* is converted to PHOS *a* by at least two mechanisms, each involving phosphorylation catalyzed by phosphorylase kinase. An important difference between the two forms of PHOS is that PHOS *a* is active in the absence of AMP whereas PHOS *b* is active only in the presence of AMP. The activation of phosphorylase kinase can occur via an elevation of free calcium level within the cytosol or via the adenylate cyclase system as activated by the interaction of the catecholamines with the plasma membrane receptor site. This system provides for two methods for initiating glycogenolysis. The calcium activation of PHOS provides a direct link between contractile activity of the muscle and its metabolism. The mechanism for calcium activation is its binding to the kinase, which alters its affinity for PHOS. The second method for PHOS activation provides for a continual activation of the system, as indicated by exercise-associated changes in concentrations of hormones in the blood. Although glycogenolysis can be initiated in the absence of catecholamine stimulation from the adenylate cyclase system [37, 97], there probably is a synergism between the "internal" and "external" activation of phosphorolysis. During some types of exercise there may be a greater reliance upon one or the other regulation. An example of a primary reliance on the calcium activation would be during short-term, high-intensity exercise or during isometric conditions when blood flow to the muscle is restricted. In other instances, such as severe emotional stress, sympathetic stimulation may precede the onset of exercise. In prolonged exercise adrenergic activation of PHOS may also be crucial. Other factors also influence the activities of PHOS. Thus, a binding of AMP to PHOS relieves the inhibition of PHOS b to the extent that its activity is sufficient to initiate phosphorolysis of glycogen. AMP also enhances PHOS a activity. In addition, Pi is needed as a reactant in glycogen degradation [21, 116]. Its concentration can be increased by the breakdown of phosphocreatine (PCr). Pi has been suggested as being a regulator of PHOS activity during exercise, but, although its concentration increases 10- to 20-fold ($\sim$1 μmol·g^{-1} to $\sim$22 μmol·g^{-1}) [77] during exercise, this magnitude of change makes it an unlikely major regulator of PHOS and glycogenolysis.

The percentage of PHOS in the a form increases at the onset of muscular contraction to an extent that PHOS a could easily provide an excessive glucose flux through the Embden–Meyerhof pathway, the result being a surplus of pyruvate and the produc-

tion of lactate (Figure 3). However, some changes occur during continued exercise to modulate this initial burst of glycogenolysis. First, although PHOS a concentration increases at the onset of exercise, as the exercise continues its percentage of the total rapidly declines. The mechanism of the remission of PHOS a to PHOS b is not understood, because it occurs while there is a continual flux of calcium through the cytoplasm as contraction continues and the concentrations of epinephrine and norepinephrine in the blood increase (Figure 4). Since degradation of PHOS a to PHOS b is catalyzed by PHOS phosphatase, there must be activation of PHOS phosphatase. The transient alkalinizing effect that occurs at the onset of contraction, produced by the hydrolysis of PCr and by other mechanisms [81], may be involved in the initial burst of PHOS a forma-

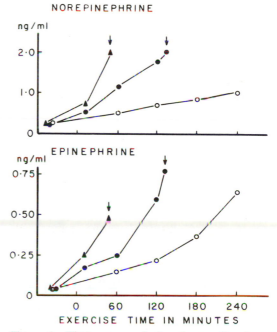

Figure 4. Time course of the changes in plasma epinephrine and norepinephrine during light ($\bigcirc$), moderately intense ($\bullet$), and heavy ($\blacktriangle$). exercise. Arrows indicate the point of exhaustion.

tion, because alkalinization activates PHOS *b* kinase, which catalyzes the PHOS *b* to PHOS *a* conversion [74, 75]. Lowering of the pH with continued activity and activation of PHOS phosphatase by an increase in free glucose concentration [8, 10] may be involved in the regression of PHOS *a* toward resting values during continued muscular activity [19, 24]. Such an effect of free glucose may be another way that the hydrolysis of the α-1,6 bonds in the glycogen molecule assists in regulating the flux of glucose through the Embden–Meyerhof pathway during exercise. A reduction of pH during exercise can not be considered as important in PHOS regulation, since the pH optimum of PHOS is about 6.1 (see below).

The large number of factors that influence PFK activity have led many to the conclusion that PFK is the prime regulator of glycolytic flux [113]. Among these "regulatory factors" are AMP, ATP, ADP (perhaps some function of their ratios), citrate, ammonium, and fructose bisphosphate. How many of these factors operate synergistically or antagonistically during exercise to control the flow of glucose units through the Embden—Meyerhof pathway is unknown. The role of ATP is to lower the affinity of the PFK for fructose-6-phosphate. Thus, reductions in the ATP concentration relieve the inhibition and promote a glycolytic flux. Also of importance is the fact that ADP, which relieves the inhibition, may increase in concentration during exercise; any combination of a decrease in ATP and an increase in ADP, which lowers the ratio of the two, enhances PFK activity. The mode of action of citrate on PFK is that it enhances the inhibition produced by ATP. Elevation of citrate level has been proposed to occur during high rates of fat oxidation, when an excessive production of citrate is released into the cytoplasm. The role of this mechanism during exercise is uncertain, since citrate also inhibits isocitrate dehydrogenase. If the concentration of citrate increases to the point where citrate is re-

leased from mitochondria, it would also inhibit mitochondrial respiration.

The initial events in the degradation of glycogen are catalyzed by enzymes frequently described as "soluble" or "cytosolic." As a point of clarification, it should be emphasized that this description of the enzymes of the Embden–Meyerhof pathway simply means that they are extramitochondrial and easily extractable. They should not be considered as floating enzymes existing within a watery mass whose only constraint is the plasma membrane (sarcolemma of muscle). The fact that these enzymes are easily extracted from muscle should not be construed as meaning that they do not exist in an ordered manner within the living cell. There is considerable evidence demonstrating that they are bound to tissue structures, perhaps in ordered arrays in which substrates and products of reactions are passed systematically between enzymes [108]. Further, variations between free and bound amount of the enzyme could be an additional mode for regulating the rate of glycolysis. This enzyme arrangement is consistent with the observation that there is little or no buildup of metabolic intermediates between the various reactions.

MITOCHONDRIAL OXIDATION OF PYRUVATE

Under most conditions, the major route for removal of pyruvate from the cytosol is by its entry into the mitochondria for oxidation to CO_2 and H_2O by the citric acid cycle and respiratory chain. The initial step in this process is the transport of the pyruvate into the mitochondria. This is accomplished by a specific translocase system within the inner mitochondrial membrane. Terminal oxidation of the pyruvate then occurs via conversion of the pyruvate to acetyl coenzyme A (CoA) via the pyruvate dehydrogenase system. The activity of this system is influenced by such intramitochondrial factors as the ATP/ADP ratio, the NADH/NAD (reduced and oxidized forms of nicotinamide adenine dinucleotide) ratio, and the acetyl CoA/AcA ratio. Thus, it is also linked to the energy demands of the contractile elements. Acetyl CoA is fed into the citric acid cycle as a result of a formation of citrate catalyzed by citrate synthase. Citrate synthase is an important control point in that its activity is markedly influenced by ATP, which decreases the synthase's affinity for acetyl CoA. Additional control points in the citric acid cycle are at isocitrate dehydrogenase and α-ketoglutarate dehydrogenase, both being nonequilibrium enzymes. The acitivity of isocitrate dehydrogenase is allosterically controlled by ADP, which produces a significant activation. It is also inhibited by NADH. Thus, this is a complex control point. Additional control points exist within the respiratory chain.

Although control of the various reactions within the mitochondria is of interest, here attention will be directed to the overall control of mitochondrial respiration within muscle cells. Clearly the energy demands, expressed by hydrolysis of ATP by the myofilaments during contraction, trigger not only the increased flux of glucose units through the Embden–Meyerhof pathway, but also the rate of substrate production, including oxygen use by the mitochondria and ATP production. The early studies of Chance and Williams [20] demonstrated that the respiratory rate of mitochondria could be controlled by the ADP. These investigations revealed that mitochondria respond to increasing concentrations of ADP in a manner similar to that of a large number of enzymes to their substrates, that is, by a hyperbolic increase in respiratory rate. From this relationship, the Michaelis constant (Km) was found to be about 25 μM. Considerable effort has been expended in trying to establish the precise regulator of mitochondrial respiratory rate under *in vivo* conditions. A number of factors have been proposed as being "the

controller," including the [ADP], the [ATP]/[ADP] ratio, and the [ATP]/([ADP]·[Pi]) ratio (the phosphate potential). In each of these expressions, the concentration of the reactant is that which is free in the cytosol and not the total concentration. Of paramount importance in all of these expressions is the fact that concentration of ATP in the cell is rather high, whereas that of the other components is low. Thus, a small change, for example in [ADP], will markedly offset the [ATP]/[ADP] ratio, whereas the [ATP] is relatively unchanged.

Creatine has also been proposed as being involved in the control of cellular respiration. This stems from the proposal of Bessman [15] that the immediate acceptor for the ATP produced within the mitochondria and translocated to the outer surface of the inner mitochondrial membrane is creatine, with the formation of PCr by mitochondrial-bound creatine kinase. A series of steps are then used to exchange the high-energy phosphate of the PCr with that of ADP to regenerate the ATP in the cytosol. Some support for the importance of the creatine-PCr shuttle comes from the observation that the concentration of creatine needed to stimulate half maximal respiration in mitochondria is one-tenth that of ADP [87]. This then represents a sensitive way for controlling mitochondria respiration and one that is still linked to the energy consumption of the system.

Both regulation of glucose flux through the Embden–Meyerhof pathway and mitochondrial respiration of skeletal muscle during exercise are directly linked to ATP demand in the contractile process. The immediate signal for this energy consumption probably is a transient rise in cytosolic [ADP], which can be sensed by both systems. The synergistic relationship between the activation of both systems for ATP production is therefore geared toward keeping a rather constant [ATP] within the muscle cell. These systems appear to fail only during very heavy exercise, when some reductions in ATP occur [57, 68].

CARBOHYDRATE UTILIZATION IN EXERCISE

The relative amount of CHO used by humans can be determined from the nonnitrogen R-value (cf. Chapter 6). The criterion that must be met for the measured R-value to represent metabolism is that the rate of CO_2 present in the expired air reflects its production from O_2 consumed in the tissue. This implies that the dynamics of the ventilatory system are not disturbed to a point where there is either release or retention of CO_2 that is not attributable to the metabolism. Several situations can produce this effect. The two most important are hyperventilation, which lowers alveolar Pco_2 to the point where CO_2 is unloaded from the blood, and metabolic acidosis produced by the release of acids, such as lactate, into the blood, which also releases CO_2 . With light to moderately heavy exercise, a steady state is usually established in about 20 minutes, at which time the R-value is representative of tissue metabolism [23]. At this point the R-value determined from the O_2 and CO_2 content of the blood, obtained from arterial and venous blood draining of an exercising limb, also agrees with the R-value based on gas exchange in the lung (43, 53, 60). In addition to R and blood-RQ measurements, other methods are available to evaluate the contribution of various substrates to energy metabolism. Included are measurement of blood flow combined with arteriovenous (av) differences for substrates and metabolites across an organ or exercising limb, tissue biopsies for determining substrates, and the use of tracer substances.

The use of these methods has demonstrated that the relative contribution of CHO to the total metabolism increases as a curvilinear function of exercise intensity at near or above the maximal oxygen uptake ($\dot{V}o_2$max), when nearly all of the energy may be derived from CHO oxidation (Figure 5). To discuss the interplay between intramuscular and extramuscular CHO use in exercise in more detail, we will consider three levels of exercise: light, moderate, and heavy (Figure 5).

Light Exercise

A light workload is defined as that which demands 30 to 40% of an individual's $\dot{V}o_2$max with a heart rate of about 110 bpm. The R-value in the early phase of this exercise is on the order of 0.80 to 0.85, and it gradually declines to just below 0.80 after several hours of exercise. Sedentary persons will not become exhausted at this exercise intensity. Muscle glycogen utilization is low, averaging less than 10 mmol glucose units $\cdot$ kg^{-1} $\cdot$ hr^{-1}. During the first couple of hours all of the glycogen depletion occurs in the slow-twitched fibers; overall depletion of the fast-twitch fibers is very minor [44] (Figure 6). No increase in blood lactate occurs. The uptake of glucose from the blood by the exercising legs gradually increases during the exercise, being ~1.5 to 2.0 mmol $\cdot$ min^{-1} after some hours of exercise [3]. This glucose uptake by the muscles, as well as by other tissues, is well matched by a release of glucose from the liver, since the arterial glucose concentration is stable throughout the exercise. A decline can only be anticipated after 3 to 4 hours or more of exercise, since the total clearance of glucose from the extracellular space amounts to 180 to 215 μmol or around 50 μmol glucose units $\cdot$ hr^{-1}, which is in the range that gluconeogenesis in the liver can produce glucose when the initial storage of glycogen in the liver is subnormal (Table 1). Exercise at this intensity can be sustained for many hours.

Moderate Exercise

Moderately heavy workloads demand 60 to 70_ of the $\dot{V}o_2$max and elicit heart rates of

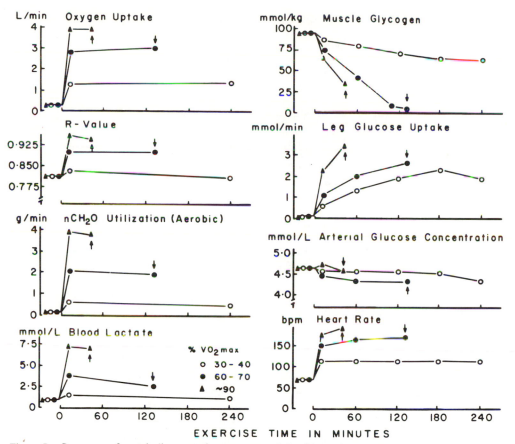

Figure 5.   Summary of metabolic events in response to light (○), moderate (●), and heavy (▲) exercise. This figure illustrates changes in heart rate, total body oxygen consumption, respiratory exchange ratio: (R-value; indicative of total fuel use), and blood lactate and changes representing metabolism in a single leg. Arrows represent the points of exhaustion.

160 to 170 bpm. The R-value will be close to 0.90 early in the exercise (Figure 5) and does not drop during exercise. Fatigue will be experienced, and after 2 to 3 hours of exercise even well-motivated subjects become exhausted.

Muscle glycogen content is reduced in a triphasic manner at this workload, being faster during the first 20 to 30 minutes of the exercise than later in the exercise. Thereafter a steady high rate of muscle glycogen utilization is observed, until muscle glycogen stores are depleted. Exercise usually can continue some time after this point is reached. Early in the exercise, glycogen

depletion occurs in the slow-twitch fibers, but some few fast-twitch fibers display depletion of glycogen (Figure 6). When a major portion of the slow-twitch fibers are glycogen depleted, both fast-twitch fiber types lose glycogen at a high rate. Of interest is the fact that blood lactate concentration is the highest after 5 to 10 minutes of exercise when the fast-twitch fiber involvement is small or nonexistent. Blood lactate level is declining and approaching the preexercise concentration later in the exercise when fast-twitch fibers are involved to a greater extent.

At this exercise intensity, the arterial blood glucose level remains fairly stable,

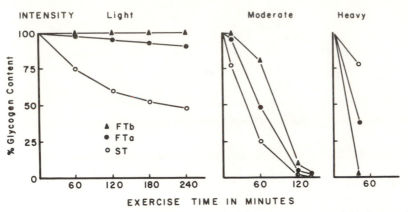

Figure 6. Time course of the relative reduction in glycogen content of the three major fiber types of human muscle during light, moderately intense, and heavy exercise. Light exercise was not continued to the point of exhaustion. See Chapter 2, Table 1 (page 11) for near-equivalent fiber type nomenclature.

being reduced by up to 0.5 mmol · L⁻¹. A decline in blood glucose concentration may be observed more frequently than at the lighter workloads, and this coincides with a fall in liver glucose output [5]. The inability of the liver to balance peripheral glucose utilization tissues probably occurs in the late stages of the exercise when glycogen-empty muscle fibers still contribute to the force development but have to rely to a great extent on extracellular fuels. At this workload exhaustion coincides with depletion of glycogen stores in both liver and muscle. Attempts to enhance the utilization of blood substrates have only minor effects [28].

Heavy Exercise

At a high exercise intensity demanding approximately 90% of the $\dot{V}O_2max$, the heart rate approaches its maximal level and the subject may become exhausted anytime between 5 and 60 minutes of exercise (Figure 5). The R-value is found to be around 0.95 throughout the exercise period. Muscle glycogen depletion is pronounced, but at exhaustion, substantial amounts of glycogen are still present in the muscle. This glycogen is located in the slow-twitch fibers, with both fast-twitch fiber types

being most commonly glycogen depleted [44] (Figure 6). This does not indicate that slow-twitch fibers are not recruited in the exercise, but rather demonstrates differences in metabolic potential between the various fiber types. More complete use of the energy stored in glycogen, that is, more oxidation of the pyruvate formed, can take place in the mitochondrial-rich slow-twitch fibers. Blood lactate concentration peaks at 5 to 10 mmol·L⁻¹ after 5 to 10 minutes of exercise and is fairly stable thereafter. In contrast to the effects of exercise at lower work levels, in high-density exercise arterial glucose concentrations may increase slightly, and insulin concentration will be markedly reduced. Glucose uptake by skeletal muscle per unit time is probably greater than at the moderate workloads, but the total amount taken up by the muscle is less, due to the shorter work time. The normal amount of glycogen stored in the liver is then sufficient to supply extracellular fluid and the peripheral tissues with the glucose for which there is a demand. Thus, CHO is available in both the muscle and the liver when exhaustion occurs, but a majority of the fast-twitch fibers are glycogen depleted.

At exercise close to or above $\dot{V}O_2max$ it is very difficult to quantitate exactly the contribution of various substrates to the energy metabolism. R- or RQ values are unreliable due to the rapidly developing metabolic acidosis and unloading of CO_2 from tissues and blood. The value of the use of tracers as well as of estimation of av differences, combined with blood flow measurements to evaluate substrate utilization, is limited due to the short work time and the fact that steady-state conditions are never reached. All indications favor exclusive use of CHO as fuel at these high work rates. A very high rate of muscle glycogen utilization is observed in the active muscle—the rate is so high that there may be a net release of glucose from the exercising limb [27, 115]. This can occur only if intracellular free glucose concentration exceeds that of the extracellular space, and would be the result of unphosphorylated glucose formed by hydrolysis of the α-1,6 bonds at the branching points of the glycogen molecule. In such cases, Glu-6-P would also accumulate in the muscle fibers, inhibiting hexokinase [31, 105] and thereby the rate at which glucose can be phosphorylated. This series of events would be more pronounced in the fast-twitch fibers, because they have the lowest hexokinase activity [105]. These fibers also experience the greatest glycogen depletion. The rapid accumulation of high concentrations of lactate in muscle and blood at maximal work is a further sign of a large dependence upon muscle glycogen as a substrate during heavy exercise.

Static Exercise

The basic mechanisms regulating CHO utilization are also at play in static contractions. However, when such contractions are sustained at a tension at which intramuscular pressure is elevated above arterial pressure, which may occur at about 20% of the maximal voluntary contraction (MVC), mechanical hindrance to blood flow will minimize the delivery and utilization of blood-borne substrates, including oxygen, as well as the role of circulating hormones and efflux of metabolites from the muscle. The highest rate of

glycogen breakdown is observed in very intense static contractions, but exhaustion occurs within such a short time that the total amount of lactate accumulated in the muscle is quite small. The highest concentrations of lactate are found when the contractions are in the range of 40 to 50% of the MVC or above. In these intense contractions it is likely that muscle glycogen is the sole substrate, as blood flow is very low or nonexistent. At lower contraction tensions, and when such static contractions are performed intermittently, an interplay is likely between the extramuscular and intramuscular supply of CHO, as in dynamic exercise.

GLUCONEOGENESIS AS AN ENERGY SOURCE DURING EXERCISE

Attempts have been made to determine the amount of glucose synthesized via gluconeogenesis in the liver during exercise in humans [3]. These studies suggest that during prolonged (240 minutes) mild exercise, the glucose released from the liver than can be attributed to gluconeogenesis represents only about 0.65 mmol $\cdot$ min^{-1}. This could account for about 8% of the total energy consumed per hour during such exercise. This fraction of the energy for exercise would be less with heavier exercise; however, current methodology has not permitted assessment of this process during heavy exercise. Thus, at present it appears that gluconeogenesis may be important only in the state of starvation, but its marginal role in prolonged exercise should not be neglected. The hormonal changes governing gluconeogenesis in exercise are described in Figure 7.

REGULATION OF INTERPLAY BETWEEN INTRAMUSCULAR AND EXTRAMUSCULAR CARBOHYDRATE UTILIZATION

The permeability of the sarcolemma for glucose is markedly increased with muscular

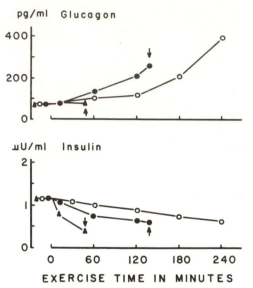

Figure 7. Time course of changes in the concentration of plasma glucagon and insulin in humans during the course of light (○), moderately heavy (●), and heavy (▲) exercise.

contraction [79]. It has been proposed that this insulin-independent glucose transport could be regulated by intracellular calcium concentration. From data on glucose uptake by the muscle, it is evident that glucose uptake gradually increases, being quite low early in the exercise and reaching a maximum later, when muscle glycogen content is lowered. Thus, there is an inverse relationship between muscle glucose uptake and rate of glycogen utilization. The link could be that the glucose formed when glycogen is broken down limits glucose uptake due to a smaller extracellular gradient for glucose. Of note is the fact that the insulin-mediated glucose uptake amounts to a very minor fraction of the total glucose uptake. In fact, insulin may not be needed—not even in a permissive dose—for glucose uptake by the muscle when it contracts.

In humans there is a very close coupling between peripheral tissue utilization of blood-borne glucose and the output of glucose from the liver, which maintains glucose concentration of the blood within narrow limits. The insulin level or insulin/glucagon ratio and glucose levels in the plasma are thought to be the stimulus for this regulation. The site for the sensor(s) could be either in the liver itself or in the hypothalamic region of the brain, with the effect being mediated via the sympathetic nervous system. Recent research suggests that a deviation (lowering) of blood glucose determines the hepatic glucose output, with insulin altering the sensitivity of this mechanism [61, 62].

LACTATE METABOLISM

As suggested previously, one important aspect of carbohydrate metabolism is the ability to oxidize the glucose molecule to lactate with the production of some ATP that is not dependent upon the uptake of oxygen. The historical development regarding the production and role of lactate in the metabolism of muscle has been reviewed by Karlsson [65]. From this discussion it appears that perhaps the earliest report of lactate in muscle was that of Berzelius, who observed it in the muscles of exhausted game animals. This was followed by numerous observations that the concentration of lactate in muscle becomes elevated with exercise. In fact, at one time it was thought that the immediate energy for the contractile process came from the production of lactate. That this was incorrect was subsequently shown by Lundsgaard [80] and Infante and Davies [59], who demonstrated that muscular contraction is powered by the hydrolysis of ATP.

There is no doubt that the ability of muscle to degrade glycogen or glucose units to lactate is important in exercise. The earlier studies of Lundsgaard demonstrated that without this source for energy production, the total work performed by the anaerobic muscle was greatly reduced. Studies with subjects lacking PFK and PHOS also demonstrate diminished exercise capacity [49]. The production of utilizable energy (ATP) derived from lactate production has several important aspects.

The mechanism(s) by which lactate production is controlled during exercise has (have) been debated for some time. The classical view is based on the fact that when muscle contracts in the absence of oxygen, there is obligatory lactate production. It has therefore been assumed that the production of lactate is consistent with oxygen in sufficiency and there is anaerobiosis within the muscle. Evidence from several different situations refutes such a claim. First, lactate accumulates in muscle and blood well before the point when oxygen delivery is inadequate to support metabolism. Second, in persons exercising at the same absolute or relative load, after training lactate accumulation in the muscle and blood is lower than before training (Figure 1). At the same absolute submaximal power production, blood flow to the muscle, a$\bar{v}$ oxygen difference, and oxygen uptake are the same regardless of whether or not lactate is produced [4]. Third, measurements of oxygen tensions within tissue suggest that lactate can be produced under fully aerobic conditions. The point is that lactate can be produced in the muscle in spite of adequate oxygen supply, but when oxygen supply is insufficient, lactate formation accelerates.

Since lactate can be produced under aerobic conditions, it must be assumed that in some situations lactate production represents a mismatch between the rate of pyruvate production and the amounts of pyruvate needed to fuel the oxidative processes carried out by the mitochondria. Under such conditions the excess pyruvate is reduced to lactate by a simple mass action effect resulting from the availability of pyruvate and NADH. Since the lactate dehydrogenase reaction is an equilibrium reaction, lactate production will occur whenever cellular mechanisms present substrates to the enzyme.

Another aspect is the rate at which lactate can be produced. This varies widely [36] and depends upon the concentration of the enzymes of the Embden–Meyerhof pathway present within the muscle, which in turn varies widely as a function of fiber types contained in muscle (see Saltin and Gollnick [105]. The maximal rate of lactate production induced by the electrical stimulation of fast-twitch fibers (those with high concentrations of enzymes of the Embden–Meyerhof pathway) of rats reportedly is about 0.5 μmol $\cdot$ g^{-1} wet weight $\cdot$ s^{-1}, and the rate for slow-twitch fibers is about half that. In human skeletal muscle, lactate has been observed to accumulate at the rate of about 0.9 μmol $\cdot$ g^{-1} wet weight $\cdot$ s^{-1} [1] during isometric contractions. Since 1.5 μmol of ATP is produced per micromole of lactate produced, the ATP production by muscle from a maximal activation of the Embden–Meyerhof pathway ranges from 0.375 to 0.75 μmol $\cdot$ g^{-1} wet weight $\cdot$ s^{-1} for slow-twitch and fast-twitch muscle fibers of rats and to 1.35 μmol $\cdot$ g^{-1} wet weight $\cdot$ s^{-1} for human skeletal muscle. The maximal rate of ATP utilization is about 3.0 μmol $\cdot$ g^{-1} $\cdot$ s^{-1}. There is an early breakdown of PCr at the onset of maximal exercise; if this were present in a concentration of 25 μmol $\cdot$ g^{-1} PCr would be depleted in 7 to 8 seconds. During very short maximal burst of exercise, such as sprinting, only a relatively small ($\sim$6–8 μmol $\cdot$ g^{-1}) increase in muscle lactate concentration would be needed to provide the required ATP. The onset of exhaustion under such conditions may not be related to elevation in muscle lactate level. It would be necessary to perform maximal effort for 40 to 50 seconds to completely load the buffering capacity of muscle beyond its limits in order to exert a major disturbance of pH.

ROLES OF AEROBIC AND ANAEROBIC ATP PRODUCTION FROM GLYCOGEN DURING MAXIMAL EFFORT

The aerobic and anaerobic energy production of ATP from muscle glycogen is important during heavy exercise. Such production can be related to reported values for ATP production and consumption during exercise. Sustained ATP production of about 55 and consumption of about 75 mmol $\cdot$ kg^{-1} wet weight $\cdot$ min^{-1} have been observed for human skeletal muscle during an isometric contraction of about 65% of maximal voluntary contractile strength [69] and isolated mouse extensor digitorum longus muscle [32]. Oxygen uptake of about 350 ml$\cdot$kg^{-1} wet weight$\cdot$min^{-1} has been measured for human skeletal muscle during dynamic exercise [4]. This would consume about 0.47 g glucose units $\cdot$ kg^{-1} wet weight $\cdot$ min^{-1} and produce about 94 mmol ATP$\cdot$kg^{-1} wet weight$\cdot$min^{-1}. To this could be added about 20 to 45 mmol of ATP [69, 84] from lactate production (15–30 mmol$\cdot$kg^{-1} and would consume an additional 1.1 to 2.7 g glucose units $\cdot$ kg^{-1} wet weight $\cdot$ min^{-1}. Thus, lactate production, while yielding about 20 to 50% as much ATP as the aerobic process, consumes 2.3 to 5.7 times more glycogen, which is a high cost for the intracellular glycogen store. These calculated glycogen consumptions by skeletal muscle may not be verifiable during normal exercise with the biopsy technique, since muscle samples obtained with this technique include fibers that vary between being inactive to maximally active. The combined maximal capacity for ATP production from aerobic and anaerobic processes of skeletal muscle during sustained exercise appears to range from 115 to 140 mmol ATP$\cdot$kg$^{-1}\cdot$min^{-1}, which is greater than that reported for isolated mouse muscle or human muscle during the isometric contractions. The reason for this disparity is unknown but could lie in the nature of the exercise.

Another important consideration concerning lactate production during muscular activity is that although it contributes to the total energy-producing capacity of muscle, it can have adverse effects resulting from the generation of protons by a lowering of the pH of the fibers. Most of the protons remain within the muscle during short bursts of activity, since the translocation rate of lactate to the vascular, to other fluid compartments, and to tissues of the body is limited. Some data are available that allow estimates of these buffering pools. Human skeletal muscle has been estimated to be able to buffer about 60 μmol H$^+$ $\cdot$ g^{-1} $\cdot$ pH^{-1} [101, 103]. The majority of the buffering capacity of resting muscle appears to be attributable to the presence of the proteins, bicarbonate and phosphate, and to carnosine. Capacity is augmented during exercise by the release of additional phosphate from the breakdown of PCr. Hydrogen ions are taken up in the process of the transfer of high-energy phosphate from PCr to ADP, and this contributes to the overall control of pH.

The reported effects of a lowering of muscle pH include alterations in the processes involved in the excitation-contraction coupling, in the contractile properties, and in the ability to sustain the flux of substrates through the major energy-producing pathways [35, 39, 84]. There is some uncertainty as to the maximal proton load that muscle can sustain without this occurring. At this time it may suffice to say that the pH of skeletal muscle during maximal exercise reportedly is in the range of 6.2 to 6.4 [54, 101–104]. On this basis, it would appear that the proton container of muscle could be filled in 40 to 70 seconds with protons generated by the Embden–Meyerhof pathway.

It should be pointed out, however, that ^{31}P nuclear magnetic resonance [33, 99, 111] has been used to estimate the pH of muscle at rest and during exercise, and pH's as low as 5.9 have been reported for healthy individuals during intense exercise. Use of these pH's in the previous calculations gives estimated work periods that can be sustained by humans that are inordinately long compared with those that can actually be accomplished. Although this method is promising and is attractive due to its noninvasive nature, it provides indirect estimates of intracellular constituents, and additional time is needed to validate results.

The concentration of lactate in blood can be evaluated rather easily, and the total that can be assimilated by this compartment is determined by the blood volume. If it is assumed that this lactate pool is in equilibrium with the total extracellular space, the latter can also be estimated. A more difficult task is evaluation of the amount of lactate that is taken up by other tissues, and thus an estimate of the total amount produced of lactate or present in the body is difficult to achieve.

LACTATE AS A FUEL FOR MUSCULAR WORK

It is an old [9] and often verified [67, 106] observation that the initial elevation in lactate concentration in blood at the onset of moderately severe, prolonged exercise is followed by a gradual decline toward resting values. These observations were extended with Jorfeldt [63] demonstrated that active muscle took up and oxidized ^{14}C-labeled lactate. Another indication of the use of lactate as a substrate for oxidative metabolism in contracting muscles is the finding of a markedly larger postexercise clearance of lactate during exercise compared with the resting state [55]. Attempts to quantitate the importance of oxidation of the lactate removed from the blood during exercise has led to a variety of estimates of the contribution of lactate to the total metabolism [27, 41]. The methodological difficulties associated with methods used to date are such that uncertainty exists as to the exact contribution the uptake and oxidation of lactate make to the metabolism of muscle [70]. When such estimates were based solely on net uptake of lactate, assessed from the venous-arterial difference in the exercising leg and the blood flow, with one leg low and the other high in glycogen content, the oxidation of lactate could account for from 2 to 8% of the total muscle metabolism [43]. It is evident that a substantial flux of lactate may occur between fibers in a contracting muscle, as measured with a tracer technique. However, such measures cannot give an estimate of the oxidative use of the lactate removed from the blood by the muscle.

On the basis of these tracer studies of lactate metabolism in exercise, it has been suggested that lactate is produced at equal rates in trained and untrained muscle, the difference in lactate concentration in blood being attributable to a larger clearance rate of lactate from the blood in the trained state. It is difficult to envisage a model to incorporate this concept within the well-established observations of a low R-value (greater fat oxidation) and a reduced rate of glycogen degradation during exercise in endurance-trained humans.

CARBOHYDRATE METABOLISM AND MUSCULAR-FATIGUE

As discussed previously, the production of lactate during exercise results in a reduction in pH of the muscle. It has been reported that PFK is very sensitive to pH [114]. In fact, it has been further reported [114] that at pH 6.9, PFK activity is almost nil. On the basis of available findings, this appears to be unlikely *in vivo*. Of importance is the fact that the pH of muscle at rest is about 7.0. The lactate concentration of muscle during heavy exercise has been reported to be in the range of 20 to 30 mmol · g^{-1} wet muscle. Using the equation that relates muscle lactate to pH [102], such a lactate concentration would produce a pH of around 6.5, which also has been measured [54]. If PFK is as inhibited as has been reported by Trivedi and Danforth [114], it would be impossible for the Embden—Meyerhof pathway to continue to the extent that lactate production could produce these low pH values and high lactate concentrations. ATP concentrations in the muscle would be susceptible to marked reductions. Moreover, since PHOS is not inhibited by a low pH (in fact its maximal activity occurs at approximately pH 6.1), it could be expected that its activity would continue during exercise with a large accumulation of Glu-1-P, Glu-6-P, and fructose-6-phosphate. However, this does not happen in frog muscle stimulated under anaerobic conditions [38, 43, 52, 68] or in humans during intense exercise [38, 43, 45]. In frog muscle, the rise in Glu-6-P was not dissimilar to the rise in fructose-1,6-bisphosphate, which suggests that there is no preferential inhibition of PFK. In these experiments the lactate concentration of the muscle was sufficient to have produced a pH of about 6.4. On the basis of these findings, it appears that the inhibitory effect of pH on PFK may not be as dramatic as reported in the earlier experiments. This is in accord with the observation that ATP resynthesis is well maintained except at very extreme conditions, that is, at repeated bursts of short-term intense exercise.

Since it appears that a lowering of muscle pH does not have as severe an effect on the regulation of PFK as has been proposed, it is possible that a decrease in pH might exert an effect on the contractile properties of muscle. This has been studied by Donaldson and Hermansen [35], who demonstrated that a lowering of muscle pH reduced the affinity for the binding of calcium to sites on the contractile proteins, thereby reducing the tension developed at a given calcium concentration. The effect appeared to be most pronounced in the fast-twitch fibers, in which a 50% reduction in tension occurred at a pH of 6.5.

In more prolonged exercise, lactate does not accumulate and the pH is not markedly reduced. Instead, availability of substrate may be crucial. In experiments in which muscle glycogen content has been either increased or decreased, prolonged exercise capacity at exercise intensities above 50 to 60% of the Vo_2max is closely related to the initial glycogen content of the muscles engaged in the exercise. Although a high glycogen content in muscle does not enable performance at a higher exercise intensity, since this is a function of cardiovascular capacity, it does enable individuals to perform exercise longer at a given submaximal pace.

The importance of local glycogen stores to muscle metabolism during heavy exercise may have several reasons, such as (a) their intracellular localization and the lack of need to transport CHO from external sites to the site of its use, (b) the slightly higher energy yield per unit of oxygen consumed, (c) the ability to derive some energy from the anaerobic phase of the Embden–Meyerhof pathway, and (d) the relative ease for translocation within the cell. Although these points are true and may be important for maximal performance, it is our opinion that the significance of muscle glycogen concentrations stems from the inability of glucose and fatty acids to cross the cell membrane rapidly enough to provide adequate acetate units for mitochondrial respiration. The best evidence supporting this concept comes for the studies of Haller et al. [49]. They studied patients with McArdle's disease, who lack muscle PHOS and thus depend entirely upon blood-borne substrates as fuels for muscular contraction. These subjects have a low work capacity, and manipulations to supply the muscle with more substrates improved the subjects' exercise tolerance. This relates well to the finding in normal individuals of reductions in maximal oxygen uptake and exercise capacity when muscle glycogen stores are reduced [6, 51].

The situation may be different when only a small fraction of the muscle mass is engaged in the exercise. Data are available from forearm [115] and from single-leg knee-extensor exercise [107]. After the first 15 to 30 minutes of exercise, glucose uptake (in the case of knee-extensor work) contributed between 30 and 50% of the total energy turnover, which amounted to 3.25 kcal·min^{-1} (another 30–50% supplied by free fatty acids that were taken up by the muscles from the blood). The total uptake of glucose by the muscle was only 14 to 15 g in 60 minutes of exercise. With 50 to 60 g of glycogen in the liver, hepatic glucose output can maintain blood glucose concentration at a normal or near-normal level for many hours under these conditions, especially in view of the capacity for glucose production via gluconeogenesis.

CARBOHYDRATE USE BY THE CENTRAL NERVOUS SYSTEM: IMPLICATION FOR USE OF EXTRACELLULAR GLUCOSE BY MUSCLE DURING EXERCISE

Under conditions of heavy exercise and almost total reliance on CHO, the total amount of glucose utilized can be in the range of 20 to 30 mmol $\cdot$ min^{-1}. Most of this will be consumed by the skeletal muscle. With the assumption that the total extracellular space of humans is 12 L and that the average glucose concentration is this fluid is 4.5 mmol $\cdot$ L^{-1}, about 55 mmol of glucose is available from this pool at any one time. Without any further augmentation, this energy pool would be exhausted in 2 to 3 minutes during heavy exercise. An adverse effect of such a depletion of the extracellular glucose stems from the fact that the nervous system is almost exclusively dependent upon glucose delivered to it by the circulatory system for its metabolism. It has been estimated that the nervous system uses about 0.38 mmol glucose $\cdot$ min^{-1}. Without a continual replenishment of glucose into the extracellular fluid, fuel for the central nervous system could last 2.5 hours. However, glucose uptake from the extracellular fluid to fuel the metabolism of the skeletal muscles during heavy exercise would deplete the supply to a point that would severely compromise the functional capacity of the central nervous system. As discussed earlier, under most conditions glucose is continually released from the liver to balance its use by peripheral tissues. However, this release is inadequate to meet total body demands for glucose during heavy exercise. The problem is solved through inhibition of glucose uptake by muscle during heavy exercise, partially as a result of reduction in the insulin concentration of the blood [16, 17, 98, 117] and by inhibition of hexokinase due to a rise in Glu-6-P and free ADP [48] in the muscle cell during heavy exercise. It is recognized that the total amount of insulin traversing the muscle is increased due to elevated blood flow. However, since hormone binding to receptor sites is concentration dependent rather than volume (concentration times blood flow) dependent, this is an effective way to reduce the insulin-dependent transport of glucose into muscle. Not only is there reduced glucose uptake by muscle during heavy exercise, but, as pointed out earlier, there may actually be release of glucose from the muscle in some circumstances.

A number of investigators report precipitous declines in blood glucose concentration during exercise with dysfunction of the central nervous system [12, 23, 76, 85], resulting in loss of visual acuity and inability to concentrate. This has been observed during moderately severe exercise sustained for several hours. During such exercise, lack of inhibition of glucose uptake can probably be attributed to failure of the levels of Glu-6-P and free ADP to become elevated within the muscle cell. Continued glucose uptake by muscle from blood will ultimately reduce total body reserves to a dangerously low point. In some studies, for example that of Christensen and Hansen [23] with humans and that of Dill and coworkers [34] with dogs, glucose feeding reversed these effects and restored working capacity. These data provide further support for the suggestion that the gluconeogenic capacity of the liver is insufficient to produce glucose rapidly enough to support the metabolism of muscle and the central nervous system.

Effect of Preexercise Ingestion of Glucose

The importance of depression in blood insulin concentration during exercise has been demonstrated by preexercise ingestion of glucose, which produces an increase in insulin level and a rapid decline in blood glucose level during exercise [2, 117]. Of interest, and of practical importance, in this regulatory system is that glucose ingestion during exercise does not produce an insulin surge, in spite of the fact that glucose is taken up into the blood stream from the gut [17].

The reason is that during exercise, insulin release is inhibited by the sympathetic nervous system [42]. Ingestion of fructose appears to elevate insulin concentration even less [70]. Oral intake of sugar during exercise has not greatly altered the rate by which muscle glycogen stores are depleted, probably because the total amount made available to the body is rather small. However, the ingested sucrose is used by the working muscles [94, 95]. Glucose has been infused directly into the blood of humans during exercise. This has maintained blood glucose levels and reduced the rate of glycogen depletion in muscle [4]. In the rat [7], infusion during exercise retarded the rate of glycogen depletion from liver and hind limb muscles during moderately severe exercise. This treatment did increase the work capacity of the animals. A similar prolongation of exercise capacity occurred in humans after oral ingestion of CHO [30], and it occurred without any modification of the relative contribution of fat and CHO in the total metabolism. Also in humans, ingestion of solid glucose by mouth at hourly intervals during prolonged exercise has been reported to produce elevations in blood glucose 20 minutes after consumption [50]. This protocol lowered the rate of depletion of muscle glycogen and enabled the subjects to improve their sprinting capacity at the end of the exercise. It also lowered the plasma free fatty acid concentrations and resulted in a greater reliance on CHO, as indicated by R-values. Intravenous infusion of glucose during exercise also has been reported to retard the release of glucose from the liver of humans [61, 62]. Preexercise ingestion of fructose has been tried as a way of conserving muscle glycogen stores. Under these conditions glycogen sparing was noted during 30 minutes of exercise at an intensity of about 75% of $\dot{V}O_2$max [78] but not during 2 hours of exercise at about 55% of $\dot{V}O_2$max [71]. Infusion of fructose into resting human subjects after an overnight fast produced an increase in muscle glycogen content similar to that following an infusion of glucose [91]. However, under these conditions the in-

crease in liver glycogen was more than 3.5-fold greater following fructose than following glucose infusion. These data are consistent with the observation that the liver takes up fructose more rapidly than glucose [91].

Several factors must be considered when examining the possible role of fructose ingestion in sparing muscle glycogen depletion during exercise [72]. An important factor is the rate of gastrointestinal absorption, which has been shown to be considerably lower (Figure 8) than that for glucose [25]. However, once fructose or glucose is absorbed, the rate of glycogen synthesis is about the same for both (Figure 9) [26]. Furthermore, when glucose or fructose were infused into humans, there was a greater increase in liver glycogen concentration compared with muscle concentration following the fructose infusion (Figures 10 and 11) [89]. In addition, the lower affinity of hexokinase for fructose than for glucose [31] and the fact that hexokinase is inhibited by fructose [48] combine to make fructose unlikely as a carbohydrate source that will retard gly-

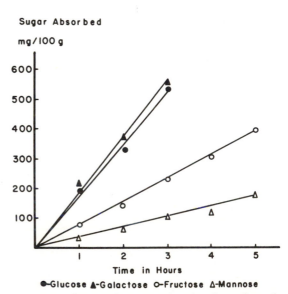

Figure 8. Comparative rates for the absorption of sugars by the rat gut. (Data from Cori, C.F. The fate of sugar in the animal body. I. The rate of absorption of hexoses and pentoses from the intestinal tract. *J. Biol. Chem.* 66:691–715, 1925.)

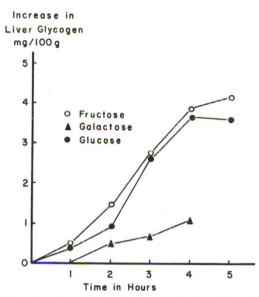

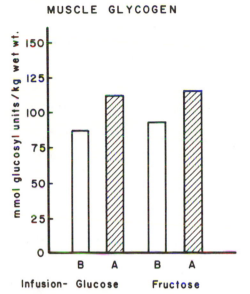

Figure 9. Rate of glycogen increase in the rat liver after absorption of different monosaccharides. (Data adapted from Cori, C.F. The fate of sugar in the animal body. III. The rate of glycogen formation in the liver of normal and insulinized rats during the absorption of glucose, fructose, and galactose. *J. Biol. Chem.* 70:577–585, 1926.)

Figure 11. Comparison of concentrations of glycogen in human skeletal muscle after infusion of either glucose or fructose. (Modified from Nilsson, L.H., and E. Holtman. Liver and muscle glycogen in man after glucose and fructose infusion. *Scand. J. Clin. Lab. Invest.* 3:5–10, 1974.

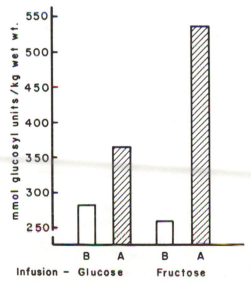

Figure 10. Comparison of concentrations of glycogen in the human liver before and after infusion of either glucose or fructose. (Modified from Nilsson, L.H., and E. Hultman. Liver and muscle glycogen in man after glucose and fructose infusion. *Scand. J. Clin. Lab. Invest.* 3:5–10, 1974.)

cogen depletion of muscle during exercise. Thus, any biochemical advantage to carbohydrate metabolism of the contracting muscle is obscure. There is a smaller insulin surge in response to fructose ingestion compared with glucose ingestion [78]. Whether this can offset the disadvantage of the slower absorption of fructose and its use by muscle is unknown. However, during exercise the insulin concentration in blood is normally depressed, and if glucose were ingested after the onset of exercise, any adverse effect from a rise in insulin would be largely negated. Thus, at the present time the evidence that fructose ingestion prior to exercise will significantly conserve muscle glucose stores is not sufficiently strong to recommend its consumption.

Effect of Beta-Blockers

As pointed out earlier, the sympathetic nervous system is involved in the regulation of CHO metabolism both in muscle and liver. Thus, it could be anticipated that treatment with β-blockers would markedly affect hepatic glucose output and muscle glycogen breakdown. This is, however, not what is generally observed. Blood glucose concentration is well maintained and muscle glucose breakdown during exercise is almost unaffected [64]. This should not be taken as an indication that the sympathetic nervous system has no role for regulating these variables at rest and exercise. Rather, it indicates that other regulatory factors can operate to produce a close to normal adjustment. The largest effect that treatment with β-blockers may have on muscle CHO metabolism is related to reduced cardiac output and subsequent reduction in blood flow to muscle during exercise. This affects lactate elimination from the muscle, resulting in increased muscle lactate concentrations. The amount of glucose offered to the muscle will also be diminished, but glucose uptake by the muscle is relatively flow independent.

DIET

The source of fuel for energy metabolism used during rest and exercise can be greatly altered by diet, as alluded to previously (Table 1). If a person consumes a high CHO diet, the R-value may approach 1.0, which indicates almost complete dependence on the oxidation of CHO. Conversely, the consumption of a CHO-poor diet results in progressively greater reliance on fat as the fuel for metabolism and a corresponding decrease in the resting R-value, which indicates decreased use of CHO. This pattern of coupling between diet and metabolism extends into exercise. Elevated storage of CHO in liver and muscle enables these organs to use more of this fuel during exercise. Further, exercise capacity is prolonged in relation to this enlarged storage of muscle glycogen. Profound changes in diet over a couple of days result only in a very small or no alteration in the concentration of enzymes in related pathways. Instead, the availability of substrate, augmented by hormonal changes, is the factor for the preferential use

of fuels observed after short-term changes in diet.

PHYSICAL TRAINING

Endurance-type physical training results in reduced dependence on CHO as fuel. This alteration in metabolic response to exercise is in part brought about by smaller changes in ATP and ADP in muscles during exercise after training [36, 66] and appears to be related to increase in the concentration of mitochondria within the trained muscle fibers. Thus, ADP, or its equivalent as creatine, can be rapidly translocated into mitochondria, and thereby the drop in any of the ratios of ATP to ADP, AMP, or Pi is kept small. The result of the adaptation to endurance training therefore is the enhanced capability of the muscle cell to match the flux of glucose units through the Embden–Meyerhof pathway to the needs of the mitochondria for pyruvate to fuel the terminal oxidative processes. Because of the small alteration in ATP and ADP, the activation of PFK would be less and pyruvate formation would be reduced. As there is no buildup of glucose monophosphate intermediates in muscle during exercise, the overall activation of glycogenolysis at the level of PHOS must also be reduced in response to training. In addition, more of the pyruvate formed is transported into the mitochondria, because they occupy a larger volume fraction in the trained muscle. The reduced lactate production found after training is therefore a reflection of the decreased flux of glucose units through the Embden–Meyerhof pathway and reduced availability of pyruvate to lactate dehydrogenase system (LDH, NADH). An explanation of the reduction in lactate formation as a result of increased mitochondrial protein concentration in skeletal muscles following endurance training has been proposed by Gollnick and coworkers (46, 47). The relationship between exercise intensity and the accumulation of NH_3 in the blood is very similar to that for lactate and exercise [18]. Moreover, this relationship shifts to the right in response to training [36]. In heavy exercise the production of NH_3 has been related to excessive accumulation of ADP, which is converted to AMP which is then deaminated to inosine monophosphate (IMP) and NH_3. This purportedly occurs to avoid excessive stimulation of metabolism by accumulation of the nucleotides. These data support the concept that training and the associated increase in mitochondria are important in forestalling a buildup of ADP and AMP at submaximal exercise intensities. It should be noted, however, that NH_3 production also can occur in prolonged moderate exercise. This production appears to be independent of AMP deamimation and may be associated with amino acid metabolism [47a].

Sparing of muscle glycogen has important practical implications, because these stores are essential for prolonged exercise capacity. This can be demonstrated in two ways. If endurance-trained and untrained subjects perform at the same submaximal power output, CHO utilization is less in the trained individuals and time to exhaustion is lengthened in relation to the difference in muscle glycogen degradation. If, instead, the trained and untrained subjects exercise at the same relative workload, work time may not be much different because CHO utilization will be quite similar in the two conditions, but the pace or total amount of work performed is highest in the trained individuals, related to differences in the Vo_2max of the individuals.

An area that has not been extensively studied is the metabolic effects of training regimens directed toward improving muscular strength or anaerobic performance capacity. Strength training could be anticipated to cause a larger dependence upon CHO as a fuel, as no adaptations occur in the muscle in respect to capillaries or mitochondrial enzymes (see Saltin and Gollnick [105]). In fact, a reduction in these variables may occur if a significant enlargement of muscle fibers is achieved. The enzymes catalyzing the reactions supplying the contractile machinery with energy are also relatively unchanged. Sprint training may, to a small extent, cause

adaptations similar to those found with endurance training. However, this appears to be related to whether training also includes activity extended over a minute or more.

Endurance training of rats in which massive hypertrophy has been induced by surgical removal of the synergistic muscle has produced changes in mitochondrial enzymes similar to the changes that occur in normal animals [100]. The rates of glycogen depletion during prolonged exercise were less in the liver and in both normal and hypertrophied skeletal muscle in the trained than in the nontrained animals. These data suggest that even in very large muscle fibers, there is no diffusion limitation for oxygen or other substrates.

Training to improve anaerobic capacity could include training to enhance the rate at which lactate can be formed and to enhance the amount of lactate or protons the muscle can accumulate. Increased concentrations of enzymes of the Embden–Meyerhof pathway may be of importance for the maximum rate of glycogen degradation and lactate formation that can be achieved, although these enzymes are found at very high concentrations in the muscle of sedentary humans. Nevertheless, training at high intensity results in a further elevation of these enzymes (see Saltin and Gollnick [105]). In addition to this effect, the buffering capacity of skeletal muscle reportedly can be increased by training (104).

SUMMARY

Carboyhydrate, as glycogen, is the major fuel stored within skeletal muscle. It occupies a key role in the energy production of exercise, and under a number of conditions its depletion may be responsbile for exhaustion. At rest and at low exercise intensities, its use is small and most of the fuel combusted may be derived from the blood. As exercise intensity increases, the contribution of carbohydrate to the total metabolism also increases, until carbohydrate may be the sole energy source during exercise intensities that approach maximal oxygen uptake. It appears that muscle relies heavily on its glycogen store during heavy exercise because of the immediate proximity of the store to the metabolic pathways and the fact that it can be metabolized both aerobically and anaerobically. During moderately heavy exercise, the time of onset of exhaustion is closely related to depletion of the glycogen store of muscle. Therefore, any adaptations that result in less use by the muscle cell during exercise or to increase storage within the cell will enhance performance capacity. Well-documented factors that are important in this regard are endurance training and dietary modifications. Endurance training produces local adaptations within muscles whereby there is a shift to greater fatty acid oxidation at a given submaximal power output. The storage of glycogen in muscle is augmented by endurance training and by a combination of exercise and diet. These adaptations work synergistically to enhance performance capacity.

REFERENCES

1. Ahlborg, B., J. Bergström, L.-G. Ekelund, G. Guarnieri, R.C. Harris, E. Hultman, and L.-O. Nordesjö. Muscle metabolism during isometric exercise performance at constant force. *J. Appl. Physiol.* 33:224–228, 1972.
2. Ahlborg, G., and P. Felig. Substrate utilization during prolonged exercise preceded by ingestion of glucose. *Am. J. Physiol.* 233:E188–E194, 1977.
3. Ahlborg, G., P. Felig, L. Hagenfeldt, R. Hendler, and J. Wahren. Substrate turnover during prolonged exercise in man: Splanchnic and leg metabolism of glucose, free fatty acids and amino acids. *J. Clin. Invest.* 53:1080–1098, 1974.
4. Andersen, P., and B. Saltin. Maximal perfusion of skeletal muscle in man. *J. Physiol. (London)* 366:233–249, 1985.
5. Armstrong, R.B., C.W. Saubert IV, W.L. Sembrowich, R.E. Shepherd, and P.D. Gollnick. Glycogen depletion in rat skeletal muscle fibers at different intensities and durations of exercise. *Pflügers Arch.* 352:243–256, 1974.
6. Åstrand P.-O., I. Hallbäck, R. Hedman, and B. Saltin. Blood lactates after prolonged severe exercise. *J. Appl. Physiol.* 18:619–622, 1963.
7. Bagby, G.J., H.J. Green, S. Katsuta, and P.D. Gollnick. Glycogen depletion in exercising rats infused with glucose, lactate, or pyruvate. *J. Appl. Physiol.* 45:425–429, 1978.
8. Bailey, J.M., and W.J. Whelan. The role of glucose and AMP in regulation of the conversion of phosphorylase *a* into phosphorylase *b*. *Biochem. Biophys. Res. Comm.* 46:191–197, 1972.
9. Bang, O. The lactate content of the blood during and after muscular exercise in man. *Skand. Arch. Physiol.* 74:51–82, 1936.
10. de Barsy, T., S. Stalmans, M. Laloux, H. De Wulf, and H.-G. Hers. The effect of glucose on the conversion of muscle phosphorylase *a* into *b* or *b'*. *Biochem. Biophys. Res. Comm.* 46:183–190, 1972.
11. Benedict, F.G., and E.P. Cathcart. *Muscular Work.* Washington D.C.: Carnegie Institute, Publication No. 187, 1913.
12. Bergström, J., L. Hermansen, E. Hultman, and B. Saltin. Diet, muscle glycogen, and physical performance. *Acta Physiol. Scand.* 71:172–179, 1967.
13. Bergström, J., and E. Hultman. Muscle glycogen synthesis after exercise: An enhancing factor localized to the muscle cells in man. *Nature* 210:309–310, 1966.
14. Bergström, J., E. Hultman. A study of the glycogen metabolism during exercise in man. *Scand. J. Clin. Lab. Invest.* 19:218–228, 1967.
15. Bessman, S.P., and C.L. Carpenter. The creatine-creatine phosphate energy shuttle. *Annu. Rev. Biochem.* 54:831–862, 1985.
16. Bohannon, V.V., J.H. Karam, and P.H. Forsham. Endocrine response to sugar ingestion in man. *J. Am. Diet. Assoc.* 76:555–560, 1980.
17. Bone, A., S.A. Malcolm, R.D. Kilgour, K.P. MacIntyre, and A.N. Belcastro. Glucose ingestion before and during intensive exercise. *J. Appl. Physiol.* 50:766–771, 1981.
18. Buono, M.J., T.R. Clancy, and J.R. Cook. Blood lactate and ammonium ion accumulation during graded exercise in humans. *J. Appl. Physiol.* 57:135–139, 1984.
19. Cartier, L.-J., and P.D. Gollnick. Sympathoadrenal system and activation of glycogenolysis during muscular activity. *J. Appl. Physiol.* 58:1122–1127, 1985.
20. Chance, B., and G.R. Williams. Respiratory enzymes in oxidative phosphorylation. I. Kinetics of oxygen utilization. *J. Biol. Chem.* 217:383–393, 1955.
21. Chasiotis, D., K. Sahlin, and E. Hultman. Regulation of glycogenolysis in human muscle at rest and during exercise. *J. Appl. Physiol.* 53:708–715, 1982.
22. Christensen, E.-H. Der Stoffwechsel und die respiratorischen Funktionen bei schwerer körperliche Arbeit. *Arbeitsphysiologie* 5:463–478, 1932.
23. Christensen, E.-H., and O. Hansen. Arbeitsfähigkeit und Ehrnährung. *Skand. Arch. Physiol.* 81:160–175, 1939.
24. Conlee, R.K., J.A. McLane, M.J. Rennie, W.W. Winder, and J.O. Holloszy. Reversal of phosphorylase activation in muscle despite continued contractile activity. *Am. J. Physiol.* 237: R291–R296, 1979.
25. Cori, C.F. The fate of sugar in the animal body. I.

The rate of absorption of hexoses and pentoses from the intestinal tract. *J. Biol. Chem.* 66:691–715, 1925.

26. Cori, C.F. The fate of sugar in the animal body. III. The rate of glycogen formation in the liver of normal and insulinized rats during the absorption of glucose, fructose, and galactose. *J. Biol. Chem.* 70:577–585, 1926.

27. Corsi, A., M. Midrio, and A.L. Granata. In situ utilization of glycogen and blood glucose by skeletal muscle during tetanus. *Am. J. Physiol.* 216:1534–1541, 1969.

28. Costill, D.L., E. Coyle, G. Dalsky, W. Evans, W. Fink, and D. Hoopes. Effect of elevated plasma FFA and insulin on muscle glycogen usage during exercise. *J. Appl. Physiol.* 43:695–699, 1977.

29. Costill, D.L., W.M. Sherman, W.J. Fink, C. Maresh, M. Witten, and J.M. Miller. The role of dietary carbohydrates in muscle glycogen synthesis after strenuous running. *Am. J. Clin. Nutr.* 34:1831–1836, 1981.

30. Coyle, E.F., J.M. Hagberg, B.F. Hurley, W.H. Martin, A.A. Ehsani, and J.O. Holloszy. Carbohydrate feeding during prolonged strenuous exercise can delay fatigue. *J. Appl. Physiol.* 55:230–235, 1983.

31. Crane, R.K., and A. Sols. The non-competitive inhibition of brain hexokinase by glucose-6-phosphate and related compounds. *J. Biol. Chem.* 210:597–606, 1954.

32. Crow, M.T., and M.J. Kushmerick. Chemical energetics of slow- and fast-twitch muscles of the mouse. *J. Gen. Physiol.* 79:147–166, 1982.

33. Dawson, M.J., D.G. Gadian, and D.R. Wilkie. Contraction and recovery of living muscles studied by ^{37}P nuclear magnetic resonance. *J. Physiol. (London)* 267:703–735, 1977.

34. Dill, D.B., H.T. Edwards, and J.H. Talbott. Studies in muscular activity. VII. Factors limiting the capacity for work. *J. Physiol.* 77:49–62, 1932.

35. Donaldson, S.K.B., and L. Hermansen. Differential, direct effects of H^+ on Ca^{2+} activated force of skinned fibres from soleus, cardiac and adductor magnus muscles of rabbits. *Pflügers Arch.* 376:55–65. 1978.

36. Dudley, G.A., and R.L. Terjung. Influence of aerobic metabolism on IMP accumulation in fast-twitch muscle. *Am. J. Physiol.* 248:C37–C42, 1985.

37. Durmmond, G.I., J.P. Harwood, and C.A. Powell. Studies on the activation of phosphorylase in skeletal muscle by contraction and by epinephrine. *J. Biol. Chem.* 244:4235–4240, 1969.

38. Edwards, R.H.T., R.C. Harris, E. Hultman, L. Kaijser, d. Vioh, and L.-O. Nordesjö. Effect of temperature on muscle energy metabolism and endurance during successive isometric contractions, sustained to fatigue, of the quadriceps muscle in man. *J. Physiol.* 220:335–352, 1972.

39. Fabiato, A., and F. Fabiato. Effects of pH on the myofilaments and the sarcoplasmic reticulum of skinned cells from cardiac and skeletal muscle. *J. Physiol. (London)* 276:233–255, 1978.

40. Gaesser, G.A., and G.A. Brooks. Glycogen repletion following continuous and intermittent exer-

cise to exhaustion. *J. Appl. Physiol.* 49:722–728, 1980.

41. Gaesser, G.A., and G.A. Brooks. Metabolic bases of excess post-exercise oxygen consumption: A review. *Med. Sci. Sports Exer.* 16:29–43, 1984.

42. Galbo, H., N.J. Christensen, and J.J. Holst. Catecholamines and pancreatic hormones during autonomic blockade in exercise. *Acta Physiol. Scand.* 101:428–437, 1977.

43. Gollnick, P.D., B. Pernow, B. Essén, E. Janson, and B. Saltin. Availability of glycogen and plasma FFA for substrate utilization in leg muscle of man during exercise. *Clin. Physiol.* 1:12–42, 1981.

44. Gollnick, P.D., K. Piehl, and B. Saltin. Selective glycogen depletion pattern in human muscle fibers after exercise of varying intensity and at varying pedalling frequency. *J. Physiol. (London)* 241:45–57, 1974.

45. Gollnick, P.D., K. Piehl, C.W. Saubert IV, R.B. Armstrong, and B. Saltin. Diet, exercise, and glycogen changes in human muscle fibers. *J. Appl. Physiol.* 33:421–425, 1972.

46. Gollnick, P.D., M. Riedy, J.J. Quintinskie, and L.A. Bertocci. Differences in metabolic potential of skeletal muscle fibres and their significance for metabolic control. *J. Exp. Biol.* 115:191–199, 1972.

47. Gollnick, P.D., and B. Saltin. Significance of skeletal muscle oxidative enzyme enhancement with endurance training. *Clin. Physiol.* 2:1–12, 1982.

47a. Graham, T.E., P.K. Pederson, and B. Saltin. Muscle and blood ammonia and lactate response to prolonged exercise hyperoxia. *J. Appl. Physiol.* In press.

48. Grossbard, L., and R.T. Schimke. Multiple hexokinases of rat tissue: Purification and comparison of soluble forms. *J. Biol. Chem.* 241:3546–3560, 1966.

49. Haller, R.G., S.F. Lewis, J.D. Cook, and C.G. Blomquist. Myophosphorylase deficiency impairs muscle oxidative metabolism. *Ann. Neurol.* 17:196–199, 1985.

50. Hargreaves, M., D.L. Costill, A. Coggan, W.J. Fink, and I. Nishibata. Effect of carbohydrate feedings on muscle glycogen utilization and exercise performance. *Med. Sci. Sports Exer.* 3:219–222, 1984.

51. Heigenhauser, G.J.F., J.R. Sutton, and N.L. Jones. Effect of glycogen depletion on the ventilatory response to exercise. *J. Appl. Physiol.* 54:470–474, 1983.

52. Helmreich, E., and C.F. Cori. Regulation of glycolysis in muscle. *Adv. Enzyme Reg.* 3:91–107, 1964.

53. Henriksson, J. Training induced adaptations of skeletal muscle and metabolism during submaximal exercise. *J. Physiol.* 217:661–675, 1977.

54. Hermansen, L., and J.-B. Osnes. Blood and muscle pH after maximal exercise in man. *J. Appl. Physiol.* 32:304–308, 1972.

55. Hermansen, L., and I. Stensvold. Production and removal of lactate during exercise in man. *Acta Physiol. Scand.* 86:191–201, 1972.

56. Hermansen, L., and O. Vaage. Lactate disappearance and glycogen synthesis in human muscle after

maximal exercise. *Am. J. Physiol.* 233: E422–E429, 1977.

57. Hultman, E., J. Bergström, and N. McLennan-Anderson. Breakdown and resynthesis of phosphorylcreatine and adenosine triphosphate in connection with muscular work in man. *Scand. J. Clin. Lab. Invest.* 19:56–69, 1967.

58. Hultman, E., and L.H. Nilsson. Liver glycogen in man: Effect of different diets and muscular exercise. In: Pernow, B., and B. Saltin (eds.). *Muscle Metabolism During Exercise.* New York: Plenum Press, 1971, pp. 143–152.

59. Infante, A.A., and R.E. Davies. Adenosine triphosphate breakdown during single isotonic twitch from sartorius muscle. *Biochem. Biophys. Res. Comm.* 9:410–415, 1962.

60. Jansson, E. On the significance of the respiratory exchange ratio after different diets during exercise in man. *Acta Physiol. Scand.* 114:103–110, 1982.

61. Jenskins, A.B., D.J. Chisholm, D.E. James, K.Y. Ho, and E.W. Kraegen. Exercise-induced hepatic glucose output is precisely sensitive to the rate of systemic glucose supply. *Metabolism* 34: 431–436, 1985.

62. Jenkins, A.B., S.M. Furler, D.J. Chisholm, and E.W. Kraegen. Regulation of hepatic glucose output during exercise by circulating glucose and insulin in humans. *Am. J. Physiol.* 250:R411–R417, 1986.

63. Jorfeldt, L. Metabolism of L (+)-lactate in human skeletal muscle during exercise. *Acta Physiol. Scand. (Suppl.)* 338, 1970.

64. Kaiser, P., P.A. Tesch, A. Thorsson, J. Karlsson, and L. Kaijser. Skeletal muscle glycolysis during submaximal exercise following acute β-adrenergic blockade in man. *Acta Physiol. Scand.* 123:258–281, 1985.

65. Karlsson, J. Lactate and phosphagen concentrations in working muscle of man. *Acta Physiol. Scand. (Suppl.)* 358, 1971.

66. Karlsson, J., L.-O. Nordesjö, L. Jorfeldt, and B. Saltin. Muscle lactate, ATP, and CP levels during exercise after physical training in man. *J. Appl. Physiol.* 33:199–203, 1972.

67. Karlsson, J., L.-O. Nordesjö, and B. Saltin. Muscle glycogen utilization during exercise after physical training. *Acta Physiol. Scand.* 90:210–217, 1974.

68. Karlsson, J., and B. Saltin. Oxygen deficit and muscle metabolites in intermittent exercise. *Acta Physiol. Scand.* 82:115–122, 1971.

69. Katz, A., K. Sahlin, and J. Henriksson. Muscle ATP turnover rate during isometric contraction in humans. *J. Appl. Physiol.* 60:1839–1842, 1986.

70. Katz, J. The application of isotopes to the study of lactate metabolism. *Med. Sci. Sports Exer.* 18:353–359, 1986.

71. Koivisto, V.A., M Härkönen, S.-L. Karonen, P.H. Groop, R. Elovainio, E. Ferrannini, L. Sacca, and R.A. Defronozo. Glycogen depletion during prolonged exercise: Influence of glucose, fructose, or placebo. *J. Appl. Physiol.* 58:731–737, 1985.

72. Koivisto, V.A., S.-L. Karonen, and E.A. Nikkilä. Carbohydrate ingestion before exercise: Comparison of glucose, fructose, and sweet placebo. *J. Appl. physiol.* 51:783–787, 1981.

73. Kraegen, E.W., D.E. James, A.B. Jenkins, and D.J. Chisholm. Dose-response curves for in vivo insulin sensitivity in individual tissues in rats. *Am. J. Physiol.* 248:E353–E362, 1985.

74. Krebs, E.G., D.J. Graves, and E.H. Fischer. Factors affecting the activity of muscle phosphorylase b kinase. *J. Biol. Chem.* 234:2869–2873, 1959.

75. Krebs, E.G., D.S. Love, G.E. Bartovold, K.A. Tayser, W.L. Meyer, and E.H. Fischer. Purification and properties of rabbit skeletal muscle phosphorylase b kinase. *Biochemistry* 3:1022–1033, 1964.

76. Krogh, A., and J. Lindhard. The relative value of fat and carbohydrate as sources of muscular energy. *Biochem. J.* 14:290–336, 1920.

77. Kushmerick, M.J. Patterns of mammalian muscle energetics. *J. Exp. Biol.* 115:165–177, 1985.

78. Levine, L., W.J. Evans, B.S. Cadarette, E.C. Fisher, and B.A. Bullen. Fructose and glucose ingestion and muscle glycogen use during submaximal exercise. *J. Appl. Physiol.* 55:1767–1771, 1983.

79. Levine, R., and M.A. Goldstein. On the mechanism of action of insulin. *Rec. Adv. Horm. Res.* 11:343–380, 1955.

80. Lundsgaard, E. Untersuchungen über Muskelkontracktionen ohne Silchsäurebildung. *Biochem. Z.* 217:162–175, 1930.

81. MacDonald, V.W., and F.F. Jöbsis. Spectrophotometric studies on the pH of muscle. *J. Gen. Physiol.* 68:179–195, 1976.

82. Maehlum, S. Muscle glycogen synthesis after glucose infusion during post-exercise recovery in diabetic and non-diabetic subjects. *Scand. J. Clin. Lab. Invest.* 38:349–354, 1978.

83. Maehlum, S., P. Felig, and J. Wahren. Splanchnic glucose and muscle glycogen metabolism after glucose feeding during postexercise recovery. *Am. J. Physiol.* 235:E255–E260, 1978.

84. Mainwood, G.W., and J.M. Renaud. The effect of acid-base on fatigue of skeletal muscle. *Can. J. Physiol. Pharmacol.* 63:403–416, 1985.

85. Marsh, M.E., and J.R. Mulin. Muscular efficiency on high carbohydrate and high fat diets. *J. Nuti.* 1:105–137, 1928.

86. McLane, J.A., and J.O. Holloszy. Glycogen synthesis from lactate in the three types of skeletal muscle. *J. Biol. Chem.* 254:6548–6553, 1979.

87. Moreadith, R.W., and W.E. Jacobus. Creatine kinase of heart mitochondria: Functional coupling of ADP transfer to the adenine nucleotide translocase. *J. Biol. Chem.* 257:899–905, 1982.

88. Needham, D.M. *Machina Carnis. The Biochemistry of Muscular Contraction in Its Historical Development.* Cambridge: Cambridge University Press, 1971.

89. Nilsson, L.H., P. Fürst, and E. Hultman. Carbohydrate metabolism of the liver in normal man under varying dietary conditions. *Scand. J. Clin. Lab. Invest.* 32:331–337, 1973.

90. Nilsson, L.H., and E. Hultman. Liver glycogen in man: The effect of total starvation or a carbohydrate-poor diet followed by carbohydrate refeeding. *Scand. J. Clin. Lab. Invest.* 32:325–330, 1973.

91. Nilsson, L.H., and E. Hultman. Liver and muscle

glycogen in man after glucose and fructose infusion. *Scand. J. Clin. Lab. Invest.* 3:5–10, 1974.

92. Olsson, K.-E., and B. Saltin. Variation in total body water with muscle glycogen changes in man. *Acta Physiol. Scand.* 80:11–18, 1970.

93. Piehl, K., S. Adolfsson, and K. Nazar. Glycogen storage and glycogen synthetase activity in trained and untrained muscle of man. *Acta Physiol. Scand.* 90:779–788, 1974.

94. Pirnay, F., J.N. Crielaard, N. Pallikarakis, M. Lacroix, F. Mosora, G. Krzentowski, A.S. Luyckx, and P.J. Lefebvre. Fat of exogenous glucose during exercise of different intensities in humans. *J. Appl. Physiol.* 53:1620–1624, 1982.

95. Pirnay, R., M. Lacroix, F. Mosora, A. Luyckx, and P. Lefebvre. Glucose oxidation during prolonged exercise evaluated with naturally labelled [^{13}C]glucose. *J. Appl. Physiol.* 43:258–261, 1977.

96. von Pettenkofer, M., and C. Voit. Untersuchungen über den Stoffverbrauch des normalen Menschen. *Z. Biol.* 2:459–573, 1866.

97. Posner, J.B., R. Stern, and E.G. Krebs. Effects of electrical stimulation and epinephrine on muscle phosphorylase, phosphorylase b kinase, and adenosine 3′, 5′ phsophate. *J. Biol. Chem.* 240:982–985, 1965.

98. Pruett, E.D.R. Glucose and insulin during prolonged work stress in men living on different diets. *J. Appl. Physiol.* 28:199–208, 1970.

99. Radda, G.K., L. Chan, R.B. Bore, D.G. Gadian, B.D. Ross, P. Styles, and D. Taylor. Clinical application of ^{31}P NMR. In *International Symposium on NMR Imaging*. Witcofski, R.L., N. Karstaedt, and C.L. Partain (eds.). Proceedings of Winston-Salem, N.C.: Bowman Gray School of Medicine, 1981, pp. 159–169.

100. Riedy, M., R.L. Moore, and P.D. Gollnick. Adaptive response of hypertrophied skeletal muscle to endurance training. *J. Appl. Physiol.* 59:127–131, 1985.

101. Sahlin, K. Intracellular pH and energy metabolism in muscle of man. *Acta Physiol. Scand. (Suppl.)* 455:1–56, 1978.

102. Sahlin, K. Effect of acidosis on energy metabolism and force generation in skeletal muscle. *Biochem. Exer.* 13:151–160, 1982.

103. Sahlin, K., R.C. Harris, B. Bylind, and E. Hultman. Lactate content and pH in muscle samples obtained after dynamic exercise. *Pflügers Arch.* 367:143–149, 1976.

104. Sahlin, K., and J. Henriksson. Buffer capacity and lactate accumulation in skeletal muscle of trained and untrained man. *Acta Physiol. Scand.* 122:331–339, 1984.

105. Saltin, B., and P.D. Gollnick. Skeletal muscle adaptability: Significance for metabolism and performance. In Peachy, L.D., R.H. Adrian, and S.R. Geiger (eds.). *Handbook of Physiology*. Baltimore: Williams & Wilkins, 1983, pp. 555–631.

106. Saltin, B., L.H. Hartley. Å. Kilbom, and I Åstrand. Physical training in sedentary middle-aged and older men. II. Oxygen uptake, heart rate, and blood lactate concentration at submaximal and maximal exercise. *Scand. J. Clin. Lab. Invest.* 24:323–334, 1969.

107. Saltin, B., B. Kiens, and G. Savard. A quantitative approach to the evaluation of skeletal muscle substrate utilization in prolonged exercise. In Benzi, B., L. Packer, and N. Siliprandi (eds.). *Biochemical Aspects of Physical Exercise*. Amsterdam: Elsevier Science Publishers, 1986, pp. 235–244.

108. Sigel, P., and D. Pette. Intracellular localization of glycogenolytic and glycolytic enzymes in white and red rabbit skeletal muscle. *J. Histochem. Cytochem.* 17:225–237, 1969.

109. Swanderdamm, J. *Johann Swammerdamm's Bibel der Natur*. Leipzig, 1752.

110. Taylor, A.W., R. Tayer, and S. Roa. Human skeletal muscle glycogen synthetase activities with exercise and training. *Can. J. Physiol. Pharmacol.* 50:411–415, 1972.

111. Taylor, D.J., P. Styles, P.M. Matthews, D.A. Arnold, D.G. Gadian, P. Bore, and G.D. Radda. Energetics of human muscle: Exercise-induced ATP depletion. *Mag. Reson. Med.* 3:44–54, 1986.

112. Terjung, R.L., K.M. Baldwin, W.W. Winder, and J.O. Holloszy. Glycogen repletion in different types of muscle and in liver after exhausting exercise. *Am. J. Physiol.* 226:1386–1391, 1974.

113. Thornheim, K., and J.M. Lowenstein. Control of phosphofructokinase from rat skeletal muscle. *J. Biol. Chem.* 251:7322–7328, 1976.

114. Trivedi, B., and W.H. Danforth. Effect of pH on the kinetics of frog muscle phosphofructokinase. *J. Biol. Chem.* 241:4110–4114, 1966.

115. Wahren, J. Human forearm muscle metabolism during exercise. IV. Glucose uptake at different work intensities. *Scand. J. Clin. Lab. Invest.* 25:129–135, 1970.

116. Wilson, D.F., K. Nishiki, and M. Erecińska. Energy metabolism in muscle and its regulation during individual contraction-relaxation cycles. *TIBS*:16–19, 1981.

117. Wirth, A., C. Diehm, H. Mayer, H. Mörl, I. Voge, P. Björntrop, and G. Schlierf. Plasma C-peptide and insulin in trained and untrained subjects. *J. Appl. Physiol.* 50:71–77, 1981.

Chapter 5

FUEL FOR MUSCULAR EXERCISE: ROLE OF FAT

Philip D. Gollnick, Ph.D., and Bengt Saltin, M.D.

Of the two main fuels stored in the human body and used for muscular exercise, fat has several characteristics which, in many situations, make it the substrate of choice. Of these characteristics the facts that fat contains more than twice the energy per unit weight that carbohydrate has and is not hydrated when stored in the body make it ideal as a fuel during sustained efforts, especially when the food supply is limited. The value of fat on such occasions was known long before measurements of respiratory exchange ratios (R-values) demonstrated that fat was the dominant substrate at rest and the preferred fuel at low-intensity exercise.

The survival and success of the first polar explorers, for example, those crossing the ice caps of Greenland and reaching the North and South Poles, were in part related to their ability to transport enough of the right kind of food while carrying a minimum weight. The Norwegian polar explorer, Nansen [35], was one of the first to realize that fat was a necessary component of the diet under such conditions. This fat was provided by the daily consumption of 350 to 400 g of pemican, the name given to a food consisting of ground beef into which fat was melted, which provided 60 to 70% of the daily energy requirement. Sledge dogs also were fed pemican, but theirs contained a higher content of fat. This demonstrates an early understanding that although the muscles of different species have similar basic characteristics and demands, they still are different.

Migrating birds, which fly for days, are another example of the beneficial energy/weight ratio of fat. In these animals, fat is the only fuel possible that provides ample energy store with a body weight that allows launch and sustained flight [68]. Migrating fish also rely on stored fats, some in the muscles themselves, for the energy to complete their journeys.

There have been many controversies in the history of investigations related to lipid combustion and muscular work. Some have been solved through the years, whereas others await resolution. One of the first questions to be resolved was whether fat must be converted to sugar before being used by the muscles [10]. Zuntz [71] and later Krogh and Lindhard [50] elaborated upon this problem and demonstrated that fat was used directly. A long time elapsed, however, before it was demonstrated how fat was transported from adipose tissue to the muscle, where it was taken up and used to supply acetyl coenzyme A (CoA) to the citric acid cycle of the mitochondria. One current controversy is to what extent other triacyglycerol (TG) pools, like those circulating in the blood or present in the muscle, contribute to the supply of free fatty acid (FFA) for mitochondrial oxidation. Indeed, several important aspects of fat combustion and exercise metabolism await resolution.

This chapter follows the same general outline as the previous one, in that we try to deal separately with the topics of fat and carbohydrate as fuels for muscular work. In most instances, however, both of these fuels are used simultaneously, although in different proportions, by active muscle, and separate consideration of use of the two fuels during exercise is in many ways artificial. We have attempted to overcome this difficulty by focusing attention on some of the factors that regulate the interplay in the use of the two energy sources during exercise.

SOME CHARACTERISTICS OF LIPIDS

The general class of compounds described as fats (or lipids) is far more diverse than is the carbohydrate class. The common factor that unites the fats is their general insolubility in water and their solubility in organic solvents. In this chapter we will address only the fats that are important as metabolic fuels. These are the FFAs and their storage form, TGs. Fatty acids have the basic chemical structure $CH_3(CH_2)_nCOOH$, with the total length of the carbon skeleton being determined by the number of CH_2 units. Various chain lengths of fatty acids exist in a nature and in the body, those of metabolic importance being from 12 to 18 carbon atoms long. Also, fatty acids have a variety of structures, some being unsaturated, that is, having the chemical linkage $CH_2-CH=CH-CH_2$ rather than the repeating CH_2-CH_2 configuration. In this chapter on energy metabolism as derived from fat, we will not be concerned with the different structures of the fatty acids but will merely make the general assumption that the oxidation of fatty acids can be represented by the oxidation of palmitic acid ($C_{16}H_{32}OOH$). This is based on the observation that palmitate turnover is representative of about 75% of the total FFA in the plasma [31]. An important property related to energy storage in lipid compared with that in carbohydrate is that carbon and hydrogen comprise about 90% of the FFA molecule compared with only about 50% for the carbohydrate molecule. Since the oxidation of the carbon and hydrogen of the molecule is responsible for energy release, the total energy stored per unit weight is much greater for fats than for carbohydrates.

As a general background, an important feature of FFAs is that at high concentrations they are toxic to cells. This toxicity is derived in part from their destabilizing effect on cell membrane structures, such as the mitochondria, which can lead to tissue damage. Thus, the total concentration of FFA within the cells is usually kept rather low.

SOURCES OF STORED BODY FAT

The body obtains fat for storage by the direct ingestion of fats in the diet and from lipogenesis from excess amounts of carbohydrate and protein in the diet. Dietary sources of fat for humans are primarily animal food products such as meats and dairy products. We mention only briefly that the amount and type of fat vary considerably with the source. For example, whereas fish may contain a great quantity of fat, the characteristics of the fat differ greatly from those of fat from sources such as feedlot fattened beef cattle and vegetable fat. Additional information relating directly to this topic can be obtained by consulting common textbooks of nutrition, such as that of Goodhart and Schels (21).

Lipid synthesis occurs in both the liver and the adipose tissue. The extent of lipogenesis depends on the total caloric intake. The principal storage site of FFA is the TG produced by condensation of 3 FFA units with glycerol. The largest accumulation of neutral fats is in the adipose tissue, but such fats are present in small amounts in other tissues. They are also transported in the blood as lipoprotein and chylomicrons. There are many forms for the transport of TG in the blood, some of which may have important implications for cardiovascular health. However, we address only the topic of energy metabolism. This aspect of lipoprotein metabolism is covered in Chapter 15.

The body has an enormous capacity to store fat; the total percentage of body weight that is fat ranges from 5 to above 50%. The percentage is usually lower in males than in females: Average values for males are between 15 and 25%, whereas for females the range is 25 to 35% fat. With an average body weight of about 60 kg for women and 80 kg for men, this results in energy storage of about 165,000 kcal for women and 150,000 kcal for men. This can be contrasted with an average total storage range of calories as carbohydrates of between 2500 and 4500 kcal. Thus, as a single energy source, the fat stores of the body exceed those of all carbohydrates by 30- to 60-fold. The magnitude of the storage of fat varies considerably within and between tissues. Adipose tissue contains the greatest lipid reserve of the body, and the subcutaneous adipose tissue is the major site of storage in humans. This reserve is dynamic and changes with the balance or lack of balance between caloric intake and expenditure. During periods of net negative caloric balance, the size of the individual adipocytes decreases, whereas under conditions of excess caloric intake the adipocytes take up FFA, store TG, and enlarge. The excess caloric expenditure associated with chronic exercise has been shown to reduce the size of adipocytes [3–5]. Thus, considerable fluctuations in total body fatness can occur as a function of alteration in nutritional status and caloric expenditure. Intraindividual and interindividual differences exist in the sites for adipose storage. Some evidence also indicates that regional differences exist in the responsiveness of adipocytes to lipolytic hormones [65].

Although most adipose tissue is subcutaneous, deposits also occur at other body locations. Of importance for this chapter are deposits lying within the confines of the muscle while remaining outside the muscle fibers. In animal muscle, such deposits are easily identified and can represent a large fraction of the tissue, for example, in meat such as beefsteak. The muscle contains lipid that is visible as white streaks between the more red tissues. Such deposits also exist in human skeletal muscle and are frequently an unwanted component in muscle biopsy samples.

Lipid is also contained within the muscle fibers. This energy pool is more difficult to assess quantitatively. The amount of TG stored in muscle fibers has been reported to range from 7 to 25 $\mu mol \cdot g^{-1}$ wet muscle with an approximately 50% difference between the fiber types (see Saltin and Gollnick [62]).

FAT UTILIZATION

Since most tissue contains only a small amount of fat that can be used for energy production, there is constant transport of FFA between adipose tissue and peripheral tissues. Transport is accomplished by binding of the FFA to the albumin of the blood (Figure 1). Thus, FFAs are constantly generated in the adipose tissue via lipolysis (hydrolysis of the TG), a process that can be initiated by the adrenergic hormones, whereafter the FFAs pass through the plasma membrane of the adipocyte, are transferred through the interstitial space, pass through the capillary wall, are bound to circulating albumin, and are carried via the circulation for use in tissues. When the albumin–FFA complex arrives at the peripheral tissue, for example skeletal muscle, this series of events is reversed, so that the FFA is transferred into the muscle cell. Obviously this TG hydrolysis process is also reversed when there is a net uptake of FFA by adipocytes. Thus, there is a dynamic equilibrium between the release and uptake of FFA by adipocytes. Although some information is available about the nature and mechanism of the transfer of FFA in and out of fat cells, how this process occurs across the plasma membrane of muscle, both heart and skeletal, is poorly understood.

Once a molecule of FFA is assimilated

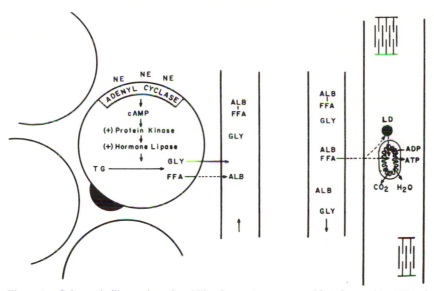

Figure 1. Schematic illustration of mobilization and transport of free fatty acids (FFA) from adipose tissue to skeletal muscle. In the adipocyte depicted, the beta-receptor is the membrane-bound adenyl cyclase that is activated by norepinephrine (NE). The cyclic adenosine monophosphate (cAMP) formed activates a protein kinase, which then activates the hormone-sensitive lipase of the fat cell. Activation of the lipase results in hydrolysis of the stored triacylglycerols to FFA and glycerol, which are transferred to the capillaries in the adipose tissue. The FFA is then bound to albumin (ALB) and carried by the blood to the muscle, where it is released and taken up. On entering the muscle, the FFA can be either transferred into the mitochondria for oxidation or stored in lipid droplets (LD) for later use. Broken lines indicate areas where translocation of FFA occurs through regions that appear to require carriers but where information about transport is scant.

into the cytosol of a muscle cell, it can be either stored as a lipid droplet or degraded to provide energy to meet the immediate energy needs (Figure 1). Most of these lipid droplets are found in close proximity to mitochondria. At rest, energy needs of the muscle are modest, and the total use of FFA is also small, with any excess being stored. Since very little of the total absolute amount of TG is stored by skeletal muscle (grams per kilogram), it is clear that the muscle is not the major organ for regulating blood lipid concentration or for storing total body fat. How the lipid droplets within muscle are formed and what determines that site of storage are unknown.

The oxidation of lipids is initiated by activation of the FFA molecule to CoA by the enzyme acyl CoA synthase (fatty acid thiokinase). This process occurs on the outer mitochondrial membrane, whereas terminal oxidation occurs within the mitochondrial matrix. Thus, the acyl CoA formed must be translocated into the mitochondria. This occurs by the acyl CoA being complexed to carnitine for transport into the mitochondria via the carnitine acyl transferase system, which is located in the inner mitochondrial membrane. On entry of the FFA into the mitochondria, the carbon skeleton of the FFA is progressively cleaved into acetyl-CoA units by a series of reactions that are collectively referred to as "β-oxidation." The acetyl unit then enters the citric acid cycle via the citrate synthase reaction and is oxidized exactly like the acetyl units that are generated from pyruvate. In fact, the citrate synthase reaction does not distinguish between acetyl units generated from fatty acids or glucose.

Knowledge about the importance of the carnitine acyl transferase system to energy metabolism during exercise comes from the study of patients with a specific deficiency for this enzyme in the mitochondrial membrane. These individuals are capable of attaining normal maximal oxygen uptakes (S. Lewis, personal communication), but their R-values are unusually high during even the lightest efforts, indicative of inability to utilize fat as a fuel. In such persons, glycogen stores are depleted more rapidly and endurance capacity is lower than in normal individuals.

The net energy yield from the complete degradation of 1 mol of a fatty acid, such as palmitate, is 129 mol of ATP, This is a net energy capture, as ATP, of about 40%, which is similar to that for glucose when it is degraded to CO_2 and H_2O. However, energy yield per liter of oxygen consumed is slightly ($\sim$5%) lower than that from oxidation of carbohydrate.

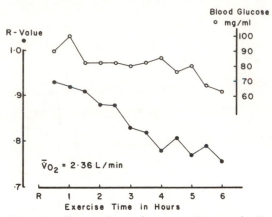

Figure 2. Changes in respiratory exchange ratio (R-value) and blood glucose during a long-lasting exercise. (Data from Edwards, H.T., R. Margaria, and D.B. Dill. Metabolic rate, blood sugar, and the utilization of carbohydrate. *Am. J. Physiol.* 108:203–209, 1934.)

CONTRIBUTION OF FAT TO ENERGY PRODUCTION OF EXERCISE

Fat metabolism, as it relates to exercise, has two important aspects: (a) Fat can only be used under aerobic conditions, and (b) since not a great deal of fat is contained within the muscle cell, it must be transported to and taken up by the muscle.

The R-value of individuals at rest who have consumed an average mixed diet is between 0.80 and 0.85. This indicates that fat contributes 50% of the total energy production. For the average person, this amounts to about 4.5 g of fat oxidized perhour. The relative contribution that fat makes to the metabolism of exercise is roughly the mirror image of the contribution from carbohydrates. Thus, during prolonged light exercise there is a progressive increase in the absolute amount of fat oxidized, which in the untrained person may peak at around 50% of Vo_2max and at that point be equivalent to a fat consumption of from 0.7 to 0.9 g·min^{-1} (Figure 2). There is a great deal of evidence from R-values in older literature that suggests that during such prolonged ex-

ercise, for example up to 8 hours, 80% or more of the energy could be derived from lipid oxidation, that is, up to 1.5 g·min^{-1} of fat is used [14] (Figure 3). From the studies of Phinney et al. [56], it can be estimated that for subjects maintained on a high-fat diet, more than 90% of the energy expended during a period of prolonged exercise will be derived from fat, a value similar to that

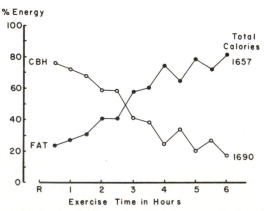

Figure 3. Comparison of the relative contribution of carbohydrate and fat to metabolism during prolonged exercise. (Data from Edwards, H.T., R. Margaria, and D.B. Dill. Metabolic rate, blood sugar, and the utilization of carbohydrate. *Am. J. Physiol.* 108: 203–209, 1934.)

reported by Christensen and Hansen [11]. As the intesity of exercise increases, there is a progressively smaller contribution of fat, both in absolute and relative terms, to the metabolism, until during very heavy exercise the amount of fat being used may be nil. The relationship between exercise intensity and the relative use of fat and carbohydrate at rest and during moderate and heavy exercise is presented in Figure 4.

TRIACYLGLYCEROL AS FUEL FOR MUSCULAR WORK

Suggestions have been made that the TGs stored in the muscle and those within the blood could serve as energy sources to fuel

muscle metabolism during prolonged work. The impetus for this suggestion comes from the observation that the uptake and oxidation of plasma FFA cannot account for all fat-derived energy. Attempts to quantitate the contribution of these TG pools of energy have produced equivocal results.

Studies on Muscle TG

Uncertainty exists over the relative role and importance of intramuscular lipid stores as energy reserves for exercise. Masoro et al. [52] could not demonstrate a major role for intramuscular TG in the muscle of monkeys during prolonged electrical stimulation. Conversely, Issekutz and Paul [38] con-

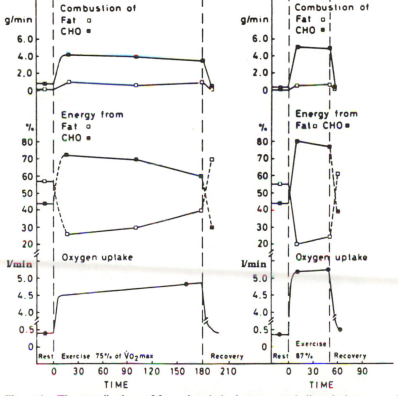

Figure 4. The contributions of fat and carbohydrate to metabolism during rest and during the conditions of moderately intense and heavy exercise. These data demonstrate the increasing reliance on fat under both exercise conditions. However, total fat combustion is much greater during moderately intense exercise.

cluded that the energy balance during prolonged exercise is such that intramuscular lipid stores must be used if one is to account for all of the substrate combusted. A number of investigators have reported decreases in neutral lipid stores of skeletal muscle in response to exercise [18, 19, 59].

Most studies with human muscle have utilized the biopsy technique to obtain tissue samples before and after exercise. Results have been mixed as to whether the TG store of skeletal muscle is used during exercise, and if so, whether it is an important energy source during exercise. There are reports of a decline in the TG concentration of human skeletal muscle after exercise varying in duration from 1 to 12 hours [8, 15]. However, a number of studies have failed to identify any major change in the triglyceride concentration of skeletal muscle after exercise [23, 42]. In some of these reports either no change was found or the magnitude of change was insufficient to account for the "missing fraction" of the energy consumed during exercise. Without doubt the diversity of these findings is related to the samples of biopsied muscle being unrepresentative of the actual muscle mass and therefore of TG content, since the assay to determine TG is sensitive and accurate. In contrast to glycogen, TG in muscle is not stored homogeneously in the fiber, and the two major muscle fibers have different TG contents (see Saltin and Gollnick [62]). This problem can be dealt with by controlling the fiber composition of the sample that is assayed, but the size of the muscle piece or the number of samples needed to solve the problem of representivity makes it difficult to perform reliable studies on humans. Fröberg and Mossfeldt [20]attempted to resolve this by using two to three large samples (20–50 mg) for the assay. They consistently observed utilization of the TG stored in muscles amounting to 2.6 to 15.8 μmol$\cdot$g^{-1} after many hours of work. As total energy turnover in this exercise was 6000 kcal or more, the contribution of muscle TG breakdown was approximately 5% of total energy turnover. Even if the muscle TG store had been completely

depleted, only 10% of the energy could have been derived from this energy source. Later studies using smaller muscle tissue samples for the assay of TG have not produced equally consistent results. An approach taken by some to determine muscle TG utilization during exercise has been to use morphometric methods to determine the size of the fat vacuoles in electron micrographs [54]. These studies have demonstrated a definite reduction in the size of the fat vacuoles, indicating use of the TG in muscle fibers during prolonged exercise. Hurley et al. [36] have reported large reductions in the TG content of human skeletal muscle following spontaneous exercise. However, the TG content and the net breakdown were larger than have ever been observed under any conditions. In fact, in these studies oxidation of all of the fat disappearing from the fibers was greater than that necessary for metabolism of the limb muscle. These studies must be replicated before any judgment can be made as to their importance.

Recently a third approach has been taken in the attempt to determine the extent of intramuscular TG—quantitative measurement of the release of glycerol from contracting muscles. Since serum TG is probably not utilized to any major degree, the glycerol is assumed to be derived by lipolysis within the muscle. Measurements indicate that with prolonged effort, muscle TG hydrolysis contributes 5 or at most 10% of the energy turnover in the later phases of a 1- to 2-hour exercise period [48, 63]. A limitation with this approach is that it does not establish whether the TG hydrolysis has occurred within or between the muscle fibers. This problem has no bearing on the question of total contribution of FFA to the energy turnover of exercise, but is important in the quantitative assessment of the relative roles of the different fat depots that contribute FFA to the pool utilized during exercise. Kiens et al. [48] have approached this problem by measuring both glycerol released from the muscle and TG depletion in groups of fibers that were dissected free from biopsy samples and cleaned prior to assay. Only a small and insignificant reduction in muscle fiber TG concentration was found following 2 hours of exercise. As glycerol release demonstrates lipolysis, these data suggest that adipocytes between fibers play a significant role in human energy production during exercise. These findings contrast with those of Hurley et al. [36], who also estimated changes in TG stores of human muscle fibers by determining TG concentration in fibers dissected from biopsy samples. As indicated earlier, the decline in the TG concentration of the fibers following exercise was larger than necessary to account for the total metabolism of the limb muscles.

Declines in muscular TG concentrations in the oxidative fibers have been noted in other species, such as the rat [43], both after swimming and running exercise, but no decline in TG concentration was detected in the moneky after prolonged electrical stimulation of the muscles [52]. Spriet, Heigenhauser, and Jones [64] also observed a decline in the TG content of rat muscle after electrical stimulation. However, in these studies intrafiber TG was not separated from extrafiber TG, and it is impossible to determine what percent of the decline in total TG occurred from within the fibers. There was also a net release of both FFA and glycerol from the stimulated muscle in these studies, and this may have occurred from adipocytes located between the muscle fibers.

From this description it appears that TGs located within the muscle fibers are used during prolonged exercise by humans but that their quantitative role is probably small. At present it has not been firmly established whether lipid droplets in the fibers or the TGs of the adipocytes between fibers, or both, contribute to TG depletion. It would appear that both energy pools are used during some types of exercise. It is hard to envisage a role for the lipid droplets in muscle other than to support metabolism.

Little is known about the regulation of lipolysis within the muscle fibers during exercise. β-Adrenergic blockade reduces the rate at which glycerol is released from the contracting muscle [16]. Infusion of a β_2-agonist exaggerates this glycerol release. Thus, it is most likely that mechanisms similar to those described in Figure 1 for regulation of the lipolysis in the fat pad operate in the muscle.

MOBILIZATION OF FFA

Dynamics of Plasma FFAs at Rest and During Exercise

At rest, the plasma FFA concentration is about 0.300 mmol·L^{-1}. At the onset of exercise there is frequently a depression in plasma FFA concentrations, which is followed by an elevation with continuing exercise [9]. The drop in plasma FFA concentration has been attributed to an initial imbalance between FFA uptake by skeletal muscle, in part as a result of a sudden increase in blood flow, and delay in activation of lipolysis and release of FFA from adipose tissue. During light and moderately heavy exercise, lipolysis is activated to the extent that after about 20 minutes, influx of FFA into the blood exceeds efflux and there is a progressive rise in plasma FFA concentrations. With prolonged exercise, plasma FFA concentrations reach values as high as 2.0 mmol·L^{-1} which approaches the limit of albumin to combine with FFA. The elevation in plasma FFA occurs both in light prolonged exercise [3] and in relatively heavy exercise (up to about 70% of $\dot{V}o_2$max) [23, 24, 57].

In man, mobilization of FFA from the adipose depots is primarily under the control of the sympathetic nervous system [32]. Thus, at rest and during exercise, lipolysis is suppressed by β-blocking agents and augmented by β-agonists. Other hormonal influences may also be involved, or at least work in concert, with catecholamines. Growth hormone has been shown to increase in concentration in the plasma of exercising human subjects [34]. However, its concentration peaks and then declines before peak plasma FFA concentration is observed. In the experiments of Hunter, Fonseka, and Passmore [34], plasma FFA and growth hormone levels did not increase when subjects consumed glucose during exercise. Thus, it appears that growth hormone may only facilitate the action of the catecholamines, perhaps by stimulation of protein synthesis [22].

Other factors can also influence the rate and magnitude of the rise in plasma FFA concentration during exercise. One is the concentration of lactate in blood, which retards the release of FFA from human adipose tissue [7, 17]. As demonstrated by Issekutz et al. [39], this is related to the degree of lactate elevation in the blood. An inhibitory effect of blood lactate concentration elevation on FFA release was found during the course of moderately intense prolonged exercise, when a rise in blood lactate concentration was induced when subjects interposed short bouts of heavy arm work into a regimen of prolonged submaximal leg work [28]. However, in both the dog and man there was a continual rise in blood glycerol concentration when plasma FFA concentration was reduced by an elevation in blood lactate concentration during exercise. These data suggest that the mechanism of action of the lactate is to provide a carbon skeleton for the formation of α-glycerophosphate within the adipocytes. This α-glycerophosphate could be used to reesterify FFAs as they are formed. Therefore, the effect of lactate is not only one of interfering with lipolysis but also of retarding release of FFAs from the fat cells.

Mobilization of FFA within adipose tissue can be accelerated by manipulating the amount of fat in the blood and by the infusion of hormones. This was demonstrated in rats by Rennie, Winder, and Holloszy [60] in experiments in which feeding of corn oil followed by injection of heparin was used to activate lipoprotein lipase, thereby increasing plasma FFA concentrations and prolonging the capacity of the animals for sustained exercise, while reducing the rate of glycogen consumption. Costill et al. [12] confirmed these results in man and also demon-

strated that ingestion of caffeine sometime before exercise elevated plasma FFA concentrations [13, 40]. When caffeine was consumed prior to exercise, the rise in plasma FFA occurred earlier after onset of exercise, but peak concentrations were not very different from those attained without treatment. Thus, it appears that this treatment might enhance mobilization of lipid and be important in evoking an earlier shift to lipid metabolism. The mechanism by which caffeine might exert its effect is associated with inhibition of phosphodiesterase, the enzyme degrading cyclic AMP. Therefore, when the adenylate cyclase system is activated to accelerate TG hydrolysis, the effect will be prolonged due to the continued presense of AMP. A possible disadvantage of caffeine ingestion is that caffeine has a stimulatory effect on phosphorylase. This could lead to greater use of glycogen, an undesirable effect. The ability of caffeine ingestion to significantly alter the metabolic response to exercise has also been questioned [69]. Also, although early elevation of plasma FFA concentration has been reported to to reduce the rate of glycogen degradation of muscle, this concept has been questioned by Ravussin et al. [58] who, on the basis of R-value, did not observe any difference in the rate of carbohydrate oxidation during prolonged moderately intense exercise. In these latter studies, comparisons were made between conditions when lipid mobilization was normal and when it was accelerated as the consequence of prior intravenous infusion of triglycerides and heparin. Moreover, there was no difference in the percentage of carbohydrate and fat oxidized in spite of the fact that plasma FFA concentration was nearly twice normal after 30 and 60 minutes of exercise.

SIGNIFICANCE OF PLASMA FFA DURING EXERCISE

A close relationship exists between plasma FFA concentration and the amount of fat being oxidized [30]. The basis for this relationship lies in the fact that uptake of FFA by muscle is dependent upon FFA concentration in the blood.

BLOOD-BORNE TRIACYLGLYCEROLS AS ENERGY SOURCES DURING EXERCISE

Blood contains significant amounts of energy in the form of TGs that are carried in a variety of forms. Attempts have been made to ascertain whether this energy reserve serves a major role as an energy source to the working muscle. Olsson et al. [55] studied this possibility by measuring the arteriovenous difference in TG content across the working forearm. They used the simple arteriovenous difference and radioactive labeled TGs. They were unable to detect uptake of TG from the blood with either method.

Reports of plasma TG use in animals are conflicting. There are several observations that prolonged exercise (1–3 hours) does not alter the TG concentration of the blood [19, 37, 67]. Conversely, there are also reports that exercise produces a decrease in the chylomicron concentration of blood and that chylomicrons are taken up by skeletal muscle during exercise [45, 51, 66]. This demonstrates the uncertainty that exists with regard to the relative contribution that plasma TGs make to the total energy metabolism of exercise. Most estimates are that at best they constitute only a minor fraction of the total substrate oxidized.

TRAINING AND FAT UTILIZATION DURING EXERCISE

As presented in Chapter 4, it is an old observation that reliance on fat as a source of energy during submaximal exercise is greater after endurance training. This was demonstrated many years ago when comparisons were made between respiratory exchange ratios of trained and nontrained person [2, 11]. Subsequently, studies were completed in which the R-value was observed to be lower after training than before training (Figure 5). This effect of training on the choice of fuel by muscle was illustrated by the training of only one leg and then having the subject perform two-legged exercise (Figure 6). The

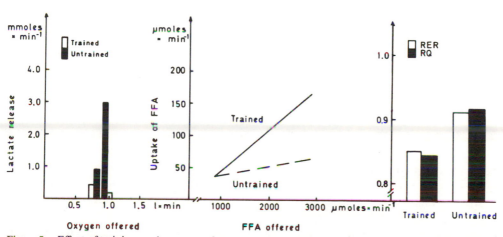

Figure 5. Effect of training on the source of energy. It can be noted that the release of lactate from exercising muscle is lower in the trained state, as are the R-and RQ values. Of additional importance is the observation that oxidation of fat in the trained state is greater when the same amount of FFA is offered (FFA concentration times blood flow) to the muscle.

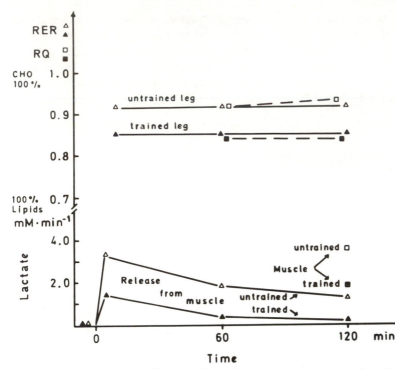

Figure 6. Comparisons of fuel use by and lactate release from the muscles of a trained and an untrained leg of a single subject. These data illustrate the importance of local changes induced by training.

questions of interest regarding this shift in the choice of fuel for exercise are, what is its importance and what is the mechanism for producing the change?

The importance of a shift to greater reliance on fat as a fuel for muscular exercise can be related to two aspects. First, since fat generally constitutes the single largest available energy pool in the body, an attempt to use this energy store to the greatest possible extent represents an intuitive "wisdom of the body." As pointed out earlier, fat is the most efficient method for energy storage devised by nature, fat having the highest energy yield of the three energy sources (fat, carbohydrate, and protein) stored in the body. Second, it has been repeatedly demonstrated that when work intensity is rather high (above ~ 50% of $\dot{V}o^2max$), there is an absolute requirement that a fraction of the fuel be derived from carbohydrate. Carbohydrate originates primarily from the glycogen

stored within the working muscles. When the glycogen reserve of muscle is depleted, the exercise either must stop or its intensity must be reduced [24, 25]. Thus, any increase in energy production that can occur from use of the lipid reserves of the body will conserve the glycogen stores, particularly those of the working muscle, and increase exercise capacity (for references, see Saltin [61]).

Although the relative importance of a shift to greater reliance on fat as a fuel for submaximal exercise can be succinctly summarized, pinpointing the mechanism that produces the response to endurance training is not so easy. A number of important adaptations occur in the body, specifically in the trained skeletal muscle; they occur in three main areas (see Saltin and Gollnick [62]).:

1. Increase in concentration of enzymes for the citric acid cycle, for fatty acid oxidation, and for the electron transport sys-

tem. The net result is an overall augmentation of those metabolic capacities that are associated with the mitochondria. Increased metabolic potential is achieved by a greater concentration of mitochondrial protein per unit weight of the muscle.

2. Increase in capillarization of muscle, with both a greater number of capillaries per muscle fiber and a decrease in the area supplied by a single capillary.

3. Increase in maximal cardiac output.

The relative importance of these changes when related to the greater reliance on fat as a fuel has been discussed in the previous chapter. Gollnick and associates [26, 27] have speculated that the increased concentration of mitochondria per unit of muscle tissue results in greater potential for translocation of cytosolic metabolites into the mitochondria. The original model that was proposed dealt with the response of different concentrations of mitochondria to adenosine diphosphate (ADP). With this model, based on a simple Michaelis–Menten type of kinetic regulation, it was shown that an increase in the concentration of mitochondria allowed the entire system to become more sensitive to metabolic regulators. This can be extrapolated to translocation of a variety of metabolic substrates and cofactors, such as pyruvate, protons from the Embden–Meyerhof pathway, fatty acids, and ADP, into the mitochondria. The net result is maintenance of conditions within the actively respiring muscle cell so as to suppress the Embden–Meyerhof pathway, to avoid excessive production of pyruvate, which can lead to production of lactate unrelated to the existence of anaerobiosis within the cell. Also germane to the problem of increasing fat utilization during exercise is that such an increase provides greater potential for translocation of fatty acids into the mitochondria via the carnitine palmityl transferase system. Taken collectively, this model can explain, at least partially, the shift toward greater fat oxidation after, compared with before, endurance training.

It is unlikely that the increase in maximal cardiac output in response to endurance training plays a significant role in the shift to a greater contribution of fat oxidation during submaximal exercise [6]. This conclusion is based on data that have demonstrated that following training, cardiac output during a standard exercise test is not different from that before training. Moreover, there may actually be a decline in blood flow through muscle during exercise in response to training [48].

Another adaptation that occurs with endurance training is the increased capillarization of muscle, which may be important for the increased use of fat during submaximal exercise [1]. Increased capillarization provides for a greater surface area for the interaction of blood-borne substrates with the muscle fibers. Since transport of FFAs from adipose tissue into blood requires that they pass through several water barriers as well as cellular membranes, this could be important. At the level of the individual muscle fiber, the greater the area of capillary that can be exposed to the muscle, the greater is the potential for exchange of intracellular and extracellular materials. One aspect that appears to limit the use of fatty acids is their transport into the fibers. An increase in the capillary supply to a muscle fiber may reduce this limitation [63]. From data available on man, it appears that mean transit time is longer after endurance training both at the same absolute and relative exercise loads. The magnitude of the increase may be 10 to 30%. The reason increased capillary density increases fat utilization may be that more capillaries are open. However, the capillaries may also be longer or have a greater diameter after training compared with before training. This adaptation becomes important when the same blood volume flows through more capillaries. In this case the time that the blood spends in the capillaries increases. This can be visualized by a hypothetical example: 150 μl of blood perfuses a single muscle fiber in 1 minute before and after training. If the fiber has four capillaries involved in perfusion, the blood flow is 37.5 μl per capillary per minute. With five capillaries per fiber, the flow rate is 30 μl per capillary per minute. Thus, the time that it takes the blood to traverse the capillary bed to produce a constant volume is increased. This longer period of time can be used for the exchange of materials between the blood and the muscular tissue.

As indicated previously, use of fatty acids as fuels is associated with their concentrations in the plasma. Keul, Doll, and Harlambie [47] observed a higher plasma FFA concentration during exercise after training compared with before training when exercise was performed at the same power output. However, the greater use of fat by muscle after training does not appear to be due to a higher concentration of FFA in plasma. In support of this conclusion are early reports that plasma FFA levels were lower in athletes than in nonathletes after voluntary runs in which the intensity of the exercise was established by the subjects [44]. In these experiments, blood lactate levels were higher in the nonathletes. Other investigators [29, 46, 48] have observed that plasma FFA concentrations are either the same or slightly lower when exercise is performed in a controlled situation in which the relative intensity of the exercise is constant. Thus, in the studies of Johnson et al. [44], this higher blood lactate level in nonathletes may have contributed to lowering of the plasma FFA concentration (see above). As shown in Figure 5, uptake and oxidation of fatty acids are greater in the trained state when the same amount of FFA is offered to the muscle by the combination of plasma concentration and total blood flow.

KETONE BODIES

Over the years there has been interest in the production and use of ketone bodies dur-
ing exercise and the influence of training on this use. As indicated in a review of this topic by Koeslag [49], a exercise-induced ketosis was observed nearly 80 years ago. It was found to be related both to the state of fitness of the person exercising and to the diet, being greater after a low carbohydrate intake. Subsequently, Johnson and colleagues [44] observed that there was no change in the concentration of ketone bodies in the blood of trained individuals in response to prolonged endurance exercise, whereas in sedentary persons a similar period of exercise resulted in an approximate 50% increase. There was no difference in the concentrations of ketone bodies in the blood of either trained or sedentary individuals following oral ingestion of sodium acetoacetate [43]. However, during exercise there was a sharp rise in total ketone body concentration in nonathletes, whereas there was no change in athletes. This was interpreted as supporting the contention that there is greater clearance of ketone bodies during exercise by athletes than by nonathletes. Subsequently, Winder, Baldwin, and Holloszy [70] demonstrated that training increases the capacity of skeletal muscle to oxidize ketone bodies. Thus, it appears that there is an adaptive response in muscle that enables it to use more ketone bodies during exercise.

DIET AND FAT USE DURING EXERCISE

Chapter 4 discussed the fact that major shifts in choice of fuel and in exercise capacity can be produced by a change in diet. As elegantly demonstrated by Christensen and Hansen [11], after short-term consumption of a diet low in fat or high in carbohydrate, work capacity was decreased or increased, respectively. In these experiments it was also evident that with the body at rest, the relative amount of fat and carbohydrate oxidized is influenced by diet. Thus, when a high-fat–high-protein diet had been consumed, the R-value was low at rest and remained low throughout exercise. However, when a high-carbohydrate diet had been consumed, the R-value indicated major carbohydrate use at rest, and this use continued into exercise even to the point of exhaustion. In these experiments, with a mixed diet the amount of carbohydrate being oxidized at exhaustion was as great as that at the onset of exercise. Collectively, these data suggest that the body can be conditioned to use a specific substrate.

There have been attempts to examine the effects of prolonged feeding of fat on the choice of fuel during exercise and the mechanism for any shift that may occur. In studies with elite bicyclists who consumed either a normal or a high-fat diet, work capacity, determined under exercise conditions requring about 60% of $\dot{V}o_2$max, was not reduced after consumption of the (low-carbohydrate) high-fat diet, [56]. In fact, subjects exercised an average of 4 minutes longer after consuming the high-fat diet. During exercise, 70% more fat was oxidized after consumption of the high-fat diet compared with the low-fat diet condition. There were no differences in blood glucose levels at rest or at exhaustion under the two dietary conditions; however, the high-fat diet produced a resting ketosis. During exercise the concentrations of ketones in the blood increased under both dietary conditons. This rise was greater after the normal diet compared with the high-fat diet, and at exhaustion ketone concentrations were greater in the low-fat diet conditons. Jansson and Kaijser [42] concluded that the consumption of a high-fat diet for an extended period results in reduced use of carbohydrate and that the relative deficit of carbohydrate is made up by a greater contribution of fat to the total metabolism [41, 42].

Miller, Bryce, and Conlee [53] examined the effect of diet in the rat by feeding a diet that contained either 11 or 78% fat for either 1 or 5 weeks. Rats maintained on the high-fat diet had a greater endurance (run time to exhaustion) than those fed a diet low in fat and high in carbohydrate. This occurred in spite of the fact that the animals fed the high-fat—low-carbohydrate diet had lower liver and muscle glycogen concentrations at rest. A smaller depletion of glycogen stores occurred in the liver and muscle of the animals fed the high-fat diet in response to exercise. A significant resting ketosis existed in the animals maintained on the high-fat diet. Not only was this ketosis not aggravated by exercise, but 3-hydroxybutyrate concentration in the blood showed a slight decline. This contrasted with a significant ketosis during exercise in the animals fed the low-fat diet. The activity of 3-hydroxyacyl CoA dehydrogenase was elevated in the muscle of the rats fed the high-fat diet. These data suggest that an adaptive response can occur in muscle in response to the chronic consumption of a high-fat diet, which appears to result in improved capacity to use fat during moderately severe prolonged exercise.

SUMMARY

Fat constitutes the largest energy store of the body. This energy reserve is primarily in the triacylglycerol stored in adipose tissue. Fat has the highest energy content per unit weight of all energy stores of the body. Fat is the preferred fuel for many tissues at rest and during light activity. However, since fat is stored primarily outside muscle cells and can only be used aerobically, its ability to fuel the metabolism of exercise is limited by the processes of lipolysis within the adipocytes and the transport to and uptake of free fatty acids (FFAs) by muscle. Lipolysis is a hormone-driven process that does not begin to produce increases in the concentration of FFAs in blood until some time after initiation of exercise. The FFAs produced by lipolysis are transported through primarily aqueous media to the muscles, where they are taken up for oxidization or storage. The transport processes appear to involve carrier substances; in the blood the carrier is the protein albumin. Mechanisms for transport across the aqueous phase of the interstitial space are largely unknown, as is the mechanism by which fatty acids cross the plasma membrane of muscle. The ability to transport fatty acids into the muscle appears to be a limiting factor for their use as an energy source during exercise. The transport processes appear to be too slow to permit fat to be a major contributor to the total energy supplied to the contracting muscle cell during heavy exercise. The process of mobilization and transport is also too slow to be of importance early in exercise. The increases in mitochondrial concentration per unit of muscle, and in capillarization, that occur with endurance training contribute to an enhanced use of fat during submaximal exercise. These adaptations are important, because they exert a glycogen-sparing effect and contribute to a greater endurance capacity.

REFERENCES

1. Andersen, P., and J. Henriksson. Capillary supply of the quadriceps femoris muscle of man: Adaptive response to exercise. *J. Physiol. (London)* 270:677–690, 1977.
2. Bang, O. The lactate content of the blood during and after muscular exercise in man. *Skand. Arch. Physiol.* 74:51–82, 1936.
3. Björntorp, B. Human adipose tissue dynamics and regulation. *Adv. Meta. Dis.* 5:277–309, 1971.
4. Björntorp, B. Effect of age, sex, and clinical conditions on adipose tissue cellularity in man. *Metabolism* 2:1091–1098, 1974.
5. Björntorp, B., G. Grimby, H. Sanne, L. Sjöström, G. Tibblin, and Wilhelmsen. Adkipose tissue cell size in relation to metabolism in weight-stable and physically active men. *Horm. Metab. Res.* 4:182–186, 1972.
6. Blomqvist, C.G., and B. Saltin. Cardiovascular adaptations to physical training. *Annu. Rev. Physiol.* 45:169–189, 1983.
7. Boyd, A.E., S.R. Giamber, M. Mager, and H.E. Lebovitez. Lactate inhibition of lipolysis in exercising man. *Metabolism* 23:531–542, 1974.
8. Carlson, L.A., L. Ekelund, and S.O. Fröberg. Concentration of triglyceride, phospholipids and glycogen in skeletal muscle and of free fatty acids and beta-hydroxybutyric acid in blood in man in response to exercise. *Eur. J. Clin. Invest.* 1:248–254, 1971.
9. Carlson, L.A., and B. Pernow. Studies on blood lipids during exercise. I. Arterial and venous plasma concentrations of unesterified fatty acids. *J. Lab. Clin. Med.* 58:833–841, 1959.
10. Chauveau, A. Source et nature du potentiel directment utilisé dans le travail musculaire d'après les exchanges respiratoires, chez l'homme en état d'abstinence, *C. R. Acad. Sci. (Paris)* 122:1163–1221, 1896.
11. Christensen, E.-H., and O. Hansen. Arbeitsfähigkeit und Ehrnährung. *Skand. Arch. Physiol.* 81:160–175, 1939.
12. Costill, D.L., E. Coyle, G. Dalsky, W. Evans, W. Fink, and D. Hoopes. Effects of elevated plasma FFA and insulin on muscle glycogen usage during exercise. *J. Appl. Physiol.* 43:695–699, 1977.
13. Costill, D.L., G.P. Dalsky, and W.J. Fink. Effects of caffeine ingestion on metabolism and exercise performance. *Med. Sci. Sports* 10:155–158, 1978.
14. Edwards, H.T., R. Margaria, and D.B. Dill. Metabolic rate, blood sugar and the utilization of carbohydrate. *Am. J. Physiol.* 108:203–209, 1934.
15. Essén, B. Intramuscular substrate utilization during prolonged exercise. *Ann. N. Y. Acad. Sci.* 301:30–44, 1977.
16. Fellenius, E. Muscle fatigue and beta-blockers: A review. *Int. J. Sports Med.* 4:1–8, 1983.
17. Fredholm, B.B. Inhibition of fatty acid release from adipose tissue by high arterial blood concentrations. *Acta Physiol. Scand.* 77 (*Suppl.* 330), 1969.
18. Fröberg, S.O. Effect of acute exercise on tissue lipids in rats. *Metabolism* 20:714–720, 1971.
19. Fröberg, S.O. Effect of training and of acute exercise in trained rats. *Metabolism* 20:1044–1051, 1971.
20. Fröberg, S.O., and F. Mossfeldt. Effect of prolonged strenuous exercise on the concentrations of triglycerides, phospholipids and glycogen in muscle of man. *Acta Physiol. Scand.* 82:167–171, 1971.
21. Goodhart, R.S., and M.E. Schels. *Modern Nutrition in Health and Disease.* 6th ed. Philadelphia: Lea & Febiger, 1980, Ch. 5, p. 150.
22. Goodman, H.M. Permissive effects of hormones on lipolysis. *Endocrinology* 86:1064–1074, 1970.
23. Gollnick, P.D., C.D. Ianuzzo, C. Williams, and T.R. Hill. Effect of prolonged, severe exercise on the ultrastructure of human skeletal muscle. *Int. Z. angew. Physiol.* 27:257–265, 1969.
24. Gollnick, P.D., B. Pernow, B. Essén, E. Jansson, and B. Saltin. Availability of glycogen and plasma FFA for substrate utilization in leg muscle of man during exercise. *Clin. Physiol.* 1:27–42, 1981.
25. Gollnick, P.D., K. Piehl, C.W. Saubert IV, R B. Armstrong, and B. Saltin. Diet, exercise, and glycogen depletion in different fiber types. *J. Appl. Physiol.* 33:421–425, 1972.
26. Gollnick, P.D., M. Riedy, J.J. Quintinskie, and L.A. Bertocci. Differences in metabolic potential of skeletal muscle fibres and their significance for metabolic control. *J. Exp. Biol.* 115:153–163, 1985.
27. Gollnick, P.D., and B. Saltin. Significance of skeletal muscle oxidative enzyme enhancement with endurance training. *Clin. Physiol.* 2:1–12, 1982.
28. Green, H.J., M.E. Houston, J.A. Thomson, J.R. Sutton, and P.D. Gollnick. Metabolic consequences of supramaximal arm work performed during prolonged submaximal leg work. *J. Appl. Physiol.* 46:249–255, 1979.
29. Gyntleberg, F., M.J. Rennie, R.C. Hickson, and J.O. Holloszy. Effect of training on the response of plasma glucagon to exercise. *J. Appl. Physiol.* 43:302–308, 1977.

30. Hagenfeldt, L., and J. Wahren. Metabolism of free fatty acids and ketone bodies in skeletal muscle. In Pernow, B., and B. Saltin, (eds.). *Muscle Metabolism During Exercise.* New York: Plenum Press, 1971. pp. 153−163.

31. Havel, R.J., L.A. Carlson, L.-G. Ekelund, and A. Holmgren. Turnover rate and oxidation of different free fatty acids in man during exercise. *J. Appl. Physiol.* 19:613−618, 1964.

32. Havel, R.J., and A. Goldfein. The role of the sympathetic nervous system in the metabolism of free fatty acids. *J. Lipid Res.* 1:102−108, 1959.

33. Havel, R J., A. Naimark, and C.R. Borchgrevink. Turnover rate and oxidation of free fatty acids of blood plasma in man during exercise: Studies during continuous infusion of palmitate-1-C¹⁴. *J. Clin. Invest.* 42:1054−1063, 1959.

34. Hunter, W.M., C.C. Fonseka, and R Passmore. Growth hormone: Important role in muscular exercise in adults. *Science* 150:1051−1053, 1965.

35. Huntford, R. *Scott and Amundsen.* London: Hodder and Stoughton, 1979.

36. Hurley, B.F., P.M. Nemeth, W.H. Martin III, J.M. Hagberg, G.P. Dalsky, and J.O. Holloszy. Muscle triglyceride utilization during exercise: Effect of training. *J. Appl. Physiol.* 60:562−567, 1986.

37. Issekutz, B., Jr., H.I. Miller, P. Paul, and K. Rodahl. Source of fat oxidation in exercising dogs. *Am. J. Physiol.* 207:583−587, 1964.

38. Issekutz, B., Jr., and P. Paul. Intramuscular energy sources in exercising normal and pancreatomized dogs. *Am. J. Physiol.* 215:197−204. 1968.

39. Issekutz, B., Jr., W.A. Shaw, and T.B. Issekutz. Effect of lactate on the FFA and glycerol turnover in resting and exercising dogs. *J. Appl. Physiol.* 39:349−353, 1975.

40. Ivy, J.L., D.L. Costill, W.J. Fink, and R.W. Lower. Influence of caffeine and carbohydrate feedings on endurance performance. *Med. Sci. Sports* 11:6−11, 1979.

41. Jansson, E. Diet and muscle metabolism in man. *Acta Physiol. Scand (Suppl.)* 487, 1980.

42. Jansson, E., and L. Kaijser. Effect of diet on the utilization of blood-borne and intramuscular substrates during exercise in man. *Acta Physiol. Scand.* 115:19-30, 1982.

43. Johnson, R.H., and J.L. Walton. The effect of exercise upon acetoacetate metabolism in athletes and nonathletes. *Q. J. Exp. Physiol.* 57:73−89, 1972.

44. Johnson, R.H., J.L. Walton, H.A. Krebs, and D.H. Williamson. Metabolic fuels during and after severe exercise in athletes and non-athletes. *Lancet* 2:452−455, 1969.

45. Jones, N.L., and R.J. Havel. Metabolism of free fatty acids and chylomicron triglycerides during exercise in rats. *Am. J. Physiol.* 213:824−828, 1967.

46. Karlsson, J., L.-O. Nordesjö, and B. Saltin. Muscle glycogen utilization during exercise after physical training. *Acta Physiol. Scand.* 90:210−217, 1974.

47. Keul, J., E. Doll, and G. Harlambie. Frei Fettsäuren, Glycerin und Triglyceride im arteriellen und femoralvenösen Blut vor und nach einem vierwöchingen körperlichen Training. *Pflügers Arch.* 316:194-204.

48. Kiens, B., B. Saltin, N.J. Christensen, and B.

Essén-Gustavsson. Skeletal muscle substrate depletion with exercise: Effect of endurance training. *Am. J. Physiol.* Submitted.

49. Koeslag, J.H. Post-exercise ketosis and the hormone response to exercise: A review. *Med. Sci. Sports Exer.* 14:327−334, 1982.

50. Krogh, A., and J. Lindhard. The relative value of fat and carbohydrate as sources of muscular energy. *Biochem. J.* 14:290−363, 1920.

51. Mackie, B.G., G.A. Dudley, H. Kaciuba-Uscilko, and R.L. Terjung. Uptake of chylomicron triglycerides by contracting skeletal muscle in rats. *J. Appl. Physiol.* 45:851−855, 1980.

52. Masoro, E.J., L.B. Rowell, R.M. McDonald, and B. Steiert. Skeletal muscle lipids. II. Nonutilization of intracellular lipid esters as an energy source for contractile activity. *J. Biol. Chem.* 241:2626−2634, 1966.

53. Miller, W.C., G.R. Bryce, and R.K. Conlee. Adaptations to a high-fat diet that increase exercise endurance in male rats. *J. Appl. Physiol.* 56:78−83, 1984.

54. Oberholzer, F., H. Claassen, H. Moesch, and H. Howald. Ultrastrukturelle, biochemische und energetische Analyze einer extremen Dauerleistung (100 km Lauf). *Schweiz. Z. Sportmed.* 24:71−98, 1976.

55. Olsson, A.G., B. Eklund, L. Kaijser, and L.A. Carlson. Extraction of endogenous plasma triglycerides by working human forearm muscle in thd fasting state. *Scand. J. Clin. Lab. Invest.* 35:231−236, 1975.

56. Phinney, S.D., B.R. Bistrian, W.J. Evans, E. Gervino, and G.L. Blackburn. The human metabolic response to chronic ketosis without caloric restriction: Preservation of submaximal exercise capacity with reduced carbohydrate oxidation. *Metabolism* 32:769−776, 1984.

57. Pruett, E.D.R. FFA mobilization during and after prolonged severe muscular work in man. *J. Appl. Physiol.* 29:809−815, 1970.

58. Ravussin, E., C. Bogardus, K. Scheidegger, B. LaGrange, E.D. Horton, and E.S. Horton. Effect of elevated FFA on carbohydrate and lipid oxidation during prolonged exercise in humans. *J. Appl. Physiol.* 60:893−900, 1986.

59. Reitman, J., K.M. Baldwin, and J.O. Holloszy. Intramuscular triglyceride utilization by red, white, and intermediate skeletal muscle and heart during exhausting exercise. *Proc. Soc. Exp. Biol. Med.* 142:628−631, 1973.

60. Rennie, M., W.W. Winder, and J.O. Holloszy. A sparing effect of increased free fatty acids on muscle glycogen content in exercising rats. *Biochem. J.* 156:647−655, 1976.

61. Saltin, B. Physiological adaptations to physical conditioning: Old problems revisited. *Acta Med. Scand. (Suppl.)* 711:11−24, 1986.

62. Saltin, B., and P.D. Gollnick. Skeletal muscle adaptability: Significance for metabolism and performance. In: Peachy, L.D., R.H Adrian, and S.R. Geiger (eds.). *Handbook of Physiology. Sec. 10: Skeletal Muscle.* Baltimore: Williams and Wilkins, 1983, pp. 555−661.

63. Saltin, B., B. Keins, and G. Savard. A quantitative

approach to the evaluation of skeletal muscle substrate utilization in prolonged exercise. In Benzi, G., L. Packer, and N. Siliprandi (eds.). *Biochemical Aspects of Physical Exercise*. Amsterdam: Elsevier Science Publisher, 1986, pp. 235–244.

64. Spriet, L.L., G.J.F. Heigenhauser, and N.L. Jones. Endogenous triacylglycerol utilization by rat skeletal muscle during tetanic stimulation. *J. Appl. Physiol.* 60:410–415, 1986.

65. Smith, U., J. Hammarstein, P. Björntorp, and J. Kral. Regional difference and effect of weight reduction on human fat cell metabolism. *Eur. J. Clin. Invest.* 9:327–332, 1979.

66. Terjung, R.L., L. Budohoski, K. Nazar, A. Kobryn, and H. Kaciuba-Uscilko. Chylomicron triglyceride metabolism in resting and exercising fed dog. *J. Appl. Physiol.* 52:815–820, 1982.

67. Therriault, D.G., G.A. Beller, J.A. Smoake, and L.H. Hartley. Intramuscular energy sources in dog during physical work. *J. Lipid Res.* 14:54–60, 1973.

68. Weis-Fogh, T. Metabolism and weight economy in migrating animals, particularly birds and insects. In Blix, G. (ed.). *Nutrition and Physical Activity*. Upsalla, Sweden: Almqvist and Wischell, 1967, pp. 84–91.

69. Winder, W.W. Effect of intravenous caffeine on liver glycogenolysis during prolonged exercise. *Med. Sci. Sports Exer.* 18:192–196, 1986.

70. Winder, W.W., K.M. Baldwin, and J.O. Holloszy. Exercise-induced increase in the capacity of skeletal muscle to oxidize ketones. *Can. J. Physiol. Pharmacol.* 53:86–91, 1975.

71. Zuntz, A. Die Quellen der Muskelkraft. *Appenheimer's Handbuch Biochemie* 4:826–855, 1911.

Chapter 6

AMINO ACID AND PROTEIN METABOLISM

Michael N. Goodman, Ph. D.

INTRODUCTION

The impact of physical activity on bodily functions and the health of the individual is quite remarkable when one considers that 20 to 30 minutes of mild to moderate exercise only 3 to 4 days per week can maintain or even increase lean body mass, reduce or delay cardiovascular disease, lower risk factors for atherosclerosis, and help in weight reduction and may also help prevent complications of certain diseases such as diabetes mellitus [32, 35, 56, 57, 64]. The mechanisms by which physical activity influences such a wide spectrum of functions are obviously complex, but hormonal changes, nutrition, and local tissue factors probably all play a role. This chapter is concerned with the effects of physical activity on amino acid and protein metabolism, with an emphasis on changes in the whole body and in skeletal muscle. In addition, the use of protein as a fuel during exercise and how such use relates to dietary requirements of protein will be discussed. Several excellent reviews on this subject have appeared previously [5, 7, 15, 19, 27, 35, 42, 51].

INFLUENCE OF PHYSICAL ACTIVITY AND NUTRITION ON MUSCLE AND BODY GROWTH

A positive correlation between total energy intake and nitrogen balance is well documented [46]. For example, surfeit energy intake can lead to a significant increase in lean body mass (i.e., skeletal muscle), which can be increased still further by physical activity [11, 21, 34, 61]. This relationship is nicely borne out in a study conducted by Torum and coworkers at the Institute of Nutrition of Central America and Panama [35]. They studied the growth of children (2–4 years of age) undergoing treatment for protein–energy malnutrition and found that children grew better in height and lean body mass when they were stimulated to be more physically active through a daily program of games that required mild to moderate levels of activity. This study supports the concept that moderate activity has a growth-enhancing effect and a favorable impact on the utilization of dietary protein.

Such a notion also extends to individuals, young or old, who are well nourished. Several studies in humans and animals have shown that mild or moderate exercise can beneficially influence the growth or size of the lean body mass or specific muscles [9, 11, 21, 34, 47, 61]. Studies in rats have shown that inactivity of muscles produced either by denervation [24] or by immobilization of hind limbs by casting [6] leads to marked atrophy. Early studies by Helander [33] showed that daily moderate exercise in rats fed *ad libitum* resulted in an increase in muscle protein content, which seemed restricted to myofibrillar proteins. In the same study, restricted activity of young rabbits decreased the percentage of myofibrillar proteins and increased that of sarcoplasmic proteins of specific muscles. Similar changes were found in muscles from 3-year-old rabbits, suggesting that many of the changes in protein metabolism during aging result, in part, from inactivity. Unfortunately, these older animals were not made to become more active to determine if the changes could be reversed.

Even when energy intake is restricted, physical activity can still have a beneficial influence on protein metabolism. Several studies in animals have demonstrated that when energy and/or protein intake is reduced, active animals accumulate more dietary nitrogen and conserve lean body mass better than do sedentary controls [47, 62]. In humans, Weltman, Matter, and Stamford [64] found that middle-aged men on a weight-reducing diet and exercising daily experienced significantly less loss of lean body mass than did those who simply restricted their energy intake. Because of this, these investigators recommended that those on slimming diets are probably well advised to be active. With very severe and prolonged caloric restriction, however, the protein sparing effects of exercise may be counterbalanced by the increased energy expenditure, and in this circumstance exercise may accelerate starvation and be harmful.

Despite this caution, physical activity can have a beneficial influence on protein metabolism in situations in which energy intake is totally restricted and endocrine influences are eliminated. Studies by Goldberg and coworkers [23] have shown that the size of skeletal muscle is affected by the pattern of muscular activity. Increased work of a muscle, especially if the work is isometric, can cause a muscle to undergo compensatory growth, while disuse leads to atrophy. Goldberg et al. showed that following tenotomy of the gastrocnemius muscle of young growing rats, the soleus and plantaris muscles increased in weight by 30 to 50% within 6 days. This response was due mainly to hypertrophy of existing muscle fibers. The hypertrophy was induced even if the rats were starved, hypophysectomized, or made diabetic, but it was not induced if the neural input to the muscle was severed. Goldberg et al. thus suggested that muscular activity takes precedence over endocrine influences on muscle size.

AMINO ACID AND PROTEIN USE DURING PHYSICAL ACTIVITY

Although the preceding section emphasized the favorable influence of activity on protein metabolism, it is now well accepted that protein (i.e., amino acids) can serve as an energy source, albeit small, during exercise. In this regard, physical activity could conceivably lead to a net catabolic effect on the body, but this has yet to be demonstrated in well-nourished individuals actively engaged in exercise.

Substrate Reserves of the Body

The substrate reserves of a normal 70-kg man are shown in Table 1. The potential energy that is available in the form of circulating substrates, primarily glucose and free fatty acids, is extremely limited, representing less than 1% of the total energy reserves. By far the greatest potential source of fuel is fat (triglyceride), which is predominantly stored in adipose tissue and accounts for about 80% of the substrate reserves. Glycogen in liver and muscle accounts for about 1 to 2% of the reserves. On the other hand, body protein contains a substantial amount of potential energy, accounting for about 17% of the energy reserves. The usefulness of protein as a fuel is limited, however, since its consumption necessitates the dissolution of structurally and functionally important tissue in the form of skeletal muscle. Protein in muscle is nevertheless labile, and amino acids can be mobilized to support hepatic gluconeogenesis during brief starvation as well as in other situations when

Table 1. BODY FUEL RESERVES IN A NORMAL 70-KG MAN IN THE POSTABSORPTIVE STATE.*

BODY FUEL	AMOUNT	
	kg	*kcal*
Fat (adipose tissue triglycerides)	12	110,000
Protein (muscle)	6	24,000
Glycogen		
Liver	0.07	280
Muscle	0.40	1,600
Glucose (body fluids)	0.02	80
Free fatty acids (body fluids)	0.004	4
Total		135,964

*Data from Cahill, G.F., T.T. Aoki, and A.A. Rossini. Metabolism in obesity and anorexia nervosa. *Nutr. Brain* 3:1–70, 1979.

glycogen and lipid fuels are exhausted or their mobilization is curtailed [13, 27].

Normal humans expend about 1.2 kcal/min at rest, a value that may rise to about 14 kcal/min during exercise. As shown in Table 1, the fuels contained in the body fluids (i.e., glucose and free fatty acids) can sustain such a high energy expenditure for only a few minutes. Consequently, during exercise humans and other mammals must rely upon the mobilization of additional substrates from tissue stores.

Carbohydrate and Lipid Usage

Early studies as far back as 1896 suggested that carbohydrates were the only fuel that could be oxidized by muscle during exercise [25, 27]. Later studies established that both carbohydrates (i.e., plasma glucose and liver and muscle glycogen) and lipids (i.e., plasma free fatty acids and muscle triglycerides) could be utilized by muscles during exercise [25, 27]. In general, the use of these fuels has accounted for almost all of the oxidative metabolism of working muscle (cf. Chapters 4 and 5).

The type and uses of fuels mobilized during exercise depend on the type of exercise, the in-

tensity and duration of exercise, and the individual's previous diet (e.g., high carbohydrate or high fat) and level of physical conditioning. The effects of many of these factors on muscle fuel metabolism are, in part, hormonally mediated. Thus, in both humans and experimental animals, insulin levels decrease and the levels of catecholamines, glucagon, growth hormone, and cortisol increase during exercise, particularly if the exercise is intense and prolonged [27].

In general, muscle glycogen is the major fuel during the early minutes of exercise, when the flow of oxygen to the working muscle does not adequately meet the demands for oxidative metabolism, and also during exercise of a very high intensity (> 85% $\dot{V}O_2$max) and short duration (1–2 minutes). When exercise is more prolonged and of low to moderate intensity, muscle glycogen is initially important as a fuel, but its use diminishes as blood glucose, free fatty acids, and intramuscular triglycerides assume more important roles. During work of long duration and high intensity (near $\dot{V}O_2$max), muscle glycogen is needed to sustain effort, and in this instance it is supplemented in great measure by plasma free fatty acids and muscle triglycerides.

Consumption of a diet rich in fat and protein reduces muscle glycogen content and produces a shift toward greater use of fat during prolonged exercise, while ingestion of a carbohydrate-rich diet increases muscle glycogen content and increases the percentage of carbohydrate used during exercise [25]. Endurance training results in greater use of lipid by muscle during exercise and leads to glycogen sparing [25].

Protein Use

The German physiologist Justus von Liebig reported in 1842 that the primary fuel for muscular contraction was derived from muscle protein, and he suggested that large quantities of meat should be eaten to replenish the supply [27]. Although his broad conclusion was later proved incorrect, his notion that extra protein should be consumed by the physically active individual has resurfaced in recent years. Estimates of the contribution of protein as a fuel during exercise have ranged from as low as 1% to as much as 15% of total energy expenditure [14, 27, 42].

It is not known if the contribution of protein to energy expenditure during exercise can exceed the upper limit so far reported. Several interesting reports indicate that it may. Slonim and Goans [58] reported that the ability of a 50-year-old man with McArdle's syndrome to perform endurance exercise markedly improved with a high-protein diet. In this genetic disease, muscle phosphorylase is deficient and glycogen cannot serve as an immediate fuel for muscle during exercise. The patient cannot tolerate intense short exercise, but can tolerate activity if it is mild and slow in onset. Presumably, in this setting plasma free fatty acids or muscle triglycerides are major fuels. This particular patient was placed on a high-protein, 2800-kcal diet consisting of 25 to 30% protein, 30 to 35% fat and 40 to 45% carbohydrate. This amount of protein (about 3 g/kg) exceeds the National Research Council's recommended dietary allowance by threefold to fourfold. Following 3 years of dietary therapy, the patient's muscle function improved clinically and he was "able to play four sets of competitive tennis, jog a mile, and run up five flights of stairs—levels of activity he had never previously accomplished" [58]. Even prior to therapy, one protein meal 45 minutes before exercise could enhance his endurance on a bicycle ergometer. It is intriguing to speculate that enhanced oxidation of amino acids by muscle during exercise was the reason for his improvement. A study by Wahren et al. [63] of another patient with McArdle's syndrome but on a normal diet supports this notion. These investigators found that during bicycle exercise of increasing intensity plasma amino acids became substantially reduced and the arteriovenous exchange of most amino acids across muscles in the working

leg became consistently more positive than in normal controls. Thus, in individuals with disorders of carbohydrate (and perhaps lipid) metabolism, amino acids may become an important fuel during exercise.

It is unfortunate that Slonim and Goans [58] and Wahren et al. [63] were not able to quantitate the amount of protein used during exercise in their patients. To quantitate the contribution of protein to the fuel mix used during exercise, past studies have relied either on measurement of urea formation during and following exercise or on changes in the metabolism of specific amino aids.

Urea Production. Since urea production is a good reflection of total body protein metabolism, many attempts have been made to quantitate the contribution of amino acids as fuel by simply measuring changes in plasma urea or urine urea output during and/or following exercise. This approach has several limitations, however. Since renal blood flow can diminish significantly during exercise, the glomerular filtration rate may fall, as may the clearance of urea. Perhaps even more critical, significant losses of urea can occur in sweat. Thus, if an individual perspires a great deal when exercising, a significant component of urea formation may go undetected.

Perhaps because of reduced renal blood flow, an increase in urine urea during or immediately after exercise has not been generally observed [17, 26, 27]. On the other hand, investigators have reported increases in plasma or serum urea and in sweat urea during exercise [14, 19, 27, 42]. For the most part, this increase has been observed in subjects who exercise for at least 1 hour or longer at 50% $\dot{V}O_2$max or greater. From the addition of urea production is serum, perspiration, and urine in these studies, about 1 to 15% of the total energy expenditure during exercise could be derived from protein breakdown. These studies reflect increased body protein breakdown during exercise, but the site of augmented protein catabolism is not clear. Some studies suggest the site may be liver [1, 19, 27], while others suggest that it may occur in muscle [19].

Amino Acid Metabolism. Another approach used to quantitate protein as a fuel during exercise is to measure the metabolism of specific amino acids. As reviewed previously [27], significant changes in amino acids in plasma as well as in muscle and liver occur during exercise. The extent and direction of these changes depend on the intensity and duration of the exercise. These measurements per se, however, provide little information about amino acid fluxes across different organs (e.g., liver and muscle). For this reason the study of Ahlborg et al. [1] is of particular importance. In this investigation, untrained male subjects were studied during 4 hours of upright bicycle exercise at light intensity (30% of $\dot{V}O_2max$). Flux of amino acids across the muscles of the working leg and the splanchnic bed and plasma levels of amino acids were measured. As is characteristic for this light exercise, at 40 minutes there was an increase in total plasma amino acids due mainly to a rise in alanine, and between 40 and 240 minutes the plasma concentrations of most amino acids, including alanine, decreased, whereas those of the branched-chain amino acids increased slightly. Prior to exercise, the leg muscles released amino acids, whereas during work there was a net uptake. The exception was alanine, which was continuously released by the muscles of the working leg. The splanchnic bed removed most amino acids during exercise and released significant amounts of branched-chain amino acids. The release of the latter from the splanchnic bed increased with the duration of exercise, probably reflecting an augmentation of protein breakdown in the liver and/or gut. It is notable that increased release of branched-chain amino acids from the splanchnic bed at 4 hours of exercise was balanced by a higher rate of removal by the muscles of the working leg. In addition, branched-chain amino acid removal was balanced by output of alanine, suggesting that the amino acids may have provided the nitrogen (amino group) for alanine formation.

In the study by Ahlborg et al. [1]. The branched-chain amino acids were removed by muscle during exercise, suggesting that these amino acids may be oxidized. Indeed, it is now well documented from studies in humans and animals that the oxidation of branched-chain amino acids, in particular leucine, increases during exercise. It is reasonable to assume that the major site of enhanced amino acid catabolism is in the working muscles [36, 38, 41, 42]. The reported contribution made by amino acid catabolism to the total energy expenditure during moderate-intensity exercise has ranged from 1 to 5% [27, 36, 42]. The marked increase in leucine oxidation by muscle during exercise seems due to specific activation of the branched-chain keto acid dehydrogenase mediated by dephosphorylation of the enzyme [3, 38]. The extent of leucine oxidation depends on the intensity and the duration of exercise [35, 45].

PROTEIN SYNTHESIS AND DEGRADATION IN THE WHOLE BODY AND MUSCLE DURING AND FOLLOWING EXERCISE

The preceding sections indicated that regular exercise can induce a catabolic rise in body protein breakdown (i.e., in urea formation). Yet there is no conclusive evidence that regular exercise leads to a net catabolic effect on the lean body mass. Quite the contrary, physical activity can protect the lean body mass under aerobic or endurance conditions and increase it under strength-building conditions (e.g., isometric exercise). For these reasons, the site of augmented protein breakdown may not be muscle. Alternatively, if it is, the body must adapt to counteract this catabolic response, perhaps during the postexercise period or even during the exercise bout. Protein content in muscle is regulated by changes in the rate of protein synthesis or protein breakdown, or both. Numerous studies in humans and animals have measured protein synthesis and protein breakdown in the whole body or specific muscles during or following exercise [reviewed in 7, 19, 27]. These studies have contributed to our understanding on how physical activity may protect or even increase muscle protein.

Protein Synthesis

Protein synthesis measured during exercise in specific muscles or in the whole body appears to follow a predictable pattern, depending on whether the activity is isotonic or isometric in nature. As shown in Table 2, under isotonic conditions, physical activity induced under a variety of conditions produced a decrease in protein synthesis in specific muscles of animals studied *in vitro* or *in vivo* or in the whole body of humans. In two studies in animals, no change was found, while in another, in which frog muscle was electrically stimulated *in vitro* for upward of 2 hours, protein synthesis in muscle increased. Under isometric conditions, in which muscle tension was increased due to stretch or tenotomy of a synergistic muscle, protein synthesis increased.

Following isotonic activity of various durations, protein synthesis in the muscles of animals or in the whole human body appears to depend on the time of the postexercise period during which the measurement is made. As shown in Table 3, immediately following activity, protein synthesis is decreased or returns to preexercise levels. Several hours after activity, protein synthesis can increase and can remain elevated for up to 24 hours.

Several factors may play a role in decreasing protein synthesis during isotonic exercise, including a fall in plasma insulin level, an increase in plasma glucocorticoid level, a decrease in muscle pH and ATP level, and an increase in muscle temperature [7, 27]. Calcium and prostaglandins may mediate the increase in protein synthesis under isometric

Table 2. PROTEIN SYNTHESIS IN SPECIFIC MUSCLES OF ANIMALS AND IN THE WHOLE HUMAN BODY DURING EXERCISE.*

SPECIES	TYPE OF ACTIVITY	DURATION OF ACTIVITY	CHANGE IN PROTEIN SYNTHESIS[‡]	REF. NO.
Rat	Electrical stimulation	10 min	↓	12
Rat	Running	40 min	↓	4
Rat	Running	40 min	–	45
Rat	Running	30–60 min	↓	19
Rat	Electrical stimulation	30–90 min	↓	48
Frog	Electrical stimulation	120 min	↓	37
Rat	Electrical stimulation	120 min	↓	2
Frog	Electrical stimulation	120 min	–	39
Frog	Electrical stimulation	> 120 min	↑	39
Rat	Work-induced hypertrophy	6 days	↑	23
Rat	Work-induced hypertrophy	4 days	↑	30
Rat	Stretch	120 min	↑	10
Rabbit	Stretch	120 min	↑	51
Chicken	Stretch	28 days	↑	40
Humans	Cycle ergometer (M)	105 min	↓	66
	Cycle ergometer (M)	120 min	↓	29
	Cycle ergometer (M)	180 min	↓	20
	Running (MOD)	225 min	↓	45,53

*Adapted from Booth, F.W., and P.A. Watson. Control of adaptations in protein levels in response to exercise. *Fed. Proc.* 44:2293–2300, 1985, with additional references.

†↑, ↓ —: increase, decrease, no change in protein synthesis, respectively.

M, mild intensity; MOD, moderate intensity.

Table 3. PROTEIN SYNTHESIS IN SPECIFIC MUSCLES OF ANIMALS AND IN THE WHOLE HUMAN BODY FOLLOWING EXERCISE.*

SPECIES	TYPE OF ACTIVITY	DURATION OF ACTIVITY	TIMING OF MEASUREMENT AFTER ACTIVITY	CHANGE IN PROTEIN SYNTHESIS†	REF. NO.
Rat	Electrical stimulation	10 min	Immediately †	–	12
Rat	Electrical stimulation	30–420 min	Immediately	–	23
Rat	Swimming	60 min	Immediately	↓	19
Chicken	Electrical stimulation	14–37 hr	Immediately	↑	8
Rat	Stretch	2–7 days	Immediately	↑	24
Rat	Running	60 min	1 hr	↑	55
Rat	Running	60 min	2–18 hr	↑	65
Guinea pig	Running	30 min	14–18 hr	↑	43
Rat	Running	120 min	24 hr	–	60
Rat	Swimming	120 min	24 hr	–	16
Humans	Running (moderate)	3.75 hr	Immediately	↑	45,53
	Swimming (moderate)	1–3 hr	12–24 hr	–	59
	Ballet dancing	1–3 hr	12–24 hr	↑	59

*Adapted from Booth, F.W., and P.A. Watson. Control of adaptations in protein levels in response to exercise. *Fed. Proc.* 44:2293–2300, 1985, with additional references.

†Immediately indicates that measurement of protein synthesis started within 30 minutes after the exercise period and, depending on the particular study, continued for up to 4 hours.

‡ ↑, ↓, –: increase, decrease, no change in protein synthesis, respectively.

conditions [7]. On the other hand, it is unclear which factors may be responsible for increasing protein synthesis in the postexercise period. An increase in amino acid transport into muscle [68], increased sensitivity of muscle to insulin [53], a fall in level of glucocorticoids [27], and modulation by prostaglandins [51] may play a role.

Protein Degradation

While changes in protein synthesis in muscles or the whole body during isotonic or isometric activity seem to comply to some predictable pattern, such is not the case with protein degradation. During exercise, especially when it is of moderate intensity and lasting 1 to 2 hours, total body protein breakdown in humans has been reported to be increased [14, 19, 27, 42, 45], decreased [20], or unchanged [66]. As an index of skeletal muscle myofibrillar protein breakdown during exercise, the output of 3-methylhistidine into the urine or its concentration in muscles has been measured. In one study, 3-methylhistidine concentration in muscle and its release from perfused rat muscle decreased during 10 minutes of electrical stimulation [12]. A similar fall in concentration was found in human muscle during endurance exercise lasting several hours [45, 53]. The output of 3-methylhistidine into the urine during exercise in humans has been reported to fall or not to change [14, 18]. Thus, in some studies muscle protein breakdown during exercise may decrease. This reponse would counterbalance the fall in protein synthesis at this time (Table 2) and conserve protein. Two studies in animals reported protein degradation in muscle to be either increased [40] or decreased [23] when exercise was isometric in nature and muscles were undergoing hypertrophy.

Immediately following a bout of exhaustive exercise in rats, protein breakdown measured in perfused muscle was found to be increased [19]. Other studies that have evaluated muscle protein breakdown following exercise are restricted to humans and have relied on measurement of urine 3-methylhistidine excretion. Immediately following heavy exercise, Decombaz et al. [17] found a decrease in 3-methylhistidine excretion. During 2 to 24 hours after moderate to heavy exercise, Calles-Escandon et al. [14] reported no change whereas Radha and Bessman [50] and Refsum, Gjessing, and Stromme [52] reported a fall in 3-methylhistidine excretion. In contrast, Dohm et al. [18] found an increase in 3-methylhistidine excretion 3 to 24 hours following moderate to heavy running, and Hickson and Hinkelmann [34] found an increase in 3-methylhistidine excretion in men undergoing daily strength-building exercise.

It is not surprising that conflicting results have been reported about 3-methylhistidine excretion following exercise. It is usually assumed that 3-methylhistidine appearing in the urine originates exclusively from actin and myosin in skeletal muscle. Significant amounts, however, can come from actin in the skin and gastrointestinal tract [18, 67]. Also, 3-methylhistidine in the diet can confound urinary measurements. Finally, it is conceivable that the renal clearance of 3-methylhistidine may change during and following exercise and in a direction that may be different from that of creatinine. In long-distance runners, urinary abnormalities are found after exercise due to a temporary hemodynamic impairment of glomerular or tubular function [22].

At present, it appears that animal studies are needed to help clarify the pattern of protein degradation in skeletal muscle immediately following and up to 24 hours after an exercise bout. For example, methodology is available for measuring total proteolysis and myofibrillar (i.e., 3-methylhistidine release) proteolysis simultaneously in perfused or incubated rat muscles [12, 23, 67]. This procedure can be applied to trained or untrained rats following a single bout of exercise.

DIETARY PROTEIN REQUIREMENTS DURING PHYSICAL ACTIVITY

As far back as 1842, von Liebig suggested that extra protein should be consumed by the physically active individual to replace that used during exercise [27]. Now, after 144 years, this issue has resurfaced primarily because of reports that endurance exercise may increase whole-body and/or muscle protein breakdown and, in particular, may increase the oxidation of leucine. As reviewed by Bier and Young [5], leucine oxidation increased threefold to fivefold in humans undergoing exercise of low to moderate intensity for several hours. The rate of leucine oxidation during the exercise period accounted for more than two-thirds of estimated minimal daily requirement for leucine. Because of this, these authors suggested that the RDA for protein and amino acids may be inadequate for individuals actively engaged in chronic moderate to heavy exercise lasting several hours or more.

Several studies have reported on the effects of chronic exercise on nitrogen balance in humans. Five studies were reviewed by Hoerr, Young, and Evans [35], and they concluded that individuals actively engaged in exercise have difficulty maintaining nitrogen balance when dietary protein intake is less than 1.0 to 1.5 g/kg body weight/day, a level of intake probably consumed by the average normal adult human. They did not find sufficient evidence to support protein intakes of 2.5 to 3.0 g/kg/day recommended previously. On the other hand, several studies by Calloway and coworkers [11, 61] have suggested that the protein requirement necessary to maintain existing lean body mass in a chronically active individual may be somewhat less than the requirement for a person who is inactive. This is thought to be a consequence of the increased energy intake generally accompanying the activity or due to an adaptive response owing to the activity itself. In another study, Hickson and Hinkelmann [34], reported that the increase in lean body mass in men undergoing daily strength-building exercise was almost the same whether the men consumed the RDA for protein (0.8 g/kg body weight/day) or three times the RDA. All of these studies seem to suggest that increased intake of protein during chronic exercise should be advised only if a net catabolic effect of exercise can be demonstrated.

At present more study is needed to determine conclusively whether chronic physical activity alters the daily requirements for protein and/or individual amino acids. It appears that past evaluation of this subject in humans has been conducted almost exclusively in adults. Future studies should include the younger population (preteens or early teens), since these subjects would be more at risk if extra protein is necessitated by chronic physical activity, because young people need protein also to sustain rapid body growth. Future studies must also bear in mind that diets high in protein-rich foods have been linked to certain human cancers [28] as well as to renal lesions leading to glomerular sclerosis [44]. Although exercise may help protect against such adverse associations with dietary protein, any recommendation to increase its consumption substantially above 1.0 to 1.5 g/kg body weight/day should be met with caution.

CONCLUDING REMARKS

Physical activity, even when it is in the form of very mild exercise, can influence in a beneficial way the growth or size of the lean body mass or specific muscles. Physical activity in young individuals can increase the rate of growth of the lean body mass, while it can protect or conserve lean body mass in older individuals even when caloric intake is moderately reduced. Thus, it appears that the activity itself beneficially influences protein metabolism in muscle specifically. Although specific changes in protein synthesis and degradation occur in muscles during and following exercise, it is not yet clear how the two processes result in these favorable effects. Because of this, an animal model to study protein synthesis and protein degradation simultaneously in muscles during and following exercise would be helpful. Finally, chronic exercise can lead to an increase in whole body protein breakdown and oxidation of specific amino acids. It is not conclusive if this warrants consumption of extra dietary protein above that of the standard American diet.

REFERENCES

1. Ahlborg, G., P. Felig, L. Hagenfeldt, R. Hendler, and J. Wahren. Substrate turnover during prolonged exercise in man. *J. Clin. Invest.* 53:1080–1090, 1974.
2. Arvill, A. Relationship between the effects of contraction and insulin on the metabolism of the isolated levator ani muscle of the rat. *Acta Endocrino.* 56:27–41, 1967.
3. Balon, T.W., J.N. Drowatzky, J.R. Claybrook, and C.L. Long. Effects of acute and chronic exercise on branched-chain aminotransferase and alpha-ketoacid dehydrogenase. *Fed. Proc.* 43:293, 1984.
4. Bates, P.C., D.J. Millward, and M.J. Rennie. Reexamination of the effect of exercise on muscle protein synthesis in the rat. *J. Physiol.* 315:27P, 1981.
5. Bier, D.M., and V.R. Young. Exercise and blood pressure: Nutritional considerations. *Ann. Intern. Med.* 98:864–869, 1983.
6. Booth, F.W. Time course of muscular atrophy during immobilization of hindlimbs in rats. *J. Appl. Physiol.* 43:656–661, 1977.
7. Booth, F.W., and P.A. Watson. Control of adaptations in protein levels in response to exercise. *Fed. Proc.* 44:2293–2300, 1985.
8. Brevet, A., E. Pinto, J. Peacock, and F.E. Stockdale. Myosin synthesis increased by electrical stimulation of skeletal muscle cell cultures. *Science* 193:1152–1154, 1976.
9. Bulbulian, R., K.K. Grunewald, and R.R. Haack. Effect of exercise duration on food intake and body composition of Swiss albino mice. *J. Appl. Physiol.* 58:500–505, 1985.
10. Buresvova, M., E. Gutmann, and M. Klicpera. Effect of tension upon rate of incorporation of amino acids into proteins of cross-striated muscle. *Experientia* 5:144–145, 1969.
11. Butterfield, G.E., and D.H. Calloway. Physical activity improves protein utilization in young men. *Br. J. Nutri.* 51:174–184, 1984.
12. Bylund-Fellenius, A., K.M. Ojmaa, K.E. Flain, J.B. Li, S.J. Wassner, and L.S. Jefferson. Protein synthesis versus energy state in contracting muscles of perfused rat hindlimb. *Am. J. Physiol.* 246:E297–E305, 1984.
13. Cahill, G.F., T.T. Aoki, and A.A. Rossini. Metabolism in obesity and anorexia nervosa. *Nutr. Brain* 3:1–70, 1979.
14. Calles-Escandon, J., J.J. Cunningham, P. Snyder, R. Jacob, G. Huszar, J. Loke, and P. Felig. Influence of exercise on urea creatinine and 3-methylhistidine excretion in normal human subjects. *Am. J. Physiol.* 246:E334–E338, 1984.

15. Cathcart, E.P. Influence of muscle work on protein metabolism. *Physiol. Rev.* 5:225–243, 1925.

16. Davis, T.A., I.E. Karl, E.D. Tegtmeyer, D.F. Osborne, S.Klahr, and H.R. Harter. Muscle protein turnover: Effects of exercise training and renal insufficiency. *Am. J. Physiol.* 248:E337–E345, 1985.

17. Decombaz, J., P. Reinhardt, K. Amantharaman, G. von Glutz, and J.R. Poortmans. Biochemical changes in a 100Km run: Free amino acids, urea, and creatinine. *Eur. J. Appl. Physiol.* 41:61–72, 1979.

18. Dohm, G.L., R.G. Israel, R.L. Breedlove, R.T. Williams, and E. Wayne Askew. Biphasic changes in 3-methylhistidine excretion in humans after exercise. *Am. J. Physiol.* 248:E588–E592, 1985.

19. Dohm, G.L., G.J. Kasperek, E.B. Tapscott, and H.A. Barakat. Protein metabolism during endurance exercise. *Fed. Proc.* 44:348–352, 1985.

20. Evans, W.J., E.C.Fisher, R.A. Hoerr, and V.R. Young. Protein metabolism and endurance exercise. *Phys. Sports Med.* 11:63–72, 1983.

21. Forbes, G.B. Body composition as affected by physical activity and nutrition. *Fed. Proc.* 44:343–347, 1985.

22. Gilli, P., E. De Paoli Vitali, G. Tataranni, and A. Farinelli. Exercise-induced urinary abnormalities in long-distance runners. *Int. J. Sports Med.* 5:237–240, 1984.

23. Goldberg, A.L., J.D. Etlinger, D.F. Goldspink, and C. Jablecki. Mechanism of work-induced hypertrophy of skeletal muscle. *Med. Sci. Sports* 7:248–261, 1975.

24. Goldspink, D.F. The influence of activity on muscle size and protein turnover. *J. Physiol.* 264:283–296, 1977.

25. Gollnick, P.D. Metabolism of substrates: Energy substrate metabolism during exercise and as modified by training. *Fed. Proc.* 44:353–357, 1985.

26. Gontzea, I., P. Sutzescu, and S. Dimitrache. The influence of muscular activity on nitrogen balance and on the need of man for proteins. *Nutr. Rep. Int.* 10:35–43, 1974.

27. Goodman, M.N., and N.B. Ruderman. Influence of muscle use on amino acid metabolism. *In* Terjung, R.L. (ed.). *Exercise and Sport Science Reviews,* Philadelphia: Franklin Insititute Press, 1982, pp.1–26.

28. Grobstein, C. Protein. In *Diet, Nutrition and Cancer.* Washington, D.C.: Research Council, National Academy Press, 1982, pp. 106–122.

29. Hagg, S., E.L. Morse, and S.A. Adibi. Effect of exercise on rates of oxidation, turnover, and plasma clearance of leucine in human subjects. *Am. J. Physiol.* 242:E407–E410, 1982.

30. Hamosh, M., M. Lesch, J. Baron, and S. Kaufman. Enhanced protein synthesis in a cell-free system from hypertrophied skeletal muscle. *Science* 157:935–937, 1967.

31. Haralambie, G., and A. Berg. Serum urea and amino nitrogen changes with exercise duration. *Eur. J. Appl. Physiol.* 36:39–48, 1976.

32. Hartung, G.H., E.J. Farge, and R.E. Mitchell. Effects of marathon running, jogging, and diet on coronary risk factors in middle-aged men. *Preven. Med.* 1:316–323, 1981.

33. Helander, E.A.S. Influence of exercise and restricted activity on the protein composition of skeletal muscle. *Biochem. J.* 78:478–482, 1985.

34. Hickson, J., and K. Hinkelmann: Exercise and protein intake effects on urinary 3-methylhistidine excretion. *Am. J. Clin. Nutr.* 41:246–253, 1985.

35. Hoerr, R.A., V.R. Young, and W.J. Evans. Protein metabolism and exercise. In White P.L., and T. Mondeika, (eds.). *Diet and Exercise: Synergism in Health Maintenance,* Chicago: American Medical Association, 1982, pp. 49–66.

36. Hood, D.A., and R.L. Terjung. Leucine metabolism in perfused rat skeletal muscle during contractions. *Med. Sci. Sports Exer.* 17:233, 1985.

37. Karpatkin, S., and A. Samuels. Effect of insulin and muscle contraction on protein synthesis in frog sartorius. *Arch. Biochem. Biophys.* 121:695–702, 1967.

38. Kasperek, G.J., G.L. Dohm, and R.D. Snider. Activation of branched-chain keto acid dehydrogenase by exercise. *Am. J. Physiol.* 248:R166–R177, 1985.

39. Kendrick-Jones, J., and S.B. Perry. Protein synthesis and enzyme response to contractile activity in skeletal muscle. *Nature* 213:406–408, 1967.

40. Laurent, G.J., M.P. Sparrow, and D.J. Millward. Turnover of muscle protein in fowl: Changes in rates of protein synthesis and breakdown during hypertrophy of the anterior and posterior latissimus dorsi muscles. *Biochem. J.* 176:407–417, 1978.

41. Lemon, P.W.R., N.G. Benevenga, J.P. Mullin, and F.J. Nagle. Effect of daily exercise and food intake on leucine oxidation. *Biochem. Med.* 33:67–76, 1985.

42. Lemon, P.W.R., and F.J. Nagle. Effects of exercise on protein and amino acid metabolism. *Med. Sci. Sports Exer.* 13:141–149. 1981.

43. McManus, B.M., D.R. Lamb, J.J. Jundis, and J. Scala. Skeletal muscle leucine incorporation and testosterone uptake in exercised guinea pigs. *Eur. J. Appl. Physiol.* 34:149–156, 1975.

44. Meyer, T.W., S. Anderson, and B.M. Brenner. Dietary protein intake and progressive glomerular sclerosis: The role of capillary hypertension and hyperperfusion in the progression of renal disease. *Ann. Intern. Med.* 98:832–838, 1983.

45. Millward, D.J., C.T.M. Davies, D. Halliday, S.L. Wolman, D. Matthews, and M. Rennie. Effect of exercise on protein metabolism in humans as explored with stable isotopes. *Fed. Proc.* 41:2686–2691, 1982.

46. Munro, H.M. Carbohydrate and fat as factors in protein utilization and metabolism. *Physiol. Rev.* 31:449–488, 1951.

47. Oscai, L.B., and J.O. Holloszy. Effects of weight changes produced by exercise, food restriction or overeating on body composition. *J. Clin. Invest.* 48:2124–2128, 1969.

48. Pain, V.M., and K.L. Manchester. The influences of electrical stimulation in vitro on protein synthesis and other metabolic parameters of rat extensor digitorum longus muscle. *Biochem. J.* 11:209–220, 1970.

49. Poormans, J.: Protein metabolism: Effects of exercise and training. *Med. Sport* 133:59-67, 1981.

50. Radha, E., and S.P. Bessman. Effect of exercise on

protein degradation: 3-methylhistidine and creatinine excretion. *Biochem. Med.* 29:96–100, 1983.

51. Ralmer, R.M., P.J. Reeds, T. Atkinson, and R.H. Smith. The influence of changes in tension on protein synthesis and prostaglandin release in isolated rabbit muscles. *Biochem. J.* 214:1011–1014, 1983.

52. Refsum, H.E., L.R. Gjessing, and S.B. Stromme. Changes in plasma amino acid distribution and urine amino acid excretion during prolonged heavy exercise. *Scand. J. Clin. Lab Invest.* 39:407–413, 1979.

53. Rennie, M.J., R.H.T., Edwards, C.T.M., Davies, S. Krywawych, D. Halliday, J.C. Waterlow, and D.J. Millward. Protein and amino acid turnover during and after exercise. *Biochem. Soc. Trans.* 8:499–501, 1980.

54. Richter, E.A., L.P. Garetto, M.N. Goodman, and N.B. Ruderman: Muscle glucose metabolism following exercise in the rat: increased sensitivity to insulin. *J. Clin. Invest.* 69:785–793, 1982.

55. Rogers, P.A., G.H. Jones, and J.A. Faulkner. Protein synthesis in skeletal muscle following acute exhaustive exercise. *Mus. Nerv.* 2:250–256, 1979.

56. Ruderman, N.B., and C.H. Haudenschild. Diabetes as an atherogenic factor. *Prog. Cardiovas. Disease* 26:373–411, 1984.

57. Schneider, S.H., L. Amorosa, A.K. Khachadurian, and N.B. Ruderman. Studies on the mechanism of improved glucose control during regular exercise in Type 2 diabetes. *Diabetologia* 26:355–360, 1984.

58. Slonim, A.E., and P.J. Goans. Myopathy in McArdle's syndrome. Improvement with a high protein diet. *N. Engl. J. Med.* 312:355–359, 1985.

59. Stein, T.P., M.D. Schluter, and C.E. Diamond. Nutrition, protein turnover and physical activity in young women. *Am. J. Clin. Nutr.* 38:223–228, 1983.

60. Tapscott, E.B., G.J. Kasperek, and G.L. Dohm. Effect of training on muscle protein turnover in male and female rats. *Biochem. Med.* 27:254–259, 1982.

61. Todd, K.S., G.E., Butterfield and D.H. Calloway. Nitrogen balance in men with adequate and deficient energy intake at three levels of work. *J. Nutr.* 114:2107–2118, 1984.

62. Viteri, F.E. In *Nuevos Conceptos Sobre Viejos Aspectos de la Des Nutricion.* Mexico City: La Academia Mexicana de Pediatria, 1974, pp. 207–229.

63. Wahren, J., P. Felig, R.J. Havel, L. Jorfeldt, B. Pernow, and B. Saltin. Amino acid metabolism in McArdle's syndrome. *N. Engl. J. Med.* 288:774–777, 1973.

64. Weltman, A., S. Matter, and B.A. Stamford. Caloric restriction and/or mild exercise: Effects on serum lipids and body composition. *Am. J. Clin. Nutr.* 33:1002–1009, 1980.

65. Wenger, H.A., J.G. Wilkinson, J. Dallaire, and T. Nihei. Uptake of ^{3}H-leucine into different fractions of rat skeletal muscle following acute endurance and sprint exercise. *Eur. J. Appl. Physiol.* 47:83–92, 1981.

66. Wolfe, R.R., R. Goodenough, M.H. Wolfe, G.T. Royle, and E.R. Nadel. Isotopic analysis of leucine and urea metabolism in exercising humans. *J. Appl. Physiol.* 52:458–466, 1982.

67. Young, V.R., and H.N. Munro. N-methylhistidine and muscle protein turnover: An overview. *Fed. Proc.* 37:2291–2300, 1978.

68. Zorzano, A., T.W. Balon, L.P. Garetto, M.N. Goodman, and N.B. Ruderman. Muscle alpha-aminoisobutyric acid transport after exercise: Enhanced stimulation by insulin. *Am. J. Physiol.* 248:E546–E552, 1985.

Chapter 7

GLUCOSE HOMEOSTASIS DURING AND AFTER EXERCISE

Ola Björkman, Ph.D., and John Wahren, M.D.

THE POSTABSORPTIVE, RESTING STATE

The period between an overnight fast and ingestion of the morning meal is generally referred to as the basal, postabsorptive state. At this time the concentrations of glucoregulatory hormones (insulin and glucagon) and substrates (glucose, amino acids, fatty acids), which were altered by meal ingestion during the preceding day, have returned to their baseline levels. Although the condition represented by the postabsorptive state is relatively unsteady, reflecting the period of metabolic transition from the fed to the fasted condition, it is a useful reference point in metabolic studies.

After an overnight fast, the return of insulin concentrations to basal levels (10–20 μU/ml) results in a substantial diminution of glucose uptake by insulin-dependent tissues such as resting muscle, adipose tissue, and liver. However, glucose uptake continues unchanged in the non-insulin-dependent tissues such as the brain, blood cells, renal medulla, and bone marrow. Total glucose utilization after an overnight fast is on the order of 0.7 to 1.0 mmol/min [3, 33]. Maintenance of blood glucose homeostasis is achieved in this state by the hepatic release of glucose at rates equal to those of tissue utilization, no other tissue or organ in the body contributing glucose to the bloodstream. The hepatic processes involved in the addition of glucose to the blood comprise glycogenolysis and *de novo* synthesis of glucose (gluconeogenesis). The relative contributions of these processes to glucose production have been estimated from measurements of net splanchnic exchange of glucose and gluconeogenic substrates [33], as well as from determinations of the rate of glycogen disappearance determined from liver biopsy samples obtained at timed intervals [22]. The results indicate that approximately 65 to 75% of basal hepatic glucose release is derived from glycogenolysis, and the remainder (25–35%) from gluconeogenesis. The hepatic glycogen store following an overnight fast is approximately 80 to 90 g [22]. This limited depot along with muscle glycogen (300–400 g) and blood glucose (20 g), is the only carbohydrate available for utilization in the basal state.

Hepatic glycogen is readily available for hepatic glucose production. The rate of glycogenolysis may vary from substantially below the basal level (more than 50% below) during meal ingestion to multiple increments in response to stress or exercise. The continuous breakdown of glycogen in the postabsorptive state exhausts the hepatic glycogen stores within 24 to 48 hours after a meal [22]. As will be discussed, during prolonged exercise, hepatic glycogen depletion occurs even sooner, due to the increased rate of glycogenolysis.

With regard to gluconeogenesis, the precursor substrates available for conversion to glucose are the glycolytic intermediates lactate, pyruvate, and glycerol and the glucogenic amino acids, primarily alanine (Figure 1). Recycling of glucose-derived lactate and pyruvate (Cori cycle) accounts for approximately 15% of hepatic glucose production [33, 34]. A further 2% is contributed by glycerol released from adipose tissue. The remaining gluconeogenesis comprises conversion of precursor amino acids, of which alanine contributes most—6 to 12% of total glucose output and 20 to 50% of the gluconeogenic component.

The predominance of alanine among amino acids in the outflow from muscle and the evidence for its synthesis from glucose-derived pyruvate in muscle tissue has led to the recognition of a glucose-alanine cycle [10, 11] analogous to the Cori cycle for lactate. The carbon skeleton of alanine is thus an end product of glucose utilization in muscle and constitutes an important precursor for hepatic glucose production. In addition, alanine serves as a nontoxic carrier of amino nitrogen from muscle to liver. The quantitative contribution made by carbon skeletons recycling along the glucose-alanine cycle is approximately 50% of that observed for the Cori cycle [11].

Unlike glycogen, which can be mobilized rapidly from the hepatic stores and released as glucose by virtue of the hepatic enzymes glycogen phosphorylase and glucose-6-phosphatase, the gluconeogenic precursors derive from peripheral tissues and must be transported to the liver for hepatic uptake and metabolism. Hepatic gluconeogenesis is therefore controlled by intrahepatic mechanisms and by the peripheral production of precursors. For these reasons, changes in the rate of hepatic gluconeogenesis are generally much more gradual than are changes in glycogenolysis. Quantitatively, gluconeogen-

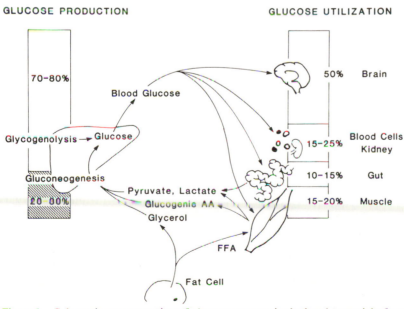

Figure 1. Schematic representation of glucose turnover in the basal (overnight-fasted) resting state in normal man. The liver is the sole site of glucose production, via glycogenolysis (75%) and gluconeogenesis (25%). The brain is the major site of glucose utilization, consuming approximately half of the output. Smaller amounts of glucose are taken up by blood cells, the renal medulla, the gut, and skeletal muscle. The last is a source of glucose precursors in the form of amino acids, primarily alanine and the glycolytic intermediaries lactate and pyruvate. The adipocyte contributes small amounts of glycerol for gluconeogenesis.

esis is less important than glycogenolysis in the postabsorptive state, but when glycogen stores are substantially depleted, gluconeogenesis becomes the dominant source for glucose production [3, 33]. The quantitative relationship between hepatic glucose production and peripheral glucose utilization in the basal, overnight-fasted state is summarized in Figure 1.

Concerning the hormonal factors responsible for hepatic glucose output in humans in the postabsorptive state, it is clear that the fall in plasma insulin from postprandial to basal concentrations is important for the stimulation of hepatic glycogenolysis and the mobilization of the precursor amino acids and energy-yielding free fatty acids necessary for gluconeogenesis. The maintenance of basal hepatic glucose output is also dependent on basal glucagon secretion, as indicated by the fall in postabsorptive blood glucose levels in response to somatostatin-induced inhibition of glucagon secretion.

In addition to glycogen in the liver and glucose in the bloodstream, an average of 300 to 400 g of glycogen is stored in muscle. Unlike liver glycogen and blood glucose, glycogen in muscle can be utilized only during exercise and primarily within the muscle itself.

Even when taken together, these stored carbohydrates represent a quantitatively minor amount of fuel. The combined caloric value of liver glycogen (80–90 g), muscle glycogen (300–400 g), and circulating blood glucose (20 g) amounts to approximately 7500 kJ, well below the total daily caloric expenditure of a normal, moderately active 70-kg adult man.

By far the largest reservoir of body fuel is in the form of fat, stored as triglyceride. In a nonobese subject, body fat amounts to 20% of total body weight [31] and has a caloric value of 550,000 to 600,000 kJ, accounting for 80% of total body fuel storage. This amount of calories equals the basal caloric requirement for approximately 2 months. In obese subjects, fat tissue may be equivalent to over 2 million kJ. Regardless of the degree

of adiposity, fat clearly represents the most expendable as well as the most plentiful fuel available to humans.

Finally, the major reservoir of body protein is in muscle tissue, amounting to approximately 6 to 8 kg [31] (exclusive of tissue water), or 160,000 kJ. This potentially rich source of energy substrate is utilized only to a minor extent during fasting or exercise. The main role of protein is to maintain body structure and muscle function; mobilization of a significant fraction as amino acids would have deleterious effects.

MUSCLE GLUCOSE UPTAKE DURING EXERCISE

The transition from rest to exercise elicits an instantaneous and dramatic increase in muscle energy metabolism. The principal substrate for the initial rise in energy turnover is muscle glycogen. However within minutes following the onset of work, blood glucose becomes a quantitatively significant substrate for muscle oxidative metabolism.

Effect of Work Intensity

To study the effect of work intensity on muscle glucose uptake, healthy subjects were examined during bicycle exercise at varying intensities, ranging from 66 to 250 W [28]. The workload was increased in a stepwise fashion every 5 to 8 minutes and leg muscle glucose uptake was measured at each workload using a catheter technique. As can be seen in Figure 2, leg muscle glucose uptake increased with increasing workload over a wide range of work intensities in a curvilinear rather than a linear fashion.

In additional studies, leg muscle glucose uptake was examined during 40 minutes of exercise at three different workloads (65, 135, and 200 W), covering a range of relative workloads from approximately 25 to 75% of $\dot{V}o_2max$ [33]. In these studies, leg muscle

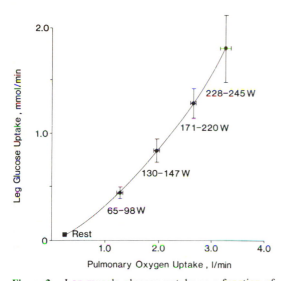

Figure 2. Leg muscle glucose uptake as a function of pulmonary oxygen uptake at rest and during exercise at different intensities. Data are expressed as mean ± standard error of the mean and have been calculated from Saltin, B., J. Wahren, and B. Pernow. Phosphagen and carbohydrate metabolism during exercise in trained middle-aged men. *Scand. J. Clin. Lab. Invest.* 33:71–77, 1974.

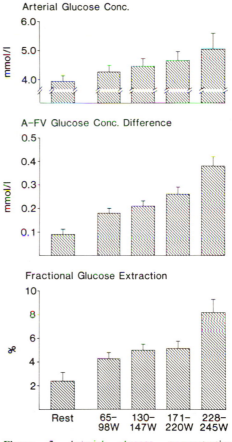

Figure 3. Arterial glucose concentration, arteriofemoral venous glucose concentration difference, and fractional extraction of glucose at rest and during leg exercise at varying intensities. Data are expressed as mean ± standard error of the mean. (Calculated from Saltin, B., J. Wahren, and B. Pernow. Phosphagen and carbohydrate metabolism during exercise in trained middle-aged men. *Scand. J. Clin. Lab. Invest.* 33:71–77, 1974.

glucose uptake rose sevenfold above the resting level at the lowest exercise intensity (65 W) and 10- and 20-fold at the higher workloads. Thus, also during exercise performed at different workloads on separate occasions, there was a curvilinear relation between workload and muscle glucose uptake.

The increased glucose uptake by contracting muscle is accompanied by a rise in muscle blood flow, the magnitude of the flow during exercise being a linear function of the workload [20]. The efficiency of muscle in extracting glucose during work—as reflected by the arteriovenous glucose difference and the fractional extraction of glucose (Figure 3)—also increases in relation to workload. However, the twofold to threefold rise in fractional glucose extraction is small compared with the 9- to 35-fold increase in glucose uptake. Thus, although muscle contraction is associated with increased efficiency in extracting glucose, the stimulation of glucose uptake in response to exercise is to a large extent dependent on an augmented availability of glucose via the rise in muscle blood flow.

Effect of Exercise Duration

The work-related increase in muscle glucose uptake that occurs in a matter of minutes after the onset of exercise continues during prolonged work and reaches a peak at 90 to 180 minutes with low-intensity exercise (30% of Vo_2max) and at 90 to 120 minutes with more strenuous work (60% of Vo_2max). When work continues beyond 2 to 3 hours, leg muscle glucose uptake falls, parallel to a gradual decrease in arterial glucose levels [2, 3].

The time course for muscle glucose uptake during prolonged exercise can be explained by a combination of changes in muscle glucose extraction and availability of glucose (Figure 4). Thus, the early exercise-induced stimulation of muscle glucose uptake occurs in the presence of small changes in arteriovenous glucose differences, since the augmented uptake is matched by an increased availability of glucose via enhanced muscle blood flow. This response is followed by a further, gradual increase in glucose uptake due to increased glucose extraction, while blood flow and glucose availability remain unchanged. The fall in muscle glucose uptake during the third and fourth hour of prolonged work reflects, not an altered efficiency of working muscle with respect to glucose uptake, but the decreased availability of glucose secondary to the falling blood glucose level.

The quantitative contribution of blood glucose to muscle oxidative metabolism can be estimated from simultaneous measurements of leg muscle oxygen and glucose uptake. Such data indicate that the proportion of oxidative metabolism that can be accounted for by uptake of glucose increases gradually with the duration of work, from 10% at 10 minutes to 25 to 30% at 40 minutes and to 35 to 40% at 90 to 120 minutes at workloads in the range of 30 to 70% of maximal oxygen uptake [33]. During exercise beyond 2 hours, the contribution of blood glucose gradually falls, to approximately 25 to 30% at 3 to 4 hours of work [3]. These data demonstrate that blood glucose is a quantitatively important source of energy for muscle oxidation.

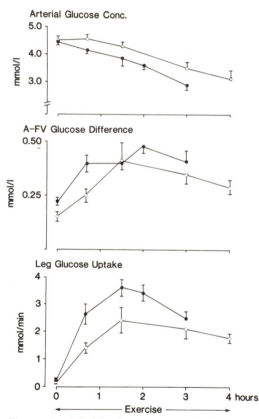

Figure 4. Arterial glucose concentration, arteriofemoral venous (A-FV) glucose difference, and estimated leg muscle glucose uptake at rest and during bicycle exercise performed at 30% of Vo_2max (open symbols and 60% of Vo_2max (filled symbols). Data are expressed as ± standard error of the mean. (Data from Ahlborg, G., P. Felig, L. Hagenfeldt, R. Hendler, and J. Wahren. Substrate turnover during prolonged exercise in man:Splanchnic and leg metabolism of glucose, free fatty acids and amino acids. *J. Clin. Invest.* 53:1080, 1974, and from Ahlborg, G., and P. Felig. Lactate and glucose exchange across the forearm, legs, and splanchnic bed during and after prolonged leg exercise. *J. Clin. Invest.* 69:45–54, 1982.

Regulation of Glucose Uptake by Exercising Muscle

Glucose utilization by muscle may be controlled at the level of glucose transport into the muscle cell or by intracellular mechanisms. Contraction alone has been shown to stimulate muscle glucose uptake in *in situ* preparations [24, 37] and it is likely, although not yet proven, that this holds true for the *in vivo* situation. Several mechanisms have been suggested to account for the stimulation of glucose uptake by contracting muscle, including a rise in intracellular calcium level, muscle hypoxia, and the energy status of the cell [19, 26, 36]. With regard to the latter possibility, studies of electrically stimulated rat hind limb show that glucose uptake is negatively related to the phosphocreatine content [27]. These results were substantiated recently by Katz and coworkers, who showed that leg muscle glucose uptake during exercise in humans over a range of work intensities (50–100% of Vo_2max) was inversely correlated with the phosphocreatine content [21]. The background to this relationship is not clear, but it is conceivable that changes in phosphocreatine levels influence the phosphorylation of certain membrane proteins associated with glucose transport.

Exercise is accompanied by a gradual fall in plasma insulin concentration. Simultaneously, muscle glucose uptake increases several-fold. It might then be supposed that insulin is not directly involved in the control of glucose uptake by working muscle. However, it should be remembered that the quantity of insulin delivered to the working muscle increases with the rise in blood flow that accompanies exercise. The insulin clamp technique has been used to study the combined effect of insulin and exercise on muscle glucose uptake. Measurements were undertaken in the resting state and during exercise, with either basal or elevated insulin levels. The results indicated that the combined effects were synergistic rather than just additive [8]. It was also found that increased insulin inflow (calculated as leg muscle insulin inflow)—whether due to increased concentration, a rise in blood flow, or a combination of the two—was significantly correlated to the increased rate of muscle glucose uptake (Figure 5). This observation suggests that the enhanced delivery of insulin to exercising muscle, resulting from the rise in blood flow, may be of importance in the stimulation of muscle glucose uptake. One may hypothesize that the increased amount of insulin delivered to the muscle in response to exercise is distributed

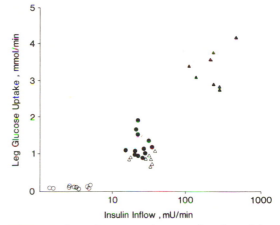

Figure 5. Leg glucose uptake as a function of log insulin inflow to the leg. Six subjects were studied at rest and during exercise alone. Four subjects were examined at rest before and during insulin infusion and during exercise and insulin infusion. Data represent individual values in the basal state at rest (n=10, ○), during insulin infusion at rest (n=8, △), during exercise alone (n=12, ●), and during exercise and insulin infusion (n=8, ▲). The two variables were significantly correlated (r−0.82, P<0.001). DeFronzo, R.A., E. Ferrannini, Y. Sato, P. Felig, and J. Wahren. Synergistic interaction between exercise and insulin on peripheral glucose uptake. *J. Clin. Invest.* 68:1468–1474, 1981.

and bound to previously unexposed insulin receptors through an opening up of previously nonperfused muscle capillaries.

With regard to intracellular mechanisms, the first step following glucose entry into the cell is phosphorylation of glucose by hexokinase. The activity of this enzyme is modulated through feedback inhibition by glucose-6-phosphate (Glu-6-P). A recent study by Katz and coworkers [21]showed that leg muscle glucose uptake during dynamic exercise at 95 to 100% of Vo_2max exceeded glucose utilization, as indicated by an accumulation of intracellular glucose. This was associated with an elevated Glu-6-P concentration. Their data therefore suggest that, during exercise at high workloads, phosphorylation of glucose rather than its transport across the cell membrane is rate limiting for glucose utilization, due to feedback inhibition of hexokinase by Glu-6-P. Other intracellular regulatory mechanisms may also influence the rate of glycolysis; for example, under conditions of increased fat oxidation, the rate of glycolysis may be reduced through interference with the phosphofructokinase and pyruvate dehydrogenase reactions [25].

HEPATIC GLUCOSE PRODUCTION DURING EXERCISE

The intensity and duration of exercise are the major determinants of both the magnitude of the rise in hepatic glucose production and the relative contributions of glycogenolysis and gluconeogenesis to this response. During exercise lasting 40 minutes, splanchnic (hepatic) glucose output increases gradually, to values twofold, threefold, and fivefold above basal when the exercise is mild (65 W), moderate (130 W), and heavy (200 W), respectively [33]. With regard to gluconeogenesis, peripheral (mainly muscle) production of precursors is increased, but this is offset by a reduction in splanchnic blood flow. As a result, the absolute rate of gluconeogenesis remains largely unchanged. The relative contribution of gluconeogenesis to glucose production falls as exercise becomes heavier. Thus, the contribution remains at the basal level (20–25%) during mild exercise but falls to 6 to 15% during moderate to heavy exercise [33]. It is thus clear that the major source of the increased glucose production during short-term exercise, especially at heavy workloads, is hepatic glycogenolysis. Since the rate of hepatic glycogen breakdown may increase fivefold above the basal level, as much as 35 to 40% of the hepatic glycogen stores are mobilized during 1 hour of strenuous exercise (assuming the hepatic glycogen content at the onset of exercise to be in the order of 75 to 90 g).

Since a significant proportion of the glycogen store is mobilized during relatively short-term exercise, it is evident that prolonged exercise (several hours) may eventually deplete the hepatic glycogen depots to the point where hepatic glycogenolysis does not suffice to keep the blood glucose level constant. This possibility was investigated, using exercise lasting 3 to 4 hours [3]. During 4 hours of exercise at 30% of $\dot{V}O_2$max, splanchnic glucose production was approximately twice the resting level. The arterial glucose concentration was unchanged during the first 90 minutes of exercise but then declined gradually, indicating that glucose production failed to keep pace with the accelerated glucose uptake in working muscle. Cumulative glucose production during 4 hours of work amounted to approximately 75 g. The estimated contribution from hepatic gluconeogenesis was approximately 20% at 40 minutes of exercise and then rose with continued exercise to 45% at 240 minutes (Figure 6). This response resulted from an augmented splanchnic uptake of gluconeogenic precursors, reflecting both

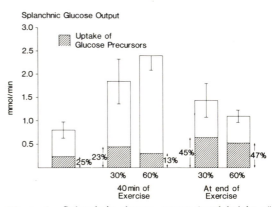

Figure 6. Splanchnic glucose output (total height of bar) and uptake of glucose precursors (calculated as glucose equivalents, crosshatched area of bar) at rest and during prolonged work performed at 30% and at 60% of $\dot{V}O_2$max. Percentage values indicate the maximal contribution of gluconeogenesis to glucose production. Uptake of glucose precursors represents the sum of lactate, pyruvate, glycerol, and amino acid uptake. In the case of the heavier exercise, amino acids were not measured and therefore not included in the calculations (mean values ± standard errors of the mean are indicated). (Data from Ahlborg, G., P. Felig, L. Hagenfeldt, R. Hendler, and J. Wahren. Substrate turnover during prolonged exercise in man: Splanchnic and leg metabolism of glucose, free fatty acids and amino acids. *J. Clin. Invest.* 53:1080. 1974, and from Ahlborg, G., and P. Felig. Lactate and glucose exchange across the forearm, legs, and splanchnic bed during and after prolonged lege exercise. *J. Clin. Invest.* 69:45–54, 1982.

increased fractional extraction and elevation in the arterial levels of these precursors. Of the 75 g of glucose produced during the 4 hours of work, approximately 15 to 20 g (or 25%) could be attributed to hepatic gluconeogenesis and the remaining 55 to 60 g (or 75%) to hepatic glycogenolysis [3].

During more intense exercise, the hepatic glycogen content declined more rapidly, as one would expect [2]. Thus, with work at 60% of $\dot{V}o_2$max the cumulative splanchnic glucose output reached 75 g at 3 hours, compared with 4 hours when exercise was performed at 30% of $\dot{V}o_2$max. As in the case of prolonged low-intensity work of long duration, splanchnic uptake of gluconeogenic precursors was increased at the end of exercise and accounted for approximately half of the glucose production, even excluding the uptake of amino acids (Figure 6).

These results indicate that a substantial proportion of the hepatic glycogen depot can be mobilized during prolonged exercise at intensities ranging from 30 to 60% of Vo_2max. Furthermore, as hepatic glycogen stores are gradually depleted during prolonged exercise, the rate of hepatic glycogenolysis diminishes. Simultaneously, hepatic gluconeogenesis is stimulated but does not fully compensate for the decrease in glycogen breakdown. As a result, splanchnic glucose production can no longer keep pace with peripheral glucose uptake and the plasma glucose concentration falls.

Regulation of Hepatic Glucose Production during Exercise

A number of hormonal changes are associated with exercise and serve to maintain an adequate supply of fuels for the exercising muscle. The plasma insulin concentration declines during exercise of any duration. The plasma glucagon level does not change during exercise of mild to moderate intensity, but it rises when exercise is heavy or prolonged and is accompanied by mild hypoglycemia [2, 3]. In addition, circulating levels of both epinephrine and norepinephrine, as well as growth hormone, rise during exercise. These hormonal changes, together with the stimulation of hepatic glucose production via direct nervous activation of hepatocytes, should be considered as possible regulatory factors in the control of hepatic glucose output during exercise.

To examine whether a fall in plasma insulin beyond the basal level is responsible for the exercise-induced stimulation of hepatic glucose production, the following investigation was performed. Healthy subjects were studied in the resting state before and during a low-rate glucose infusion (2 mg/min/kg) and during exercise with continued glucose administration [13]. The hepatic-vein catheter technique was employed. In the resting state, glucose infusion elevated the glucose level by 1 mmol/L and the peripheral insulin level rose two-fold. This degree of hyperinsulinemia was accompanied by an almost complete inhibition of splanchnic glucose output (Figure 7). During exercise with unchanged glucose infusion, glucose production rose by degrees (Figure 7), with some lag but with much the same magnitude compared with controls. Plasma insulin was maintained at or above basal levels, and plasma glucagon levels did not change. These data suggest that a normal exercise-induced rise in glucose production may occur even when insulin does not fall below the basal level. It should be noted that the insulin concentration fell gradually during exercise also in the glucose-infused subjects. It is conceivable that this fall played a permissive role in the stimulation of hepatic glucose output (perhaps by allowing other counter-regulatory hormones to augment hepatic glucose production).

Additional studies were undertaken to examine the role of basal glucagon levels in the regulation of glucose production during exercise. Somatostatin was infused to produce hypoglucagonemia, whereupon brief exercise of moderate intensity was performed. The hypoglucagonemia was induced either 10 minutes or 60 to 120 minutes before the

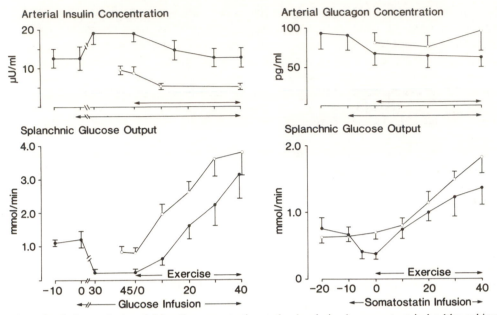

Figure 7. Left panel: Arterial insulin concentration and splanchnic glucose output in healthy subjects before and after intravenous glucose infusion (2 mg/kg/min) during leg exercise (filled symbols). Results from control studies when exercise was performed without glucose infusion are also shown (open symbols). Right panel: Arterial glucagon concentration and splanchnic glucose output in healthy subjects before and after intravenous somatostatin infusion (9 μg/min) during leg exercise (filled symbols). Results from control studies without somatostatin infusion are indicated by the open symbols (mean values ± standard errors of the mean are given). (Data from Felig, P., and J. Wahren. Role of insulin and glucagon in the regulation of hepatic glucose production during exercise. *Diabetes* 28:71–75, 1979 and from Björkman, O., P. Felig, L. Hagenfeldt, and J. Wahren. Influence of hypoglucagonemia on splanchnic glucose output during leg exercise in man. *Clin. Physiol.* 1:43–57, 1981.

start of work. In both circumstances, the exercise-induced rise in glucose production was similar to that in controls, despite significantly reduced plasma glucagon levels [7] (Figure 7). The absolute rate of splanchnic glucose production was lower, because glucose output had already been suppressed at rest. Moreover, with somatostatin infusion and insulin replacement during exercise, the rise in splanchnic glucose production was also normal [7]. These studies indicate that basal glucagon levels are not essential for the exercise-induced rise in hepatic glycogenolysis. Whether the contribution of gluconeogenesis during exercise—the main source of glucose production during exercise after prolonged fasting [6] as well as in the later stages of prolonged (3–4 hours) exercise [2, 3] is dependent on the presence of basal or

elevated glucagon levels remains to be determined.

Both glucose infusion and hypoglucagonemia limited the absolute rate of glucose production during exercise by an amount equal only to that by which production was suppressed prior to exercise. Thus, although a normal, exercise-induced increment in glucose production occurs even when the plasma concentration is unchanged and the basal glucagon level declines, the total rate of glucose production during work seems to be dependent on the prevailing plasma insulin and glucagon concentrations, as well as the rate of glucose production at the start of exercise. Since small changes in insulin [12] and acute alterations in glucagon [14, 32] influence hepatic glucose production at rest, it is conceivable that insulin and glucagon play a modulatory role in the regulation of glucose production during exercise. These hormones may be involved in regulating that proportion of glucose production during exercise that is needed to provide the brain and nonexercising tissues with glucose, while the rise in glucose production above the resting level occurs independently of insulin and glucagon to match the energy requirements of the contracting muscle.

In contrast to the results obtained in humans, studies in dogs indicate that glucagon plays an important role in the regulation of hepatic glucose output during exercise [38]. When dogs exercise after somatostatin-induced hypoglucagonemia, the normal increase in hepatic glucose production does not occur. Species differences are likely to account for most of the apparent controversy. Thus, in the normal dog, the plasma glucagon concentration increases parallel to the exercise-induced rise in hepatic glucose production. The potent stimulatory effect of exercise on glucagon secretion in dogs is further emphasized by the observation that somatostatin infusion during exercise does not completely suppress glucagon levels. In humans, on the other hand, the plasma glucagon level does not increase during exercise unless the work is either very strenuous or lasts at least 90 minutes [2, 3], and the rise is effectively suppressed by somatostatin infusion at a quarter of the rate used in the dog studies [7]. Moreover, due to these differences in glucagon response, a significant correlation is found between the glucagon/insulin molar ratio and the increment in hepatic glucose production during work in dogs [38]. This does not hold in humans, as shown by the rise in glucose production in the face of unchanged glucagon levels and a very slow decline in insulin. Further work in this area is needed because neither the studies in humans nor those in dogs have succeeded in defining the role of glucagon in the regulation of hepatic glucose production during work.

Studies designed to examine the role of circulating catecholamines have shown that neither beta-adrenergic nor alpha-adrenergic blockade interferes with the exercise-induced rise in glucose production in normal humans [30]. However, these studies involved exercise performed in the overnight fasted state without elicitation of hypoglycemia. Under experimental conditions in which exercise is associated with an exaggerated catecholamine response, such as during prolonged fasting [6] and prolonged exercise accompanied by hypoglycemia [2, 3], the elevated catecholamine levels may play an important role in glucose production.

Although one should not exclude the possibility that hormones (including growth hormone and cortisol) other than insulin, glucagon, and catecholamines may be involved in the control of hepatic glucose production during exercise, it is unlikely that they play a major stimulatory role in this respect. In fact, since changes in circulating hormone levels (insulin, glucagon, and catecholamines included) fail to explain the exercise-induced rise in glucose production, it has been suggested that this rise is caused by direct stimulation of hepatocytes via nervous activation. Support for this view has been provided by animal studies in which electrical stimulation of the splanchnic nerves stimulated glycogen phosphorylase activity [15, 29], leading to glycogen depletion and hyperglycemia [9]. There is evidence to suggest that human liver cells have abundant sympathetic innervation and that electrical stimulation of the splanchnic nerves in humans does result in increased glucose production [23]. The possible importance of this phenomenon for the exercise-induced rise in hepatic glucose production remains to be determined.

GLUCOSE METABOLISM DURING POSTEXERCISE RECOVERY PHASE

Cessation of physical exercise elicits a marked redistribution of the cardiac output. Blood flow to the previously exercising limbs decreases, while the perfusion of the splanchnic area rises to the basal level. The transition from exercise to the resting state is characterized by the initiation of resynthesis of the glycogen stores in muscle and by stimulation of hepatic gluconeogenesis. The hormonal regulation of these responses is dependent on the duration of the preceding exercise. Recovery after short-term and prolonged exercise will be described in the following.

Recovery After Short-Term Exercise

Following the interruption of short-term exercise (40 minutes or less), glucose uptake by muscle falls rapidly but remains threefold to fourfold above the resting level for at least 40 minutes [35]. In the absence of increased lactate or alanine release, and since free fatty acid concentrations are elevated, presumably resulting in increased FFA uptake and oxidation, these findings support ongoing resynthesis of muscle glycogen.

Splanchnic glucose output falls gradually after the end of exercise, reaching basal levels within 40 minutes (Figure 8). This decrease comes entirely from inhibition of hepatic glycogenolysis, since there is augmented splanchnic uptake of gluconeogenic precursors, particularly lactate, pyruvate, and glycerol. During the recovery phase, splanchnic uptake of these precursors exceeds the rates observed during exercise and is twofold to fourfold greater than in the basal state. This rise in precursor utilization is the combined result of increased splanchnic blood flow, elevated arterial levels, and increased fractional extraction. The net effect is a doubling of the proportion of glucose output attributable to hepatic gluconeogenesis compared with the basal state [35]. In addition, during the early recovery phase, arterial FFA levels reach a peak of approximately twice the exercise value, thereby increasing the availability of FFA to the liver and presumably facilitating gluconeogenesis.

During recovery after short-term exercise, there is significant lactate uptake by muscle

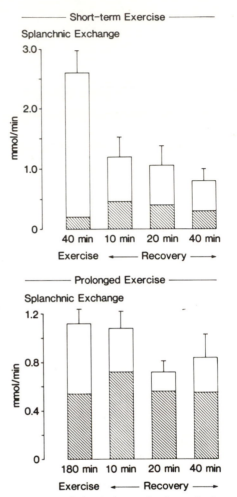

Figure 8. Splanchnic production of glucose (total height of bar) and uptake of glucogenic precursors (hatched area) at the end of exercise and during recovery from short-term (upper panel) and prolonged (lower panel) exercise. (Data from Ahlborg, G., and P. Felig. Lactate and glucose exchange across the forearm, legs, and splanchnic bed during and after prolonged leg exercise. *J. Clin. Invest.* 69:45–54, 1982, and from Wahren, J., P. Felig, R. Hendler, and G. Ahlborg. Glucose and amino acid metabolism during recovery after exercise. *J. Appl. Physiol.* 34:838–845, 1973.

in association with elevated lactate levels [35]. This uptake has been suggested to contribute to muscle glycogen synthesis [18]. The simultaneous uptake of lactate across the splanchnic area and by previously exercising muscle and only a gradual fall in lactate levels during the recovery period indicate ongoing net lactate production. The site and source for this production are unknown, but stimulation of glycogenolysis in previously resting muscle may be an important factor, as demonstrated following prolonged exercise (see below).

The hormonal changes during the recovery period are characterized by a rapid increase in insulin levels within the first 2 to 10 minutes of the recovery phase [35]. The elevated muscle glucose uptake during recovery after short-term exercise can therefore be attributed in part to the stimulatory effect of insulin. Of particular interest is the greater rise in insulin concentration in portal venous plasma compared with arterial plasma. In combination with the observed rise in splanchnic blood flow, these observations suggest increased hepatic insulin availability, possibly mediated via cessation of inhibitory adrenergic signals, as reflected by a return of norepinephrine concentrations to basal levels [16]. In view of the marked sensitivity of hepatic glycogenolysis to insulin, the rise in insulin level is the most likely determinant of the postexercise decline in hepatic glucose output to basal levels. In contrast, glucagon levels remain unchanged during the recovery period and may thereby contribute to the augmented hepatic uptake of gluconeogenic precursors. Metabolic and hormonal changes after short-term exercise are summarized in Figure 9.

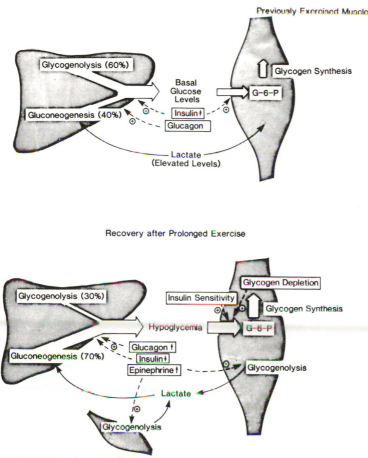

Figure 9. Schematic representation of the metabolic and hormonal changes during recovery after short-term (upper panel) and prolonged (lower panel) exercise.

Recovery After Prolonged Exercise

The fluxes of glucose and the levels of glucoregulatory hormones are quite different at the end of prolonged exercise (>2 hours). Short-term exercise reduces hepatic and muscular glycogen stores only to a limited extent and the glucose concentration stays at the basal level. In contrast, after 2 to 3 hours of exercise, the glycogen depots of both these tissues are substantially depleted and hypoglycemia gradually ensues. Furthermore, circulating levels of glucagon and catecholamines undergo greater elevations, and insulin concentrations fall more markedly, during prolonged compared with short-term exercise.

As observed during recovery after short-term work, glucose uptake by previously working muscle declines rapidly but remains three to five times greater than before exercise [2, 4]. However, in contrast to the situation in recovery from short-term work, this stimulation of glucose uptake cannot be attributed to insulin, since the insulin levels remain suppressed. These findings suggest that after prolonged exercise there is an increase in tissue insulin sensitivity in the exercised muscle. Splanchnic glucose output falls following cessation of exercise due to a decrease in hepatic glycogenolysis. Hepatic gluconeogenesis remains at its elevated level. As a result, the proportion of glucose production accounted for by uptake of gluconeogenic precursors increases from 50% to 65 to 80% during the recovery period (Figure 8).

A persistent suppression of the insulin level is accompanied by a continuation of the greater elevations in glucagon and catecholamines [2], suggesting that the hormonal responses after prolonged work play a role in the maintenance of glucose availability for the brain by stimulating hepatic gluconeogenesis (the only source of glucose production under these conditions). The augmented catecholamine levels during and after prolonged work have been suggested to stimulate glycogen breakdown [1], resulting in lactate production from resting muscle both during and after exercise. On the basis of these observations it has been suggested that repletion of the glycogen stores in previously exercising muscle may occur by release of lactate from previously resting muscle and subsequent transformation to glucose in the liver for muscle glucose uptake [2, 4] (Figure 9).

As indicated in Figure 9, prolonged exercise is followed by significant release of lactate also from the muscle that was previously active. It is possible that this lactate release reflects epinephrine-stimulated glycogen breakdown in muscle fibers with intact or only partially depleted glycogen stores (presumably fast-twitch fibers). This explanation would therefore be compatible with the hypothesis that glycogen breakdown and repletion may occur simultaneously in the same muscle, and it also raises the possibility of a redistribution of glycogen from nondepleted to depleted fibers within the muscle.

GLUCOSE METABOLISM DURING EXERCISE AND FASTING

When fasting continues beyond the postabsorptive state (12 to 14 hours after a meal), a number of adaptive hormonal and metabolic alterations occur. The insulin level falls gradually, while the glucagon concentration increases. These changes in pancreatic hormones are accompanied by stimulation of lipolysis as well as of hepatic gluconeogenesis and ketogenesis. The hepatic glycogen stores are gradually depleted, and after 2 to 3 days of food deprivation, the glycogen depots are almost totally exhausted [22]. As a result, hepatic glucose production is entirely dependent on hepatic gluconeogenesis, and the rate of glucose output is only 40% of that after an overnight fast [6]. The arterial glucose level is also reduced (-30%) compared with the overnight fasted situation [6].

Bicycle exercise following 60 hours of fasting is reported to elicit a gradual rise in splanchnic glucose production [6]. However, both the exercise-induced increase and the absolute rate of glucose production during exercise are markedly lower compared with exercise in the overnight fasted state (Figure 10). In contrast to the control situation, in which augmented hepatic glycogenolysis accounted for the major proportion of the exercise-induced rise in glucose production, in the 60-hour fasted state the rise was entirely covered by increased uptake of gluconeogenic precursors. The available evidence thus indicates that the adaptation to prolonged (2–3 days) starvation includes exercise-induced stimulation of hepatic gluconeogenesis, which partly compensates for the inability to mobilize hepatic glycogen.

Despite the diminished splanchnic glucose production in th 60-hour fasted state, the arterial glucose concentration rises significantly during exercise [6]. This observation is compatible with a decreased peripheral glucose uptake during exercise in the fasted state. Since brain glucose uptake does not decline appreciably within 2 to 3 days of fasting [5], reduced peripheral glucose utilization primarily reflects lowered muscle glucose uptake, as indicated by direct measurements of glucose uptake by contracting muscle in obese humans undergoing therapeutic starvation for 3 to 4 weeks [17]. In these studies, forearm glucose uptake was approximately 50% lower than in postabsorptive normal controls, both at rest and during 30 minutes of exercise.

Inasmuch as glucose utilization by working muscle was lower during prolonged fasting, alternative fuels must have been utilized. Direct evaluation of FFA uptake by contracting forearm muscle has indicated greater uptake following prolonged starvation (2 weeks) than after an overnight fast [17]. In view of the doubling of FFA levels already after 60 hours of fasting, it is likely that a shift toward increased utilization of FFA occurs within 2 to 3 days of fasting. Other alternative substrates for energy production under these conditions include ketone bodies, muscle glycogen, and muscle triglycerides, but the relative importance of these fuels remains to be examined.

Interestingly, exercise in the 60-hour fasted state is accompanied by increased levels of lactate and pyruvate, indicating increased peripheral production of these substrates [6]. This response probably reflects stimulation of anaerobic glycolysis in muscle due to increased epinephrine levels and to inhibition of pyruvate oxidation, which is known to occur under circumstances of accelerated fat oxidation [25]. Moreover, in view of the blunted muscle glucose uptake, it is possible that increased breakdown of muscle glycogen contributes to the augmented levels of pyruvate and lactate. This increased breakdown may have occurred in resting as well as in exercising muscle, as previously demonstrated during exercise in the overnight fasted state [2, 4].

Regardless of the site and source of the

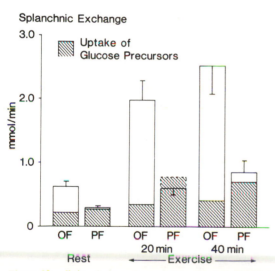

Figure 10. Splanchnic exchange of glucose (total height) of bars) and gluconeogenic precursors (hatched area) at rest and during exercise at a relative intensity of 55 to 60% of Vo_2max in overnight-fasted (OF) and prolonged (60-hour)-fasted (PF) healthy subjects. Data are calculated as glucose equivalents. Uptake of gluconeogenic precursors represents the sum of lactate, pyruvate, glycerol, and alanine uptake. Mean values ± standard errors of the mean are indicated. (Björkman, O., and L.S. Eriksson. Splanchnic glucose metabolism during leg exercise in 60-hour-fasted human subjects. *Am. J. Physiol.* 245 (*Endocrinol, Metab.* 8):E443–E448, 1983.

increased output of lactate and pyruvate, this response suggests that the terminal oxidation of glucose in muscle is minimized in the fasted state, resulting in an increased supply of precursors for hepatic gluconeogenesis. Thus, during exercise in the prolonged fasted state, muscle may be regarded as performing a dual role in the maintenance of glucose availability for the brain: both attenuated peripheral glucose uptake and accelerated delivery of substrates for hepatic gluconeogenesis.

ACKNOWLEDGMENTS

This work was supported in part by the Swedish Medical Research Council (3108). Dr. Björkman was a recipient of fellowships from the Swedish Medical Research Council and the Swedish Academy of Science.

REFERENCES

1. Ahlborg, G. Mechanism for glycogenolysis in nonexercising human muscle during and after exercise. *Am. J. Physiol.* 248:E540–E545, 1985.
2. Ahlborg, G., and P. Felig. Lactate and glucose exchange across the forearm, legs, and splanchnic bed during and after prolonged leg exercise. *J. Clin. Invest.* 69:45–54, 1982.
3. Ahlborg, G., P. Felig, L. Hagenfeldt, R. Hendler, and J. Wahren. Sustrate turnover during prolonged exercise in man: Splanchnic and leg metabolism of glucose, free fatty acids and amino acids. *J. Clin. Invest.* 53:1080, 1974.
4. Ahlborg, G., P. Felig, and J. Wahren. Splanchnic and peripheral glucose and lactate metabolism during and after prolonged arm exercise. *J. Clin. Invest.* 77:690–699, 1986.
5. Björkman, O., G. Ahlborg, J. Wahren, and P. Felig. Changing patterns of brain ketone, glucose and lactate metabolism within a 60 h fast in man. (Abstract). *Diabetologia* 23:156, 1982.
6. Björkman, O., and L.S. Eriksson. Splanchnic glucose metabolism during leg exercise in 60-hour-fasted human subjects. *Am. J. Physiol.* 245 (*Endorcrinol. Metab.* 8):E443–E448, 1983.
7. Björkman, O., P. Felig, L. Hagenfeldt, and J. Wahren. Influence of hypoglucagonemia on splanchnic glucose output during leg exercise in man. *Clin. Physiol.* 1:43–57, 1981.
8. DeFronzo, R. A., E. Ferrannini, Y. Sato, P. Felig, and J. Wahren. Synergistic interaction between exercise and insulin on peripheral glucose uptake. *J. Clin. Invest.* 68:1468–1474, 1981.
9. Edwards, A.V. The glycogenolytic response to stimulation of the splanchnic nerves in adrenalectomized calves, sheep, dogs, cats and pigs. *J. Physiol.* 213:741–759, 1971.
10. Felig, P., T. Pozefsky, E. Marliss, and G.F. Cahill Jr. Alanine: Key role in gluconeogenesis. *Science* 167:1003, 1970.
11. Felig, P., and J. Wahren. Amino acid metabolism in exercising man. *J. Clin. Invest.* 50:2703–2714, 1971.
12. Felig, P., and J. Wahren. Influence of endogenous insulin secretion on splanchnic glucose and amino acid metabolism in man. *J. Clin. Invest.* 50: 1702–1711, 1971.
13. Felig, P., and J. Wahren. Role of insulin and glucagon in the regulation of hepatic glucose production during exercise. *Diabetes* 28:71–75, 1979.
14. Felig, P., J. Wahren, and R. Hendler. Influence of physiological hyperglucagonemia on basal and insulin-inhibited splanchnic glucose output in normal man. *J. Clin. Invest.* 58:761–765, 1976.
15. Freude, K.A., L.S. Sandler, and F.J. Zieve. Electrical stimulation of the liver cell: Activation of glycogenolysis. *Am. J. Physiol.* 240 (*Endocrinol. Metab.* 3):E226–E232, 1981.
16. Hagberg, J.M., R.C. Hickson, J.A. McLane, A.A. Ehsani, and W.W. Winder. Disappearance of norepinephrine from circulation following strenuous exercise. *J. Appl. Physiol.* 47:1311–1314, 1979.
17. Hagenfeldt L., and J. Wahren. Human forearm muscle metabolism during exercise. VI. Substrate utilization in prolonged fasting. *Scand. J. Clin. Lab. Invest.* 27:299–306, 1971.
18. Hermansen, L., and O. Vaage. Lactate disappearance and glycogen synthesis in human muscle after maximal exercise. *Am. J. Physiol.* 233 (*Endocrinol. Metab.* 5):E422–E429, 1977.
19. Holloszy, J., and H.T. Narahara. Enhanced permeability to sugar associated with muscle contraction: Studies of the role of Ca^{2+}. *J. Gen. Physiol.* 50:551–562, 1967.
20. Jorfeldt, L., and J. Wahren. Leg blood flow during exercise in man. *Clin. Sci.* 41:459–473, 1971.
21. Katz, A., S. Broberg, K. Sahlin, and J. Wahren. Leg glucose uptake during maximal dynamic exercise in man. *Am. J. Physiol.* 251 (*Endocrinol. Metab.* 14): E65–E70, 1986.
22. Nilsson, L.H., and E. Hultman, Liver glycogen in man: The effect of total starvation or a carbohydrate-poor diet followed by carbohydrate refeeding. *Scand. J. Clin. Lab. Invest.* 32:325, 1973.
23. Nobin, A., B. Falc, S. Ingemansson, J. Jarhult, and E. Rosengren. The sympathetic innervation of the liver in man: Possible role in blood glucose regulation. *Eur. Surg. Res.* (*Suppl.* 1) 9:170, 1977.
24. Plough, T., H. Galbo, and E.A. Richter. Increased muscle glucose uptake during contractions: No need for insulin. *Am. J. Physiol.* 247 (*Endocrinol. Metab.* 10):E726–E731, 1984.
25. Randle, P.J., E.A. Newsholme, and P.B. Garland. Regulation of glucose uptake by muscle. *Biochem. J.* 93:652–665, 1964.

26. Randle, P.J., and G.H. Smith. Regulation of glucose uptake by skeletal muscle. 1. The effects of insulin, anaerobiosis and cell poisons on the uptake of glucose and release of potassium by isolated rat diaphragm. *Biochem. J.* 70:490–500, 1958.

27. Rennie, M.J., J.-P. Idström, G.E. Mann, T. Schersten, and A.-C. Bylund-Fellenius. A paired-tracer dilution method for characterizing membrane transport in the perfused rat hindlimb. *Biochem. J.* 214:737–743, 1983.

28. Saltin, B., J. Wahren, and B. Pernow. Phosphagen and carbohydrate metabolism during exercise in trained middle-aged men. *Scand. J. Clin. Lab. Invest.* 33:71–77, 1974.

29. Shimazu, T., and A. Amakawa. Regulation of glucogen metabolism in liver by the autonomic nervous system. VI. Possible mechanism of phosphorylase activation by the splanchnic nerve. *Biochem. Biophys. Acta* 385:242–256, 1975.

30. Simonson, D.C., V. Koivisto, R.S. Sherwin, E. Ferrannini, R. Hendler, A. Juhlin-Dannfeldt, and R.A. Defronzo. Adrenergic blockade alters glucose kinetics during exercise in insulin-dependent diabetics. *J. Clin. Invest.* 73:1648–1658, 1984

31. Snyder, W.S., et al. (eds.). *Report of the Task Group on Reference Man.* ICRP Publication No. 23. New York: Pergamon Press, 1975.

32. Wahren, J., S. Efendic, R. Luft, L. Hagenfeldt, O. Bjorkman, and P. Felig. Influence of somatostatin on splanchnic glucose metabolism in postabsorptive and 60-hours fasted humans. *J. Clin. Invest.* 59:299–307, 1977.

33. Wahren, J., P. Felig, G. Ahlborg, and L. Jorfeldt. Glucose metabolism during leg exercise in man. *J. Clin. Invest.* 50:2715, 1971.

34. Wahren, J., P. Felig, E. Cerasi, and R. Luft. Splanchnic and peripheral glucose and amino acid metabolism in diabetes mellitus. *J. Clin. Invest.* 51:1870–1878, 1972.

35. Wahren, J., P. Felig, R. Hendler, and G. Ahlborg. Glucose and amino acid metabolism during recovery after exercise. *J. Appl. Physiol.* 34:838–845, 1973.

36. Walker, P.M., J.P. Idström, T. Scherstén, and A.-C. Bylund-Fellenius. Glucose uptake in relation to metabolic state in perfused rat hindlimb at rest and during exercise. *Eur. J. Appl. Physiol.* 48:163–176, 1982.

37. Wallberg-Henriksson, H., and J.O. Holloszy. Contractile activity increases glucose uptake by muscle in severely diabetic rats. *J. Appl. Physiol.* 57:1045–1049, 1984.

38. Wasserman, D.H., H.L.A. Lickley, and M. Vranic. Interactions between glucagon and other counterregulatory hormones during normoglycemic and hypoglycemic exercise in dogs. *J. Clin. Invest.* 74:1404–1413, 1984.

Chapter 8

METABOLIC CONSEQUENCES OF ENDURANCE EXERCISE TRAINING

John O. Holloszy, M.D.

Endurance exercise training, such as prolonged, intense running or cycling, results in adaptations that make possible a remarkable increase in exercise capacity. This increase is manifested in the ability to perform more exercise in a given time interval and to perform strenuous exercise of a given intensity for a longer time. Underlying this training-induced increase in exercise capacity are a unique combination of adaptations in the skeletal muscles, the cardiovascular system, and the autonomic nervous system and in certain of the hormonal responses to exercise.

The cardiovascular adaptations include a volume overload type of cardiac hypertrophy, an increase in capillary density in the trained muscles, a larger blood volume, and an enhanced ability to lower peripheral resistance during strenuous exercise. These adaptations, by making possible a greater stroke volume and maximum cardiac output, play a major role in the increase in maximum oxygen uptake capacity ($\dot{V}O_2max$) that occurs in response to endurance exercise training. The adaptations in skeletal muscle involve an increase in the capacity for aerobic metabolism made possible by an adaptive increase in mitochondrial content as well as a number of other enzymatic adaptations that may contribute to the altered metabolic response to exercise in the trained state. In contrast to strength training, endurance training usually does not cause muscle hypertrophy or an increase in strength. The autonomic nervous system and neuroendocrine adaptations to endurance exercise training include increased vagal tone at rest and a blunted catecholamine response to submaximal exercise.

This chapter will deal with certain of the metabolic consequences of the adaptations to endurance training.

CARBOHYDRATE UTILIZATION

Studies in which serial biopsies of the quadriceps muscle were obtained on men performing prolonged, strenuous endurance exercise have provided evidence that depletion of muscle glycogen stores is associated with development of severe fatigue that forces either cessation of exercise or a decrease in exercise intensity [22]. There is also evidence that the length of time for which strenuous endurance exercise can be continued may be increased by raising muscle glycogen concentration, and vice versa [2]. It appears that, although oxidation of fatty acids can provide essentially all of the energy needed for light exercise, muscle glycogen is indispensable for the performance of prolonged, strenuous exercise.

It is still not clear why a supply of muscle glycogen is indispensable for strenuous exercise (requiring approximately 60% or more of $\dot{V}O_2max$) but not for light exercise. One possibility is that substrate supply may become limiting when glycogen stores are depleted during heavy exercise. Perhaps the rates of free fatty acid and glucose uptake by muscle, together with the rate of intramuscular triglyceride hydrolysis, may be able to keep pace with the muscles' energy demands during light exercise but not during heavy exercise. This would make provision of pyruvate via glycogenolysis essential.

In this context, a finding of great importance relative to the mechanisms by which training increases endurance is that humans deplete their muscle glycogen stores less rapidly during the same exercise when they are trained than when they are untrained [48]. Studies on rats have given similar results, and have further shown that liver glycogen is depleted less rapidly in the trained state [17]. In rats at different levels of training, ranging from 10 to 120 minutes of running per day, there was an inverse relationship between the respiratory capacity of leg muscles and the total amount of glycogen utilized during the same exercise test [17]. The slower utilization of carbohydrate during exercise of the same absolute intensity in the trained state is compensated for by a proportional increase in fat oxidation. This is reflected in a lower respiratory exchange ratio (R-value) [48].

Endurance exercise training results in an increase in $\dot{V}O_2max$, making it possible for an individual to exercise at higher work rates in the trained than in the untrained state. Despite the fact that a higher work rate is required to attain the same relative rate of oxygen consumption (i.e., the same percentage of $\dot{V}O_2max$) in the trained state, the rate of glycogen depletion is the same or slower and the R-value is lower in the trained compared with the untrained state at the same relative work rate [22, 48]. It appears that the increase in energy requirement caused by the greater work rate needed to attain the

same relative $\dot{V}O_2$ following training is met entirely by a proportional augmentation of fat oxidation.

As discussed in detail in subsequent sections, the increased oxidation of fat in the trained state is likely a consequence of the increase in muscle mitochondria and may play a major role in bringing about the decreased utilization of carbohydrate during exercise of the same absolute intensity. In addition, biochemical consequences of the adaptations to endurance training, in particular the increase in mitochondria, could result in a smaller activation of phosphofructokinase, and therefore reduce the rate of glycolysis, at the same exercise intensity in the trained state. However, the biochemical mechanisms responsible for the slower depletion of muscle glycogen at the same exercise intensity in the trained compared with the untrained state are still poorly understood, largely because of lack of information regarding how glycogenolysis is controlled in contracting muscle.

In view of the vast amount of information available regarding the properties of the enzymes involved in regulating glycogenolysis, one would expect the regulation of glycogen breakdown in contracting muscles to be well understood. This once appeared to be the case. It is generally accepted that when muscle is stimulated to contract, the Ca^{2+} released from the sarcoplasmic reticulum increases the activity of phosphorylase kinase *b* sufficiently to convert phosphorylase *b* to the active *a* form, resulting in glycogenolysis [16]. It was assumed that the rate of glycogen degradation is determined by the frequency of muscle contraction, with the Ca^{2+} released in response to each excitation causing activation of phosphorylase and a burst of glycogenolysis. However, this interpretation has proven to be incorrect.

Recent studies have shown that phosphorylase activation by the Ca^{2+} mechanism reverses and glycogenolysis stops within the first few minutes of prolonged stimulation of muscle contraction [5, 8, 43, 46]. This reversal occurs even under stimulation conditions that result in little or no fatigue [8, 43]. There is evidence that these findings on muscles stimulated to contract *in situ* have relevance to normal exercise. In a study on rats running at a constant, moderate speed to which they were accustomed, it was found that after a brief initial period of glycogenolysis, muscle glycogen stabilized at 50 to 60% of the initial concentration and did not decline further during a 2-hour run. In a recent study, rats that performed 40 minutes of intermittent strenuous running to deplete muscle glycogen were able to partially replete their leg muscle glycogen stores while continuing to run for an additional 90 minutes at a moderate pace (22m/min up a 15% incline), when they were given glucose feedings by stomach tube at 30-minute intervals during the 90-minute run [10].

It appears from these and related findings [cf. 10] that when exercise is performed in the fed state at a constant rate and at a moderate intensity at which plasma catecholamine levels are minimally elevated, glycogenolysis shuts off after a brief period and other substrates provide the muscles' energy needs. On the other hand, it is well documented that strenuous exercise to the point of exhaustion can result in almost complete depletion of muscle glycogen [2, 22, 48]. If, as available evidence indicates, the Ca^{2+}-mediated activation of phosphorylase is transient [5, 8, 10, 43, 46] and the *b* form of phosphorylase is not physiologically active [16], how is the progressive depletion of muscle glycogen during exhausting exercise brought about?

One possibility is that the other mechanism for phosphorylase kinase activation, a catecholamine-mediated increase in cyclic adenosine monophosphate (cAMP), may be responsible for stimulating glycogenolysis during strenuous, prolonged exercise [cf 46]. Epinephrine adminstration has been shown to reactivate phosphorylase and glycogenolysis by its β-adrenergic activity in rat fast-twitch and slow-twitch muscles after deactivation has occurred during prolonged stimulation of contraction [43]. The plasma cat-

echolamine response to the same absolute exercise intensity is markedly blunted by endurance exercise training [51]. In this context, it seems reasonable that reduced β-adrenergic stimulation of glycogenolysis may contribute to the slower depletion of glycogen during exercise of the same intensity in the trained compared with the untrained state.

However, other factors are also involved in bringing about slower glycogen utilization in the trained state. One is the increased reliance on oxidation of fat as a source of energy during submaximal exercise. As reviewed in the next section, increased oxidation of fatty acids has a powerful carbohydrate-sparing effect during exercise, resulting in slower depletion of glycogen in both muscle and liver [24, 45]. The mechanisms responsible for the glycogen-sparing effect of fat oxidation remain to be elucidated—this phenomenon can not be explained on the basis of current knowledge regarding the factors that regulate glycogenolysis in contracting muscle.

FAT OXIDATION

One of the most important alterations in the metabolic response to submaximal exercise induced by endurance exercise training is increased reliance on fat oxidation as a source of energy. Since the increase in muscle mitochondria induced by endurance training results in comparable increases in the capacities to oxidize fat and carbohydrate [28], it seems reasonable to ask why trained individuals oxidize proportionately more fat and less carbohydrate than do untrained persons. This phenomenon appears to be explained, at least in part, by the functioning of the "glucose-fatty acid cycle" first described by Randle and coworkers [42] in heart muscle. These investigators showed that glucose uptake, glycolysis, glycogenolysis, and pyruvate oxidation are inhibited in the heart by oxidation of fatty acids. This inhibition is mediated, at least partly, by the accumulation of citrate, which inhibits phosphofructokinase activity and results in accumulation of glucose-6-phosphate (Glu-6-P), which inhibits hexokinase. However, a number of studies on skeletal muscle failed to show an inhibitory effect of fatty acids on glucose metabolism, leading some investigators to conclude that the glucose-fatty acid cycle is limited to heart muscle and does not function in skeletal muscle [cf. 45].

However, this conclusion did not seem consistent with the observation that the progressive rise in plasma free fatty acid (FFA) concentration during prolonged exercise is associated with a decrease in R-value, indicating a change in the carbon source for oxidative metabolism from carbohydrate to fat. The decrease in R-value is evident long before glycogen stores are depleted. This observation, which suggests that the increase in plasma FFA concentration during exercise results in increased oxidation of fatty acids with inhibition of carbohydrate utilization, led to a reevaluation of whether glucose-fatty acid cycle activity is present in skeletal muscle.

One experimental approach was to elevate plasma FFA by feeding a fat meal followed 3 hours later by injection of heparin. It was found that such elevation slows the rate of glycogen depletion in muscle during standardized bouts of treadmill running in both humans [11] and rats [24, 45]. Studies on rats further showed that elevation of plasma FFA concentration slows liver glycogen depletion during exercise [24, 45] and markedly increases endurance as reflected in run time to exhaustion [24]. The increase in endurance appears to be a consequence of the sparing effect of increased FFA utilization on muscle and liver glycogen [24].

The finding that elevation of plasma FFA concentration slows hepatic glycogen depletion during exercise suggests a slowing of glucose uptake by muscle. This effect was confirmed in studies utilizing a well-oxygenated perfused rat hindquarter preparation. Glucose uptake and lactate production by well-oxygenated rat hind limb muscles

were inhibited approximately 30%, both at rest and during muscle contraction, when a high concentration of a fatty acid was included in the perfusion medium [44]. Inclusion of oleate in the perfusion medium also significantly protected against glycogen depletion in the fast-twitch and slow-twitch red types of muscle during contractile activity induced by sciatic nerve stimulation [44]. The concentrations of citrate and Glu-6-P were both increased in red muscle perfused with oleate.

It is clear from the results of these and similar studies that, as in the heart, oxidation of FFA inhibits glucose uptake and glycolysis and has a glycogen-sparing effect in skeletal muscle. In view of this evidence for glucose-fatty acid cycle activity in skeletal muscle, it seems probable that the greater oxidation of fatty acids in the trained compared with the untrained state plays a major role in bringing about the concomitant decrease in the rate of carbohydrate utilization. As described above, one mechanism for increasing the rate of fat oxidation is elevation of the concentration of FFA to which the muscles are exposed; in the physiological range, there appears to be a linear relationship between plasma FFA concentration and the rate of removal and oxidation of plasma FFA [18]. However, carefully controlled studies on the same subjects before and after they have adapted to an intense endurance exercise training program have shown that plasma FFA concentration is usually lower in the trained than in the untrained state during prolonged submaximal exercise of the same moderate absolute intensity (e.g., 60% pretraining Vo_2max) [51].

The lower plasma FFA levels in the trained state could be due to either increased utilization or decreased production. Available evidence supports the interpretation that a slower rate of fatty acid release from adipose tissue is responsible. Blood glycerol concentration during prolonged exercise of the same intensity is also lower in the trained than in the untrained state [51]. This finding suggests that the rate of production of fatty acids is decreased, because changes in plasma glycerol level usually reflect changes in the rate of lipolysis in adipose tissue [23]. Preliminary results of ^{13}C-palmitate turnover studies during prolonged exercise of the same intensity before and after 12 weeks of endurance exercise training support this interpretation [13]. Endurance exercise training results in a marked blunting of the plasma catecholamine response to submaximal exercise [51]. This decrease in sympathoadrenal activity could account for a decreased stimulation of lipolysis in adipose tissue during exercise of the same intensity in the trained compared with the untrained state.

There is usually a linear relationship between plasma FFA concentration and the rate of plasma FFA oxidation [18]. The finding that plasma FFA concentration is lower during submaximal exercise in the trained than in the untrained state suggests that the rate of oxidation of plasma FFA may be reduced in the trained state; this interpretation is supported by the finding of a slower rate of ^{13}C-palmitate oxidation [13]. Despite this evidence for decreased plasma FFA utilization, intense endurance training results in a large increase in the amount of energy derived from fat (calculated from the R-value) [20, 51]. These findings raised a question regarding the source of the additional fatty acids utilized during exercise in the trained state.

Muscle triglyceride concentration can decrease sufficiently during prolonged exercise to provide a considerable portion of the FFA oxidized [4]. Therefore, in view of the lower plasma FFA levels in the trained state, it seemed possible that increased lipolysis of muscle triglycerides might provide the fatty acids that account for the increased oxidation of fat during exercise in the trained state. To evaluate this possibility, the effect of adaptation to endurance exercise training on muscle triglyceride depletion during prolonged exercise was examined in a recent study [34]. Previously sedentary indivduals performed 12 weeks of strenuous endurance exercise training. Before and after

training they performed a 2-hour-long exercise test at an intensity that required approximately 60% of $\dot{V}O_2$max before training. Prior to and at the end of the 2 hours of exercise, muscle bipsies were obtained for measurement of triglyceride concentration. The results of this study showed that depletion of muscle triglyceride stores during the same prolonged exercise test was about twice as great in the same individuals when they were trained compared with when they were untrained [34]. The depletion of muscle triglycerides was sufficiently great to account for the larger amount of fat oxidized (estimated from the R-value and $\dot{V}O_2$) in the trained state.

To summarize, it seems reasonably well established that the increased oxidation of fat in the trained state can, by means of the glucose-fatty acid cycle, play a major role in bringing about the slower utilization of carbohydrate during submaximal exercise, and preliminary studies suggest that the greater utilization of fat during prolonged submaximal exercise of the same intensity in the trained compared with the untrained state, is fueled by increased lipolysis of muscle triglycerides.

This leaves us with the question, what are the mechanisms responsible for the greater oxidation of fatty acids in the trained state? One possibility that seems to be clearly ruled out by the finding that training results in a lower plasma FFA concentration at the same absolute exercise intensity is a greater availability of exogenous fatty acids. It seems well documented that the rate of plasma FFA oxidation is a function of concentration [18]. However, the rate at which muscle oxidizes fatty acids is not directly determined by plasma FFA concentration, but by the concentration of fatty acids in the cytoplasm to which the mitochondria are exposed, as well as the concentration of mitochondria (i.e., the capacity to oxidize fatty acids) and, perhaps, also by availability of competing substrates [cf. 29, 39]. Plasma FFA concentration, of course, is only one of the factors determining cytoplasmic fatty acid concentration.

Endurance exercise training results in a

large increase in the capacity of muscle to oxidize fatty acids; this increase is mediated by training-induced increases in the enzymes of the pathway of fatty acid oxidation [39]. If the intracellular concentration of fatty acids during exercise is similar in the trained and untrained states, the adaptive increase in mitochondria, and thus in the enzymes responsible for fatty acid oxidation, may, by itself, be responsible for the greater oxidation of fat in the trained state [29, 39]. An additional possibility is that increased lipolysis of muscle triglycerides may result in a higher cytoplasmic fatty acid concentration in the trained state, which would contribute to the increase in the rate of fat oxidation. Evaluation of this possibility will be difficult, because determination of the fatty acid concentration to which the mitochondria are exposed in the cytoplasm involves major technical problems.

The increased utilization of fat as an energy source with the concomitant sparing of glycogen stores during exercise has obvious benefits for the trained individual. However, it is not clear at present whether increased utilization of muscle triglyceride, in preference to plasma FFAs, has any physiological advantages of just represents a compensatory mechanism made necessary by decreased β-adrenergic stimulation of lipolysis in adipose tissue.

LACTATE PRODUCTION

It is well documented that exercise of the same submaximal intensity results in a smaller increase in blood and skeletal muscle lactate concentrations in the trained than in the untrained state [cf. 28]. The increase in lactate concentration during submaximal exercise was once thought to be smaller in the trained state because of improved delivery of oxygen to the working muscles. The belief that the working muscles are better supplied with blood in the trained than in the untrained state during submaximal exercise of moderate intensity was based on the misconception that because lactate is the end prod-

uct of anaerobic glycolysis, lactate appearance must reflect oxygen deficiency. Actually, well oxygenated muscles can produce large amounts of lactate [9, 36].

The finding that well-oxygenated skeletal muscle produces lactate during contractile activity is not surprising. There are four possible pathways that pyruvate can take in contracting muscle: (a) oxidation via the citrate cycle in the mitochondria, (b) conversion to lactate by the reaction catalyzed by lactate dehydrogenase, (c) conversion to alanine by means of the glutamate pyruvate transaminase reaction, and (d) conversion to malate by means of the reaction catalyzed by malic enzyme. The nicotinamide adenine dinucleotide (NADH) formed in the cytoplasm during glycolysis can be oxidized either by the mitochondria or by lactate dehydrogenase. Since mitochondria are normally impermeable to NADH, the reducing equivalents from NADH must be transported into the mitochondria via either the malate–aspartate or the glycerol–phosphate shuttle systems. [38].

There is no known mechanism for protecting pyruvate and NADH from lactate dehydrogenase and channeling them exclusively into the mitochondria in skeletal muscle. Lactate formation will occur whenever NADH and pyruvate are available to skeletal muscle lactate dehydrogenase. The relative rates at which pyruvate and NADH are oxidized in the mitochondria or used to form lactate depends on the capacity of the mitochondria and the shuttle systems for NADH to compete with lactate dehydrogenase for the pyruvate and NADH formed during glycolysis.

In view of the high level of lactate dehydrogenase activity and the relatively low content of mitochondria, particularly in the fast-twitch skeletal muscle fibers, it seems clear that well-oxygenated skeletal muscle must produce lactate during times when there is a rapid rate of glycolysis. However, the possibility that muscle hypoxia may occur during strenuous exercise under some conditions has not been ruled out. Regardless of whether or not hypoxia occurs, available evidence indicates that the lower lactate production in the trained compared with the untrained state is not attributable to better oxygenation of the skeletal muscles.

Evidence against the belief that the working muscles are better supplied with oxygen during submaximal exercise in the trained state is provided by the finding that blood flow per gram of muscle is actually lower in trained than in untrained men at the same absolute work rate [cf. 7, 28]. This is due to less diversion of blood flow from the skin, liver, and other organs during submaximal exercise in the trained compared with the untrained state. The working muscles compensate for the lower blood flow in the trained state by extracting more oxygen, resulting in a larger arteriovenous oxygen difference [7]. Since O_2 tension must be less in the muscles than in venous blood, a lower concentration of oxygen in the venous blood leaving the muscles provides evidence that the concentration of oxygen in the working muscles is lower, not higher, in the trained state.

In an early study, it was found that blood lactate concentration at the same relative exercise intensity was unchanged after a training program that induced an 18% increase in $\dot{V}_{O_2}$max [47]. However, other studies have clearly shown that exercise of the same relative intensity results in a smaller increase in lactate concentration in both muscle [37] and blood [21, 33] in people restudied after a period of intense training that results in large increases in $\dot{V}_{O_2}$max. This effect of training is shown in Figure 1.

The difference between the results of these studies may relate to the use of different forms of exercise in the exercise testing (cycle ergometer) and training (jogging) in the early study [47]. Metabolic adaptations to training are specific to the muscles involved in the training, and adaptations induced by jogging are much more evident during jogging than during cycling, and vice versa. In the more recent study, in which the training was much more intense and involved both running and cycling, the response to submaximal exercise of the same

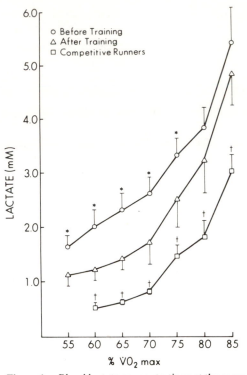

Figure 1. Blood lactate concentrations at the same relative exercise intensities between 55 and 85% of maximal oxygen uptake capacity ($\dot{V}_{O_2}$max) in eight initially sedentary men aged 29 ± 1 year who were studied before and after a strenuous 12-week-long endurance exercise training program. Included for comparison are the values obtained on eight competitive middle- and/or long-distance runner. (From Hurley, B.F., J.M. Hagberg, W.K. Allen, D.R. Seals, J.C. Young, R.W. Cuddihee, and J.O. Holloszy. Effect of training on blood lactate levels during submaximal exercise. *J. Appl. Physiol.* 56:1260-1264, 1984.)

relative intensity was evaluated during running [33].

A variety of approaches have been used in studies relating lactate concentration and exercise intensity to endurance performance. The lactate concentration and exercise intensity identified as correlating with endurance performance, which have variously been termed "lactate threshold," "onset of blood lactate accumulation," or "maximal steady state," have differed widely, even in studies using the same terminology [cf. 33]. Despite these differences, it seems clear from the results of these studies that there is a good correlation between the exercise intensity required to elicit a given lactate concentration in the 1.5 to 4 mM range and endurance performance.

It has been shown that a considerably higher relative work rate is required to attain a given lactate level in the trained than in the untrained state (Figure 1). For example, a lactate concentration of 2.5 mM occurred at 68% of $\dot{V}o_2$max before training, and at 75% of $\dot{V}o_2$max after 12 weeks of training. Eight highly trained competitive runners required an even higher relative exercise in intensity (83% of $\dot{V}o_2$max) to attain a blood lactate level of 2.5 mM. Similar differences are usually seen in endurance performance capacity, with highly trained individuals being able to exercise for 2 hours at 75 to 85% of $\dot{V}o_2$max in the activity in which they are trained whereas the majority of highly motivated, untrained people generally cannot exercise at more than 65% of $\dot{V}o_2$max for 2 hours.

Muscle biopsy studies have provided evidence that the lower blood lactate concentration during submaximal exercise in the trained state is secondary to a lower lactate concentration in the exercising muscles [37]. Furthermore, studies in which subjects trained only one leg have clearly shown that endurance exercise training results in decreased lactate production by the exercising muscles [20]. This was evidenced by a smaller lactate production by the trained than by the untrained leg during exercise with both legs. Another mechanism that could theoretically contribute to the smaller increase in blood lactate concentration during exercise in the trained state is increased rate of lactate removal. Whether training induces adaptations that result in increased lactate removal remains to be determined.

At the same absolute exercise intensity, and perhaps even at the same relative work rate, lower lactate production in the trained state could be due, in part, to increased oxidation of fat, with partial inhibition of glycolysis. However, other factors must also be involved. In the study of Hurley et al. [33], in which training increased the relative exercise intensity required to raise blood lactate to a given concentration, the R-value was similar at the exercise intensities that resulted in a blood lactate concentration of 2.5 mM before and after training. Therefore, as the result of the higher energy expenditure after training (41.0 ml·kg^{-1}·min^{-1} after compared with 29.4 ml·kg^{-1}·min^{-1} before), the calculated carbohydrate oxidation rate was 31% higher in the trained than in the untrained state during exercise that elicited a blood lactate concentration of 2.5 mM.

It thus appears that during exercise that resulted in the same blood lactate concentration, the rate of glycolysis was considerably higher after training. Therefore, for a similar rate of lactate production to occur in the untrained and trained states under these conditions, a small proportion of the pyruvate formed must be converted to lactate in the trained state. Two of the adaptations to endurance training that could result in channeling of a larger proportion of the pyruvate produced via glycolysis into the mitochondrial oxidative pathway and less into lactate formation are the increase in muscle mitochondrial content and the increase in the capacity of the malate–aspartate shuttle. These will be reviewed in the next section. Both of these adaptations increase the ability of the mitochondria to compete with lactate, dehydrogenase for pyruvate and NADH.

ADAPTATIONS IN MUSCLE

Types of Skeletal Muscle

The majority of the skeletal muscles in those mammalian species in which adaptations to endurance exercise training have been studied are a mixture of three types of muscle fiber. These are the slow-twitch red (or type I) fibers, the fast-twitch red (or type IIa) fibers, and the fast-twitch white (or type IIb) fibers. In rats, in which the adaptive response to exercise has been studied extensively, the slow-twitch red fibers have a moderately high respiratory capacity, low glycogenolytic and glycolytic capacities, and low myosin adenosine triphosphatase (ATPase) activity and are fatigue resistant; the fast-twitch red fibers have a high respiratory capacity, high glycogenolytic and glycolytic capacities, and high myosin ATPase activity, and the fast-twitch white fibers have a low respiratory capacity, high glycogenolytic and glycolytic capacities, and high myosin ATPase activity and fatigue rapidly [cf 28]. Detailed studies of the enzymatic adaptations of the different skeletal muscle fiber types in rats have provided insights regarding the plasticity of mitochondrial composition [cf. 28, 41]. However, although the mitochondrial enzyme adaptations in mixed muscles follow the same general pattern and have similar physiological consequences in rodents and humans, it is now evident that the specific information obtained from detailed studies of the different fiber types in rodents is not always applicable to human muscle.

In rats, the capacity to oxidize pyruvate and fatty acids, and the levels of the majority of mitochondrial enzymes, are roughly twice as high in the fast-twitch red fibers as in the slow-twitch red fibers, and four fold to eight-fold higher in fast-twitch red than in fast-twitch white fibers [cf. 28]. Exceptions are the mitochondrial enzymes involved in ketone oxidation, which are highest in the slow-twitch red fibers [50], and mitochondrial α-glycerophosphate dehydrogenase, which is highest in the fast-twitch white muscle fibers in the rat [52].

In contrast to the rat, in humans it is the slow-twitch red fibers that have the highest content of mitochondria. In untrained individuals, mitochondrial enzyme levels are approximately twice as high in slow-twitch fibers as in fast-twitch fibers [cf. 29]. Furthermore, the difference in mitochondrial content between fast-twitch red fibers and fast-twitch white fibers is very much smaller in humans than in rats. Although it is usually convenient to classify the muscle fibers into three, or in the case of humans

sometimes two, types, it should be realized that there is a wide spectrum of enzyme activities in fibers classified as belonging to the same type in muscles of the same individual.

In rats, strenuous endurance training, such as running at 31 m/min up to a 15% grade, does not result in a general conversion of fast-twitch white into fast-twitch red fibers; the large differences (fourfold to eightfold) in mitochondrial enzyme activities between the superficial (white) and deep (red) portions of the gastrocnemius and quadriceps muscles are still present in the trained state [1, 14, 19, 50].

In contrast, in men who have adapted to strenuous endurance training, it is often impossible to detect fast-twitch white fibers. It appears that there may be an essentially complete conversion of fast-twitch white to fast-twitch red fibers in response to endurance training in humans [6, 35]. Furthermore, mitochondrial enzyme levels tend to increase to a greater extent in the fast-twitch fibers than in the slow-twitch red fibers in response to very strenuous endurance training, so that the difference in mitochondrial content between slow- and fast-twitch fibers is largely or even completely eliminated in highly trained people.

Cross-innervation studies and studies involving chronic electrical stimulation have shown that in rodents, the fast-twitch fibers have the potential for essentially complete conversion to slow-twitch fibers [cf. 41]. It was once thought that normal exercise does not result in conversion of fast-twitch to slow-twitch fibers. However, it has recently been reported that very prolonged daily running (210 minutes at 27 m/min up to a 15% grade) can result in conversion of some fast-twitch red fibers to slow-twitch red fibers in rat skeletal muscle [41]. This increase was evidenced by an increase in the proportion of fibers with the staining characteristics of slow-twitch red fibers in the deep (i.e., red) portion of the vastus lateralis, and a change in myosin light-chain pattern, with a decrease in fast-type and increase in slow-type myosin light chains.

The majority of elite long-distance runners have a high proportion of slow-twitch red fibers in the muscles of their legs. At present it is not known whether this is due to an increase in the proportion of slow-twitch red fibers induced by long-distance running or to a selection process in which individuals with a high proportion of slow-twitch red fibers find that they have a natural ability for long-distance running.

Muscle Mitochondria

Since oxygen delivery to, and utilization by, skeletal muscle during submaximal exercise of the same absolute intensity is not increased by endurance training, it seemed possible that other adaptations within the muscles themselves might play a major role in bringing about the lower lactate levels, the slower rate of glycogen depletion, the lower R-value, and the greater endurance seen in the trained state [cf. 26]. One line of evidence that stimulated investigation of this possibility came from comparative studies of muscles of sedentary and active animals, such as the laboratory rabbit and the wild rabbit. In these studies it was found that muscles of active wild animals have a higher capacity for aerobic metabolism than do the same muscles of their sedentary domestic counterparts [cf. 25].

In this context, a series of studies was conducted to evaluate the possibility that endurance exercise training can induce an increase in the capacity of skeletal muscle for aerobic metabolism. Young rats were trained by means of a program of treadmill running in which the speed and duration of running were progressively increased until after 3 months the rats were running for 120 min/day, 5 days/week, up a 15% grade at 31 m/min, with short intervals of more rapid running interspersed at 10-minute intervals during the exercise session. This program resulted in a major training effect as evidenced by a large increase in endurance [25].

The capacity of whole homogenates and of the mitochondrial fraction of leg muscles to oxidize pyruvate [25] and fatty acids [1, 39] roughly doubles in rats that have adapted to the 2-hour/day running program. The capacity of muscle to oxidize ketones is also increased [50]. Mitochondria from muscles of the trained animals exhibit a high level of respiratory control and tightly coupled oxidative phosphorylation, providing evidence that the increase in mitochondrial electron transport capacity is associated with a rise in the capacity to generate ATP via oxidative phosphorylation [25, 39].

Underlying these increases in the respiratory capacity of skeletal muscle are increases in the levels of the enzymes of the citric acid cycle [31]; the components of the respiratory chain involved in the oxidation of NADH and succinate [25, 31] the mitochondrial coupling factor 1 [40]; the enzymes responsible for the activation, transport, and β-oxidation of long-chain fatty acids [1, 39]; and the enzymes involved in ketone oxidation [50].

The concentrations of the cytochromes and of total mitochondrial protein are increased in leg muscles of exercise-trained rats, providing evidence that the increase in mitochondrial enzymes is due to an increase in enzyme protein. Electron microscopic studies have provided evidence that increases in both the size and number of mitochondria are responsible for this increase in the mitochondrial content of skeletal muscle [cf. 29]. However, this adaptation to endurance exercise involves not just an increase in mitochondria but also an alteration in mitochondrial composition. Some mitochondrial enzymes increase twofold or more, others increase 30 to 60%, some do not increase at all when activity is expressed per gram of muscle, and some, because of the increase in mitochondrial protein, are decreased when expressed per milligram of mitochondrial protein.

The enzymes that do not increase include mitochondrial creatine kinase, adenylate kinase [40], and mitochondrial α-glycerophosphate dehydrogenase [31]. The finding that mitochondrial α-glycerophosphate dehydrogenase activity does not increase with training contrasts with the effect of thyrotoicosis. Thyrotoxicosis, which also induces an increase in muscle mitochondria, results in large increases in mitochondrial α-glycerophosphate dehydrogenase activity in red types of muscle [52]. The alterations in skeletal muscle mitochondria induced by endurance exercise make skeletal muscle mitochondria more like heart mitochondria in their enzyme pattern [26].

Mitochondria are normally impermeable to NADH. The pathways for transferring the reducing equivalents from cytoplasmic NADH formed during glycolysis into the mitochondria in skeletal muscle are the α-glycerophosphate and the malate–asparate shuttles [38]. In contrast to the capacity of the α-glycerophosphate shuttle, which does not increase [30], large increases occur in the levels of the enzymes of the malate–asparate shuttle in both the mitochondria and cytoplasm in skeletal muscle in response to endurance exercise training [27]. This increase in the capacity to transfer reducing equivalents into the mitochondria could play a role in bringing about the slower rate of lactate production during submaximal exercise in the trained compared with the untrained state by increasing the ability of the mitochondria to compete with lactate dehydrogenase for the NADH and pyruvate formed by glycolysis.

Studies of the turnover of cytochrome c and other mitochondrial enzymes have provided evidence that an exercise-induced increase in the rate of synthesis of mitochondrial proteins, rather than a decrease in degradation rate, is responsible for the increase in mitochondrial proteins [3]. The increase in mitochondrial enzymes in skeletal muscle in response to endurance exercise is a rapid process. In rats subjected to a constant daily exercise stimulus, the half-time of the increase in cytochrome c concentration and in the levels of activity of a number of mitochondrial marker enzymes is approximately 7 days [3]. The increase in cytochromes and other mitochondrial enzymes is preceded by an increase in δ-aminolvulinic acid synthetase activity [32]. δ-Aminolevulinic acid synthetase is the rate-limiting enzyme in heme synthesis, and it has been speculated that the increase in level of activity of this enzyme may play an important role in the process by which exercise induces an increase in muscle mitochondria.

In contrast to skeletal muscle, heart muscle is continually active and does not undergo an increase in the concentrations of mitochondrial enzymes, which are already very high [26]. However, although respiratory capacity per gram of muscle is unchanged, the total mitochondrial content of the heart is increased in proportion to the degree of exercise-induced cardiac hypertrophy [26].

Although the adaptation of human skeletal muscle to endurance exercise has not been studied in as great detail, it is clear from measurements made on muscle biopsies in numerous studies that, as in rats, endurance training can induce large increases in the respiratory capacity of muscle in humans [cf. 29]. These studies have demonstrated increases in the size and number of muscle mitochondria as well as increases in the levels of activity of marker enzymes of the pathway for fatty acid oxidation, the citrate cycle, and the respiratory chain.

Myoglobin

There is a significant increase in the myoglobin content of leg muscles of rats subjected to programs of prolonged treadmill running [26]. It has been shown in studies *in vitro* that myoglobin increases the rate of oxygen transport through a fluid layer. It seems likely that myoglobin also facilitates oxygen utilization in muscle *in vivo* by increasing the rate of oxygen diffusion through the cytoplasm to the mitochondria. Interestingly, in contrast to rats, highly trained humans do not have elevated myoglobin concentrations in their skeletal muscles [12]; the physiological significance of this species difference is not clear at present.

Enzymes of Glycolysis and Glycogenolysis

In contrast to the mitochondrial enzymes, the enzymes involved in glycolysis and glycogenolysis generally undergo only minor changes in skeletal muscle in response to endurance exercise [6, 28]. Two exceptions are hexokinase and lactate dehydrogenase. Hexokinase is unique among the glycolytic enzymes in that its activity roughly parallels respiratory (not glycolytic) capacity in the different types of muscle. In this context, it is interesting that exercise training, which induces an increase in mitochondrial content of skeletal muscle, also results in an increase in hexokinase activity [cf. 6, 28]. However, in contrast to the mitochondrial enzymes, in which the half-time of the increase in response to a constant exercise stimulus is about 7 days [3], hexokinase activity can increase in response to a single prolonged bout of exercise [cf. 28]. Total lactate dehydrogenase activity is generally somewhat lower in skeletal muscle of trained individuals, and has been shown to decrease with training [49] and increase with detraining [6]. More important, endurance training appears to induce an increase in the proportion of the heart type of lactate dehydrogenase (H-LDH) and a decrease in the muscle type of lactate dehydrogenase (M-LDH) in skeletal muscle [49]. This shift in LDH isozyme pattern could contribute to the lower lactate production seen in the trained state by decreasing the ability of LDH to compete with the mitochondria for the NADH and pyruvate formed in glycolysis.

Decrease in Mitochondrial Enzymes with Detraining

The effect of stopping training on mitochondrial enzymes in skeletal muscle has been studied both in rats and humans. In rats, a number of mitochondrial marker enzymes increased approximately twofold in leg muscles in response to a 15-week-long program of treadmill running. Following cessation of training, the concentration of cytochrome c and the levels of activity of citrate synthase and 3-ketoacid coenzyme A (CoA) transferase decreased exponentially toward sedentary control values with a half-time of about 7 days, and had returned to baseline between 4 and 5 weeks [3].

In people who have trained for only 8 to 12 weeks, the increase in mitochondrial enzyme levels appears to be lost in about 6 weeks after training is stopped [cf. 29]. It is not clear why reversal of the adaptive increase in mitochondria was somewhat slower in humans that in rats; one possibility is that restriction of activity was more severe in the rats housed in individual cages than in the human subjects going about their normal daily activities.

In contrast to the rather rapid loss of mitochondrial adaptations in muscles of people who have trained for only 2 or 3 months, in individuals who have been training strenuously for many years the increase in mitochondrial content appears to be more persistent. [6, 12, 29]. In a study on the effects of cessation of endurance training in subjects who had been exercising regularly for 6 to 20 years, the levels of a number of mitochondrial marker enzymes decreased significantly over a 12-week period but were still about 50% higher than in sedentary control subjects in mixed muscle [6].

Analysis of single muscle fibers revealed that this persistent elevation of mitochondrial enzyme levels above control values was much more pronounced in the fast-twitch (type II) fibers than in the slow-twitch (type I) fibers after 12 weeks of inactivity [6]. This observation suggests that many years of endurance training may induce long-lasting adaptations, such as changes in the firing frequency of the nerves innervating the fast-twitch fibers or in the recruitment pattern of these fibers. Although lactate threshold declined significantly, it too was still significantly higher in the subjects after 12 weeks of detraining than in untrained controls [12].

MECHANISMS THAT MAY BE RESPONSIBLE FOR MEDIATING ALTERED METABOLIC RESPONSES TO SUBMAXIMAL EXERCISE IN THE TRAINED STATE

If substrate and oxygen availability are not limiting, the rate of substrate flux through the citrate cycle and the rates of electron transport and oxidative phosphorylation during submaximal exercise are determined by the muscle cells' requirement for energy. During muscle contractile activity, the major factor determining the energy requirement is the rate of ATP hydrolysis at the cross-bridges formed between actin and myosin. The mechanism by which oxygen consumption is closely geared to work rate involves the tight coupling of oxidative phsophorylation to electron transport.

The primary factor regulating mitochondrial respiration appears to be the concentration of ADP [cf 19]. When muscle contracts, ATP is hydrolyzed, the concentrations of ATP and phosphocreatine decline, and the concentrations of adenosine diphosphate (ADP) and inorganic phsophate increase. The steady-state concentration of ADP attained in muscle during submaximal exercise is determined by the energy requirement of the muscle and, in turn, determines the rates of electron transport and oxygen consumption. Thus, after the onset of contractile activity that requires less than the muscle cells' maximal capacity for aerobic metabolism, ADP concentration must increase until a steady state is attained at which the rate of ATP formation by oxidative phosphorylation (and glycolysis) balances the rate of ATP hydrolysis. At the same time, the concentrations of high-energy phosphagens, ATP and PCr fall, until the steady-state level of respiration is attained, resulting in the muscle "oxygen deficit."

Oxygen consumption is the same in the trained and untrained states at the same absolute submaximal work rate. The increase in ADP concentration in response to a given submaximal work rate must therefore be smaller in trained than in untrained muscle. The reason is that with more mitochondria, that is, more respiratory chains per gram of muscle, oxygen utilization per respiratory chain must be "turned on" to a smaller extent in order to attain the same rate of oxygen consumption per gram of muscle in trained as in untrained muscle working at the same rate. In other words, the greater the number of mitochondrial respiratory chains, the lower must be the rate of O_2 utilization per respiratory chain in order to maintain a given rate of oxygen consumption per gram of muscle. Therefore, because of the increase in mitochondria, ATP and PCr concentrations decrease less, and ADP, inorganic phosphate (Pi), and creatine must increase less in response to the same submaximal exercise when a muscle is trained than when it is untrained.

Adenylate kinase activity results in conversion of some of the ADP formed during muscle contraction to AMP, part of which is deaminated by adenylate deaminase to form inosine monophosphate (IMP) and ammonia [cf. 28, 29]. As a consequence of a smaller rise in ADP, the concentrations of AMP, IMP, and ammonia are lower in trained muscle during submaximal exercise [15].

The intracellular concentrations of ATP, Pi, AMP, ADP, and ammonia play important roles in controlling the rate of glycolysis. ATP inhibits phosphofructokinase, and this inhibition is countered by Pi, ADP, AMP, and ammonia. Therefore, as a consequence of lower levels of Pi, ADP, AMP and ammonia, glycolysis should be activated to a smaller extent at a given work rate in trained than in untrained muscle. This mechanism could play a role in accounting for the slower rates of carbohydrate utilization and of lactate production during submaximal exercise in the trained than in the untrained state.

Additional factors that may contribute to the slower lactate production are the adaptive decreases in total lactate dehydrogenase activity, with a shift in isoenzyme pattern toward the heart lactate dehydrogenase, and the increase in the capacity of the malate–aspartate shuttle in muscle that occurs in response to endurance training. These adaptations should, together with the increase in mitochondria, enhance the ability of the mitochondria to compete with lactate dehydrogenase for pyruvate.

A second likely consequence of the adaptive increase in mitochondria is that work rates that exceeded the capacity of some of the muscle fibers for aerobic metabolism in the untrained state become "submaximal" following adaptation to intense endurance training. This adaptation is especially likely to occur in the fast-twitch white muscle fibers, which have the lowest content of mitochondria in the untrained state. Exercise intensities that exceeded the respiratory capacity of such muscle fibers and resulted in rapid lactate accumulation and fatigue prior to training may be within the fibers' capacity for aerobic metabolism after they have adapted to endurance training. As a consequence, the adaptations to endurance exercise may make possible prolonged steady-state contractile activity during which ATP hydrolysis is balanced by oxidative phosphorylation, at work rates that could be maintained for only short bursts by muscle fibers that had a low content of mitochondria when untrained.

A factor that plays a key role in making possible the slower utilization of muscle glycogen and blood glucose during submaximal exercise after training is the greater oxidation of fat. The concentration of plasma FFAs available to muscle, which is an important factor in determining the rate of plasma FFA utilization, is generally lower in the trained than in the untrained state at the same absolute submaximal work rate. However, the intracellular concentration of FFA available to the mitochondria is unknown, and the possibility that the intracellular FFA concentration is higher in trained than in untrained muscle during submaximal exercise has not been ruled out.

If it is assumed that intracellular FFA concentration in muscle is similar in the trained and untrained states, the difference in the rate of FFA oxidation must be a consequence of the adaptations induced by exercise. The overall rate of substrate oxidation is determined by the rate of ATP hydrolysis, which is a function of the work rate. However, the relative proportions of carbohydrate and fat oxidized are determined by substrate (i.e., FFA and pyruvate) availability, by the relative activities of the rate-limiting enzymes in the pathways for generating acetyl CoA from carbohydrate and fatty acids, and by a number of regulatory mechanisms. Of these regulatory mechanisms, the most important probably are less activation of glycolysis as a consequence of smaller changes in the levels of the high-energy phosphate compounds, Pi, and ammonia at the same submaximal work rate after muscle has adapted to training with an increase in mitochondria, and the inhibitory effects of FFA oxidation on glucose uptake and glycolysis. The increases in the levels of the enzymes of the fatty acid oxidation pathway make possible the provision of a larger proportion of the energy required during strenuous exercise by means of fat oxidation.

CONCLUSION

Endurance exercise training induces a number of adaptations in skeletal muscle. Probably the most important of these is an increase in mitochondria with an increase in respiratory capacity. One consequence of the adaptations induced in muscle by endurance exercise is that the same work rate requires a smaller percentage of the muscles' maximum respiratory capacity and therefore results in less disturbance in homeostasis. A second consequence is increased utilization of fat, with a proportional decrease in carbohydrate utilization, during submaximal exercise. These metabolic consequences of the adaptations of muscle to endurance training play important roles in the increases in endurance and in the ability to exercise at a higher percentage of Vo_2max in the trained state by slowing glycogen depletion and reducing lactate production (i.e., raising "lactate threshold").

ACKNOWLEDGMENTS

This research was supported by National Institutes of Health Research Grants AG-00425 and AM-18986 and by Institutional National Research Service Award AG-00078.

REFERENCES

1. Bladwin, K.M., G.H., Klinkerfuss, R.L. Terjung, P.A. Mole, and J.O. Holloszy. Respiratory capacity of white, red and intermediate muscle: Adaptive response to exercise. *Am. J. Physiol.* 222:373-, 1972.
2. Bergstrom, J., L. Hermansen, E. Hultman, and B. Saltin. Diet, muscle glycogen and physical performance. *Acta Physiol. Scand.* 71:140–150, 1967.
3. Booth, R.W., and J.O. Holloszy. Cytochrome c turnover in rat skeletal muscles. *J. Biol. Chem.* 252:416–419, 1977.
4. Carlson, L.A., L.-G. Ekelund, and S.O. Froberg. Concentration of triglycerides, phospholipids and glycogen in skeletal muscle and of free fatty acids and β-hydroxybutyric acid in blood in man in response to exercise. *Eur. J. Clin. Invest.* 1:248–254, 1971.
5. Chasiotis, D., K. Sahlin, and E. Hultman. Regulation of glycogenolysis in human skeletal muscle at rest and during exercise. *J. Appl. Physiol.* 53:708–715, 1982.
6. Chi, M.M.-Y., C.S. Hintz, E.F. Coyle, W.H. Martin III, J.L. Ivy, P.M. Nemeth, J.O. Holloszy, and O.H. Lowry. Effects of detraining on enzymes of energy metabolism in individual human muscle fibers. *Am. J. Physiol.* 244:C276–C287, 1983.
7. Clausen, J.P. Circulatory adjustments to dynamic exercise and effect of physical training in normal subjects and in patients with coronary artery disease. *Prog. Cardiovasc. Dis.* 18:459–495, 1976.
8. Conlee, R.K., J.A. McLane, M.J. Rennie, W.W. Winder, and J.O. Holloszy. Reversal of phosphorylase activation in muscle despite continued contractile activity. *Am. J. Physiol.* 237:R291–R296, 1979.
9. Connett, R.J., T.E.J. Gayeski, and C.R. Honig. Lactate accumulation in fully aerobic, working, dog gracilis muscle. *Am. J. Physiol.* 246:H120–H128, 1984.
10. Constable, S.H., J.C. Young, M. Higuchi, and J.O. Holloszy. Glycogen resynthesis in leg muscles of rats during exercise. *Am. J. Physiol.* 247:R880–R883, 1984.
11. Costill, D.L., E. Coyle, G. Dalsky, W. Evans, W. Fink, and D. Hoopes. Effects of elevated plasma FFA and insulin on muscle glycogen usage during exercise. *J. Appl. Physiol.* 43:695–699, 1977.

12. Coyle, E.F., W.H. Martin III, S.A. Bloomfield, O.H. Lowry and J.O. Holloszy. Effects of detraining on responses to submaximal exercise. *J. Appl. Physiol.* 59:853–859, 1985.
13. Dalsky, G., W. Martin, B. Hurley, D. Matthews, D. Bier, J. Hagberg, and J.O. Holloszy. Oxidation of plasma FFA during endurance exercise. *Med. Sci. Sports Exer.* 16:202, 1984.
14. Dudley, G.A., W.A. Abraham, and R.L. Terjung. Influence of exercise intensity and duration on biochemical adaptations in skeletal muscle. *J. Appl. Physiol.* 53:844–850, 1982.
15. Dudley, G.A., and R.L. Terjung. Influence of aerobic metabolism on IMP accumulation in fast-twitch muscle. *Am. J. Physiol.* 248:C37–C42, 1985.
16. Fischer, E.H., L.M.G. Heilmeyer Jr., and R.H. Haschke. Phosphorylase and the control of glycogen degradation. *Curr. Top. Cell Reg.* 4:211–251, 1971.
17. Fitts, R.H., F.W. Booth, W.W. Winder, and J.O. Holloszy. Skeletal muscle respiratory capacity endurance and glycogen utilization. *Am. J. Physiol.* 228:1029–1033, 1975.
18. Hagenfeldt, L. Turnover of individual free fatty acids in man. *Fed. Proc.* 34:2236–2240, 1975.
19. Harms, S.J., and R.C. Hickson. Skeletal muscle mitochondria and myoglobin, endurance, and intensity of training. *J. Appl. Physiol.* 54:798–802, 1983.
20. Henriksson, J. Training-induced adaptations of skeletal muscle and metabolism during submaximal exercise. *J. Physiol.* 270:661–675, 1977.
21. Hermansen, L. Lactate production during exercise. In Pernow, B., and B. Saltin (eds.). *Muscle Metabolism During Exercise.* New York: Plenum Press, 1974, pp. 401–407.
22. Hermansen, L., E. Hultman, and B. Saltin. Muscle glycogen during prolonged severe exercise. *Acta Physiol. Scand.* 71:129–139, 1967.
23. Hetenyi, G. Jr., G. Perez, and M. Vranic. Turnover and precursor-product relationships of non-lipid metabolites. *Physiol. Rev.* 63:606–607, 1983.
24. Hickson, R.C., M.J. Rennie, R.K. Conlee, W.W. Winder, and J.O. Holloszy. Effects of increased plasma fatty acids on glycogen utilization and endurance. *J. Appl. Physiol.* 43:829–833, 1977.
25. Holloszy, J.O. Biochemical adaptations in muscle: Effect of exercise on mitochondrial oxygen uptake and respiratory enzyme activity in skeletal muscle. *J. Biol. Chem.* 242:2278–2282, 1967.
26. Holloszy, J.O. Biochemical adaptations to exercise: Aerobic metabolism. In Wilmore, J. (ed.). *Exercise and Sport Sciences Reviews.* New York: Academic Press, 1973, pp. 45–71.
27. Holloszy, J.O. Adaptation of skeletal muscle to endurance exercise. *Med. Sci. Sports* 7:155–164, 1975.
28. Holloszy, J.O., and F.W. Booth. Biochemical adaptations to endurance exercise in muscle *Annu. Rev. Physiol.* 38:273–291, 1976.
29. Holloszy, J.O., and E.F. Coyle. Adaptations of skeletal muscle to endurance exercise and their metabolic consequences. *J. Appl. Physiol.* 56:831-838, 1984.
30. Holloszy, J.O., and L.B. Oscai. Effect of exercise on α-glycerophosphate dehydrogenase activity in

skeletal muscle. *Arch. Biochem. Biophys.* 130:653–656, 1969.

31. Holloszy, J.O., L.B. Oscai, I.J. Don, and P.A. Mole. Mitochondrial citric acid cycle and related enzymes: Adaptive response to exercise. *Biochem. Biophys. Res. Commun.* 40:1368–1373, 1970.

32. Holloszy, J.O., and W.W. Winder. Induction of δ-aminolevulinic acid synthetase in muscle by exercise or thyroxine. *Am. J. Physiol.* 236:R180–R183, 1979.

33. Hurley, B.F., J.M. Hagberg, W.K. Allen, D.R. Seals, J.C. Young, R.W. Cuddihee, and J.O. Holloszy. Effect of training on blood lactate levels during submaximal exercise. *J. Appl. Physiol.* 56:1260–1264, 1984.

34. Hurley, B.F., P.M. Nemeth, W.H. Martin III, J.M. Hagberg, G.P. Dalsky, and J.O. Holloszy. Muscle triglyceride utilization during exercise: Effect of training. *J. Appl. Physiol.* 60:562–567, 1986.

35. Jansson, E., and L. Kaijser. Muscle adaptation to extreme endurance training in man. *Acta Physiol. Scand.* 100:315–324, 1977.

36. Jobsis, F.F., and W.N. Stainsby. Oxidation of NADH during contractions of circulated mammalian skeletal muscle. *Resp. Physiol.* 4:292–300, 1968.

37. Karlsson, J., L.-O. Nordesjo, L. Jorfeldt, and B. Saltin. Muscle lactate, ATP, and CP levels during exercise after physical training in man. *J. Appl. Physiol.* 33:199–203, 1972.

38. Lehninger, A.L. Oxidative phosphorylation, mitochondrial structure and the compartmentation of respiratory metabolism. In *Biochemistry,* 2nd ed. New York: Worth, 1976, pp. 509–542.

39. Mole, P.A., L.B. Oscai, and J.O. Holloszy. Adaptation of muscle to exercise: Increase in levels of palmityl CoA synthetase, carnitine palmityltransferase, and palmityl CoA dehydrogenase and in the capacity to oxidize fatty acids. J. Clin. Invest. 50:2323–2330, 1971.

40. Oscai, L.B., and J.O. Holloszy. Biochemical adaptations in muscle. II. Response of mitochondrial adenosine triphosphatase, creatine phosphokinase, and adenylate kinase activities in skeletal muscle to exercise. *J. Biol. Chem.* 246:6968–6972, 1971.

41. Pette, D. Activity-induced fast to slow transitions in mammalian muscle. *Med. Sci. Sports Exer.* 16:517–520, 1984.

42. Randle, P.J., P.B. Garland, C.N. Hales, and E.A. Newsholme. The glucose fatty-acid cycle: Its role in insulin sensitivity and the metabolic disturbances of diabetes millitus. *Lancet* 1:785–789, 1963.

43. Rennie, M.J., R.D. Fell, J.L. Ivy, and J.O. Holloszy. Adrenaline reactivation of muscle phosphorylase after deactivation during phasic contractile activity. *Biosci. Rep.* 2:323–331, 1982.

44. Rennie, M.J., and J.O. Holloszy. Inhibition of glucose uptake and glycogenolysis by availability of oleate in well-oxygenated perfused skeletal muscle. *Biochem. J.* 168:161–170, 1977.

45. Rennie, M.J., W.W. Winder, and J.O. Holloszy. A sparing effect of increased plasma fatty acids on muscle and liver glycogen content in the exercising rat. *Biochem. J.* 156:647–655, 1976.

46. Richter, E.A., N.B. Ruderman, H. Gavras, E.R. Belur, and H. Galbo. Muscle glycogenolysis during exercise: Dual control by epinephrine and contractions. *Am. J. Physiol.* 242:E25–E32, 1982.

47. Saltin, B., L.H. Hartley, A. Kilbom, and I. Astrand. Physical training in sedentary middle-aged and older men. II. Oxygen uptake, heart rate and blood lactate concentration at submaximal and maximal exercise. *Scand. J. Clin. Lab. Invest.* 24:323–334, 1969.

48. Saltin, B., and J. Karlsson. Muscle glycogen utilization during work of different intensities. In Pernow, B., and B. Saltin (eds.). *Muscle Metabolism During Exercise.* New York: Plenum Press, 1971, pp. 289–299.

49. Sjodin, B. Lactate dehydrogenase in human skeletal muscle *Acta Physiol. Scand.* 436:9–18, 1976.

50. Winder, W.W., K.M. Baldwin, and J.O. Holloszy. Enzymes involved in ketone utilization in different types of muscle: Adaptation to exercise. *Eur. J. Biochem.* 47:461–467, 1974.

51. Winder, W.W., R.C. Hickson, J.M. Hagberg, A.A. Ehsani, and J.A. McLane. Training-induced changes in hormonal and metabolic responses to submaximal exercise. *J. Appl. Physiol.* 46:766–771, 1979.

52. Winder, W.W., and J.O. Holloszy. Response of mitochondria of different types of skeletal muscle to thyrotoxicosis. *Am. J. Physiol.* 232:C180–C184, 1977.

Chapter 9

DIETARY INTAKE PRIOR TO AND DURING EXERCISE

Eric Hultman, M.D., and Lawrence L. Spriet, Ph.D.

INTRODUCTION

The conversion of chemical to mechanical energy in the skeletal muscles of the body enables humans to perform large amounts of external work. The chemical energy is provided through dietary intake of foodstuffs and their subsequent uptake and metabolism by the muscles. The relationship between dietary intake and exercise has been of interest for at least 3000 years, but the nature of dietary fuels has been scientifically studied for only the last 150 years. Before we discuss the importance of dietary intake to exercise, we will review the nature and source of the substrates metabolized during varying types, intensities, and durations of exercise.

SUBSTRATE UTILIZATION DURING EXERCISE

Historical Introduction

Pettenkofer and Voit suggested as early as 1862, using measurements of urinary nitrogen output, that protein was not a major source of fuel during exercise in healthy well-fed humans [2]. Zuntz and colleagues (1894) reported that work was performed through the combustion of both fat and carbohydrate (CHO), while Chauveau's group (1896) maintained CHO was the sole energy source for muscular contraction [2]. Their work

was based on measurements of the respiratory exchange ratio (R-value, ratio of CO_2 output and O_2 uptake measured at the mouth) and the knowledge that the respective R-values for oxidation of fat and CHO were 0.7 and 1.0. A series of later studies by Krogh and Linhard (1920) and Christensen and Hansen (1939) using similar techniques, produced many important findings and strongly suggested that both fat and CHO were utilized during exercise [11, 43]. In light- to moderate-intensity work, the relative amounts of fat and CHO utilized depended mainly on the diet. As this intensity of work was prolonged, the energy contribution from fat increased, presumably due to a decreased CHO supply [11]. A high-fat diet in the days prior to the exercise decreased performance capacity, while CHO-rich food increased exercise endurance. As the exercise intensity increased above a certain workload, coinciding with the onset of blood lactate accumulation, the contribution of CHO began to increase, reaching nearly 100% at maximal work intensities.

However, calculations based on R-values are only approximate and give no information about the source of the fat and CHO fuels being utilized. The majority of the body's fat is stored in adipose tissue as triacylglycerol. The breakdown of adipose tissue triacylglycerol releases free fatty acids (FFAs), which are transported to the muscles via the plasma. Esterified fat circulating in plasma can be hydrolyzed to release FFAs. Triacylglycerol stored in the muscles is a third source of FFAs. Carbohydrate is stored as glycogen in muscles and liver. Glucose, derived predominantly from liver glycogenolysis and in small part from gluconeogenesis, is delivered to the muscles via the blood. As techniques became available for directly measuring fuel utilization later in the 20th century, researchers were able to examine the accuracy of the early indirect studies and identify the sources of fuels utilized during exercise.

Plasma Free Fatty Acids

Infusions of ^{14}C-labeled FFAs and the rapid appearance of $^{14}CO_2$ in the expired air of humans during low to moderate exercise demonstrated the muscle's ability to metabolize circulating FFA [33]. Additional research revealed that FFAs were carried in the plasma bound to albumin, with a transport maximum of approximately 2 mmol·L^{-1}; FFAs released from adipose tissue were the quantitatively important source; and esterified FFAs in the form of circulating triacylglycerol did not contribute significantly to the plasma FFA content or metabolism of body tissues. Work by Hagenfeldt and Wahren [29] demonstrated a linear relationship between FFA delivery and muscle uptake during prolonged moderate exercise. This suggested that the factors regulating adipose tissue FFA release also governed rate of muscle FFA oxidation.

At exercise intensities of up to about 70% of maximal oxygen uptake ($\dot{V}O_2$max) prolonged beyond 30 to 40 minutes, FFA release from adipose tissue progressively increases, resulting in greater utilization of fat. During a study of humans cycling for 4 hours at 30% of $\dot{V}O_2$max, the energy contribution from FFA was 37% during the initial 40 minutes and 62% during the final hour [1]. The maximum O_2 uptake that can be sustained entirely from FFAs is 50 to 55% of $\dot{V}O_2$max in untrained subjects, and rises to

about 65% following training due to an increased capacity to oxidize FFAs [35]. As the exercise intensity increases, the contribution of plasma FFAs to energy production decreases. In untrained subjects, FFAs continue to contribute significantly to energy production during prolonged exercise up to workloads of approximately 70% of $\dot{V}O_2$max. In trained athletes, this value is as high as 80 to 85% of $\dot{V}O_2$max. Because of the time delay in the mobilization of FFAs from adipose tissue at the onset of exercise, circulating FFAs appear of little value during intense short-term exercise.

Muscle Triacylglycerol

During prolonged moderate to heavy exercise, intramuscular triacylglycerol stores also provide significant amounts of FFAs for oxidation. Decreases in the triacylglycerol content of muscle occurred during prolonged cross-country ski racing, cycling, and running at 55 to 80% of $\dot{V}O_2$max [15, 26, 27]. Some evidence exists suggesting that FFAs derived from local triacylglycerol stores also contribute to energy production during near-maximal work. Essén [20] found a 20% decrease in muscle triacylglycerol concentration following only 5 minutes of cycling at 100% of $\dot{V}O_2$max. The exact importance of intramuscular fat as a fuel source during intense exercise remains unclear, but it appears to be quantitatively far less important than muscle glycogen.

Muscle Glycogen

The reintroduction by Bergström and Hultman of the needle biopsy technique for sampling human skeletal muscle made possible direct examination of the importance of muscle glycogen during exercise [3, 36]. In one of the first studies on this topic, untrained subjects cycled intermittently for as long as possible at about 80% of $\dot{V}O_2$max in a sequence of 15 minutes of work and 15 minutes of rest [6]. Muscle glycogen utilization was greatest during the first 15-minute work bout and then decreased successively such that glycogen concentration plotted against time decreased in a semilogarithmic fashion (Figure 1). During cycling sustained for as long as possible at a variety of workloads, glycogen utilization in the vastus lateralis muscle increased in a near exponential fashion as a function of the exercise intensity, as shown in Figure 2 [34, 54]. Representative utilization rates at 50, 100, and 150% of $\dot{V}O_2$max were 0.7, 3.4, and 10.0 mmol·kg⁻¹·min⁻¹, respectively. Carbohydrate in the forms of blood glucose and muscle glycogen contributed less than one-half of the total substrate used at workloads below 50% of $\dot{V}O_2$max. Muscle glycogen became the dominant substrate at workloads above 50% $\dot{V}O_2$max, whereas glucose uptake

was quantitatively less important. The depletion of muscle glycogen stores appeared to limit prolonged exercise at workloads between 65 and 85% of $\dot{V}O_2$max. At workloads above 75% of $\dot{V}O_2$max, muscles were unable to substitute CHO for fat even when glycogen stores were emptied. Following aerobic endurance training, the rate of muscle glycogen utilization is reduced at a given submaximal workload up to 80% of $\dot{V}O_2$max, due to greater oxidation of plasma FFAs [35]. Glycogen utilization rates in the vastus lateralis muscle during ice skating at 50 and 120% of $\dot{V}O_2$max were similar to those found during cycling (Figure 2) [28]. During prolonged running at 70 to 80% of $\dot{V}O_2$max, glycogen was utilized at rates of 1.0 and 1.3 mmol·kg⁻¹·min⁻¹ in soleus and gastrocnemius muscles, respectively (Figure 2) [7, 55]. Recent studies of sprint cycling and running sustained for only 30 seconds reported glycogen utilization rates as high as 32 to 36 mmol·kg⁻¹·min⁻¹[10, 45].

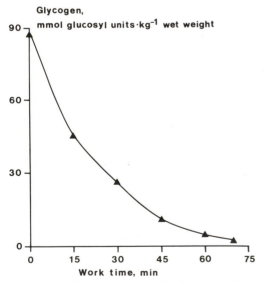

Figure 1. Glycogen content in the vastus lateralis muscle as a function of cycling time at 80% of maximal oxygen uptake capacity ($\dot{V}O_2$max). Data points are the mean values determined on 10 subjects. For each subject, exercise was performed repeatedly in periods of 15 minutes separated by 15-minute rest periods. At exhaustion, muscle glycogen stores were virtually depleted. (Data from Bergström, J., and E. Hultman. A study of the glycogen metabolism during exercise in man. *Scand. J. Clin. Lab. Invest.* 19:218–228, 1967.)

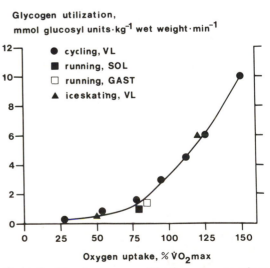

Figure 2. Muscle glycogen utilization rates at various work intensities during different types of exercise. VL, vastus lateralis muscle; SOL, soleus muscle; GAST, gastrocnemius muscle. (Data from references 17, 26, 31, 52, and 53.)

Plasma Glucose

During light to moderate exercise (30–70% of Vo_2max) sustained for longer than 1 to 2 hours, glucose uptake by the working muscles represents a significant energy source. For example, during prolonged walking at 45% of Vo_2max, exogenous glucose provided up to 55% of the CHO metabolized and 24% of the total energy expenditure [52], whereas only 12% of the required energy during prolonged running at 70% of Vo_2max was derived from exogenous glucose [12]. The liver attempts to maintain the blood glucose concentration during prolonged exercise mainly through glycogenolysis and to a small degree through gluconeogenesis. In spite of this, blood glucose level may fall to 50% of normal or less during prolonged exercise in the well-fed state [38]. Since an adequate blood glucose concentration is required to maintain central nervous system integrity, this inability of liver glucose output to match peripheral utilization is the cause of fatigue in some individuals. Direct measurements of glycogen in liver biopsy samples demonstrated that 1 hour of heavy exercise reduced glycogen from an overnight-fast level of about 270 $mmol \cdot kg^{-1}$ to 125 $mmol \cdot kg^{-1}$ [38]. In addition, 1 day without food was sufficient to deplete liver glycogen stores to values below 50 $mmol \cdot kg^{-1}$, which resulted in early onset of hypoglycemia during prolonged exercise.

Protein

The quantitative role of protein as an energy substrate in the well-fed state is minor, especially during short-term intense exercise. With prolonged exercise, protein may contribute at the most 5 to 10% of total energy turnover, judging from increases in the extracellular level of urea nitrogen and in the urinary output of urea during the rest period following exercise [53]. Measurements of the uptake and release of amino acids over the working muscles and splanch-

nic area, and of the metabolism of isotopically labeled amino acids also indicate a contribution to energy turnover during exercise [22]. Utilization of protein as a fuel during exercise most likely represents a general effect in which the normal protein synthesis rate of about 300 g/day is decreased during prolonged exercise [47] and some of the amino acids released through normal protein degradation are directed to the working muscle cells. During recovery from prolonged exercise, the protein synthesis rate increases [47].

ENERGY STORES AND EXERCISE

Fat

In the well-fed healthy individual, the store of FFAs in the form of triacylglycerol in adipose tissue is by far the largest energy source in the body (Table 1). It is unlikely that an increase in fat stores would enhance endurance performance even during very extended periods of exercise. The limitation to exercise at low workloads does not appear to be due to lack of fat substrate. However, enhancing the mobilization of fat stores prior to or during prolonged moderate to heavy exercise decreases the rate of CHO utilization. This CHO sparing may lead to enhanced endurance, as discussed later in this chapter.

Carbohydrate

Maintenance of normal body CHO stores through proper dietary intake is essential to ensure optimal exercise performance. At workloads above 85 to 90% of $\dot{V}o_2max$, the by-products of anaerobic metabolism inhibit muscular contraction and/or energy production before local glycogen stores are depleted. However, if repeated intense work bouts are required over the course of a few hours, as in ice hockey or soccer, adequate glycogen stores are essential for optimal per-

Table 1. ENERGY STORES IN A WELL-FED MAN*

ENERGY SOURCE	CONCENTRATION (mmol·kg^{-1})	ENERGY PER MOLE (kJ)	ENERGY STORED IN BODY (kJ)
Carbohydrate			
Muscle glycogen	80–100	2,850	6,400–8,000
Liver glycogen	300–500	2,850	1,550–2,600
Plasma glucose†	5	3,150	49
Fat			
Adipose tissue TG	-	30,500	275,000
Intramuscular TG	10–15	30,500	8,500–12,800
Plasma FFAs	0.3–0.6	10,150	9–18

TG, triacylglycerol; FFAs, free fatty acids.
*Assuming a moderately active 70-kg man with 40% of body weight as muscle (28 kg), a liver weight of 1.8 kg, a plasma volume of 3 L, and 9 kg of adipose tissue. Endurance-trained individuals store approximately 125 to 150 mmol·kg^{-1} as muscle glycogen and 400 to 700 mmol·kg^{-1} as liver glycogen.
†mmol · L^{-1}.

formance. During prolonged exercise at 65 to 85% of $\dot{V}o_2$max, muscle glycogen depletion can limit exercise; during extended exercise at lower intensities, liver glycogen depletion leads to hypoglycemia if no CHO is taken during the work. There are several reasons why CHO is a more versatile and important fuel than fat during muscular exercise: (a) Only carbohydrate can be metabolized anaerobically. This is important during transition periods, such as from rest to exercise or from one workload to a higher one, and during intense work, during which all the required energy cannot be provided aerobically. (b) The aerobic combustion of CHO is about 10% more efficient than the combustion of fat in terms of oxygen utilized per kilojoule of energy released. (c) Carbohydrate can be provided as a substrate for aerobic metabolism at a rate approximately double that of fat [46].

However, as Table 1 shows, the capacity for energy production from CHO is much lower than from fat. Although muscle and liver glycogen concentrations are somewhat elevated in trained athletes (Table 1, footnote), CHO depletion during prolonged exercise remains a problem. This limited storage capacity is the reason why the di-etary intake of CHO prior to and during exercise is of paramount importance to both active individuals and trained athletes.

Protein

There is no evidence that any specific body protein store available for exercise can be increased by diet. Also, as previously discussed, the role of protein as an energy substrate in the well-fed state is minor during exercise. For these reasons, dietary protein intake and exercise will not be discussed further in this chapter, except for the following comments. No evidence exists to suggest that athletes require more than the normal percentage of kilojoules derived from protein, even during periods of heavy resistance training. A normal diet should consist of 55 to 60% of the required kilojoules from CHO, 25 to 30% from fat, and 10 to 15% from protein. If a sedentary 70-kg adult consumes 10,500 kJ/day, the protein intake would be 60 to 90 g or approximately 1 g/kg of body weight. If this person begins to engage in heavy exercise regularly, the protein requirement is not significantly increased. The daily energy intake may increase by 200 to 400 kJ, but most of this increase is usually composed of CHO.

MUSCLE GLYCOGEN, DIET, AND EXERCISE PERFORMANCE

Diet

The first quantitative studies to examine the relationships among diet, exercise, and muscle glycogen stores were performed by Bergström and Hultman in 1966–1967. The feeding of a CHO-rich diet or a CHO-poor diet, or even total starvation, had relatively little effect on the glycogen content of human quadriceps femoris muscles at rest [37].

In another study [35], 7 days of a CHO-poor diet (fat and protein) decreased glycogen content by 31% in one subject, while 5 subsequent days of a CHO-rich diet replen-

ished glycogen to 110% of the prediet value (Figure 3A). Five days of total starvation reduced the glycogen concentration of another subject by only 40%. Both subjects, however, refrained from exercise during the CHO-poor dietary period.

Exercise and Diet

Following glycogen-depleting exercise there were remarkable differences in the rate of glycogen resynthesis and the final content attained, depending on the dietary regimen used [35]. Following exercise that reduced muscle glycogen concentration from 90.2 to 1.8 mmol·kg^{-1}, five subjects were fasted for 1 day. Glycogen levels rose to only 14.7 and 22.7 mmol·kg^{-1} after 4 and after 24 hours, respectively. A subsequent CHO-poor diet in two subjects for 5 to 6 days produced a

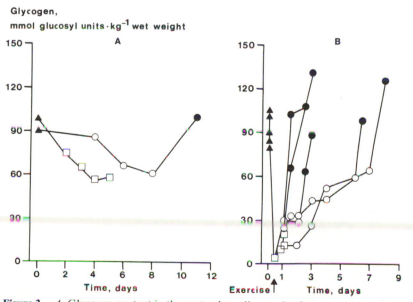

Figure 3. *A.* Glycogen content in the vastus lateralis muscle after a mixed diet (▲) and during 5 days of total starvation (□) in one subject and during 8 days of carbohydrate-poor diet (○) followed by a carbohydrate-rich diet (●) in another subject. *B.* Muscle glycogen content before and after exercise. Before exercise the diet was mixed (▲) and in the following days either total starvation (□) or a carbohydrate-poor diet (○) was used, followed by 1 or 2 days of carbohydrate-rich diet (●) (35). Note the slow rate of glycogen resynthesis when the diet is carbohydrate poor compared with the rate when the diet is rich in carbohydrate. (Data for both A and B from Holloszy, J.O., and E.F. Coyle. Adaptations of skeletal muscle to endurance exercise and their metabolic consequences. *J. Appl. Physiol.* 56:831–838, 1984.)

glycogen resynthesis rate of only 7.4 mmol·kg⁻¹·day⁻¹. In the remaining three subjects, a CHO-rich diet for 2 days rapidly replenished glycogen stores to normal (one subject) or greatly in excess of normal values (two subjects). The glycogen resynthesis rate was 73.6 mmol·kg⁻¹·day⁻¹ (Figure 3B).

A one-leg exercise model was used to deplete muscle glycogen content in the muscles of one leg but not in the other [5]. The two subjects then ate a CHO-rich diet for 3 days. Glycogen increased in the depleted muscles to 120, 193, and 230% of normal resting levels after 1, 2, and 3 days, respectively, while only small increases in glycogen content occurred in the muscles of the resting leg (Figure 4A). Following one-leg exercise, two additional subjects fasted for 2 days before consuming a CHO-rich diet for 4 days [37]. In the exercised legs, glycogen resynthesis was low during the fast but quickly increased with the CHO-rich diet, producing glycogen content about twice normal (Figure 4B). In the nonexercised legs, glycogen decreased to 63% of the post-exercise level during the fast and increased to 139% of the same level with the CHO-rich diet. Similar results were obtained in exercised and nonexercised legs of subjects following 3 days of a CHO-poor diet followed by 3 days of a CHO-rich diet (Figure 4C). these studies demonstrated that glycogen resynthesis to supernormal levels was a local phenomenon, restricted only to the exercised muscles.

Diet and Exercise Performance

The work of Christensen and Hansen [11], described in a previous section, demonstrated the importance of diet on the capacity to perform prolonged cycle exercise. A CHO-rich diet for 3 to 7 days resulted in a work time of 210 minutes at a fixed workload compared with only 80 minutes following a fat diet. Bergström and coworkers [4] directly examined the relationship between initial muscle glycogen content, varied by di-

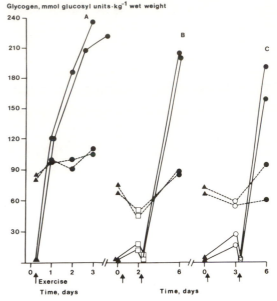

Figure 4. One-leg exercise studies showing the muscle glycogen content of the exercised (————) and rested (-------) legs. in two subjects. A. Biopsy specimens were obtained immediately after the exercise (▲) and during 3 days when subjects were fed a carbohydrate-rich diet (●). B, C. The diet was total starvation (□) for 2 days following exercise (B) or, carbohydrate-poor (○) for 3 days following exercise (C). In B and C this was followed by a second one leg exercise bout (↑) and a carbohydrate-rich diet (●). (Data for A from Bergström, J.L., E. Hermansen, E. Hultman, and B. Saltin. Diet, muscle glucogen and physical performance. *Acta Physiol. Scand.* 71:140–150, 1967.)

etary manipulation following exercise-induced depletion, and the capacity for prolonged intense exercise. Six subjects cycled to exhaustion at 75% of V̇o₂max on three occasions, each separated by 3 days. A normal mixed diet was given prior to the first endurance ride, a CHO-poor diet before the second ride, and a CHO-rich diet prior to the third. All diets contained the same number of kilojoules. The mixed, CHO-poor, and CHO-rich diets produced initial glycogen concentrations of 118, 42, and 227 mmol·kg⁻¹, respectively. The corresponding endurance times were 126, 59, and 189 minutes. A good correlation existed between initial glycogen content and cycle time (Figure 5), and exhaustion coincided with glycogen depletion regardless of the preceding dietary regimen. The sequence of exercise and different dietary regimens in this study was later adapted as a procedure to induce glycogen supercompensation.

In a similar study carried out in field conditions, 10 subjects ran a 30-km cross-country race on two occasions separated by 3 weeks. Each race was preceded by a mixed or CHO-rich diet [41]. Initial glycogen concentrations and race times following the mixed diet were 109 mmol·kg⁻¹ and 143 minutes, respectively; after the CHO-rich diet they were 216 mmol·kg⁻¹ and 135.3 minutes. The higher glycogen concentrations were associated with the maintenance of a faster running speed during the second half of the race.

Conclusions

These studies confirm the important role that diet plays in optimizing initial muscle glycogen content and subsequent exercise performance. They also identify three dietary regimens that produce elevated muscle glycogen stores. These have been referred to as "carbohydrate loading" or "supercompensation" regimens:

1. Change from a mixed to a CHO-rich diet for 3 to 4 days prior to exercise or competition.
2. Deplete muscle glycogen stores with near-exhaustive exercise, and follow this with a CHO-rich diet for 3 to 4 days.
3. Deplete muscle glycogen stores with near-exhaustive exercise, and follow this with a CHO-poor diet for 3 days, a second near-exhaustive exercise bout, and finally a CHO-rich diet for 3 days.

All three regimens begin with a mixed diet and suggest that exhaustive exercise not be performed during the CHO-rich diet. It is also important that the exercise used to deplete muscle glycogen before the start of the CHO-rich diet taxes the same muscle

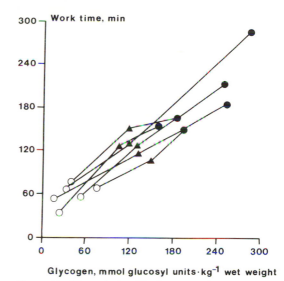

Figure 5. The relationship between the initial glycogen content in vastus lateralis muscle and work time. Six subjects cycled to exhaustion at a work load corresponding to 75% of Vo₂max. Each subject worked three times. The first experiment was preceded by a mixed diet (▲), the second by a carbohydrate-poor diet (○), and the third by a carbohydrate-rich diet (○). The energy content of the diets were identical. (Data from Bergström, J., and E. Hultman. Synthesis of muscle glycogen in man after glucose and fructose ingestion. *Acta Med. Scand.* 182:93–107, 1967.)

groups needed in the upcoming exercise event.

In active or untrained subjects, regimen 3 produces the highest muscle glycogen concentrations and regimen 1 the lowest. In athletes undergoing contstant training, regimen 1 is usually not possible, since any switch from a mixed to a CHO-rich diet will be preceded by a training bout, making this regimen similar to regimen 2. Regimen 3 is of limited value for athletes, since effective training is difficult during the CHO-poor diet and two exhausting bouts of exercise are not generally to be recommended so close to a competition. Well-trained athletes have higher muscle glycogen concentrations than do untrained subjects, which makes the effects of supercompensation less pronounced. Athletes also benefit equally from regimen 2, which requires only moderate dietary manipulations, compared with the more stressing regimen 3 [55].

It should also be noted that for every 10 mmol of glycogen stored in muscle, 4.4 g of water and 0.73 of potassium ions are stored. As an example, increasing the glycogen stores from 100 to 200 mmol·kg⁻¹ in 18 kg of the body's muscle will increase muscle water content by 800 g and postassium by 130 mmol. The extra glycogen will weigh 300 g, producing a total body increase of 1.1 kg. This extra weight and volume have been associated with feelings of muscle heaviness and stiffness, and may affect muscle performance by producing early fatigue.

LIVER CARBOHYDRATE METABOLISM, DIET, AND EXERCISE PERFORMANCE

Few studies have directly examined liver metabolism in humans, due to the invasive techniques required to obtain the appropriate measurements. However, Nilsson and Hultman performed a series of studies in the early 1970s [38, 48–51] that provided a substantial amount of information regarding interactions among liver CHO metabolism, diet, and exercise. The Menghini technique was used to obtain liver biopsies, and liver vein catheterization permitted measurements of the uptake or release of metabolites across the splanchnic region.

Diet

Following an overnight 12- to 16-hour fast, mean liver glycogen content in eight healthy subjects was 270 mmol·kg⁻¹ (range 90–500 mmol·kg⁻¹)[48]. The liver glycogen store proved to be extremely labile even in the resting state, unlike the situation in muscle. Biopsies taken during short-term starvation revealed a glycogen utilization rate of 0.3 mmol·kg⁻¹·min⁻¹, which would deplete the entire liver store in one day [50]. In two subjects fasted an entire day, liver

glycogen content decreased from 155 to 24 and 345 to 48 mmol·kg⁻¹. Further starvation in one subject produced values of 15 and 21 mmol·kg⁻¹ following a second and third day, respectively.

Starvation or a CHO-poor diet increases the amount of gluconeogenic substrates delivered to the liver (amino acids and glycerol), due to an increase in both fat and protein degradation. However, this was not sufficient for *de novo* synthesis of liver glycogen. Following an overnight fast, a fat and protein diet of 8400 kJ/day could not prevent liver glycogen from dropping to low levels, and produced no increase in glycogen during a 10-day period [50]. When the diet was changed to CHO-rich, there was an immediate 1-day increase in glycogen content, up to 500 to 600 mmol·kg⁻¹. These studies demonstrated that CHO intake through the diet on a daily basis is necessary for the preservation of the liver glycogen store. The muscle glycogen supercompensation regimens previously discussed also ensure that high glycogen levels are present in the liver prior to competition.

Blood glucose concentration during starvation or with a CHO-poor diet decreased only slightly, from 5.2 to 4.3 mmol·l⁻¹, after 10 days during which no exercise was performed [50]. Liver glucose output decreased during this time by 60%, precisely the share normally derived from glycogen degradation [49]. The maintenance of blood glucose concentration was the result of an increased output of ketone bodies from the liver [49] and a shift from glucose to ketone-body oxidation by the brain.

Exercise and Diet

Glucose output from the liver increases during exercise. During prolonged cycling by four subjects at approximately 70% of V̇o₂max, a continuous increase in glucose output occurred from a resting value of 1 to a cycling value of 5 mmol·min⁻¹ just prior to exhaustion. The average glucose output over the entire exercise period was 2.4 mmol·min⁻¹[36].

In a separate experiment, liver glycogen content decreased at a rate of 2.1 mmol·kg⁻¹·min⁻¹ during 1 hour of heavy cycling in 14 subjects [38]. The majority of the glucose output from the liver was derived from glycogen, with only a small fraction from gluconeogenesis. When exercise was performed following a CHO-poor diet (low liver glycogen content), glucose output from liver glycogenolysis was necessarily low, and increased gluconeogenesis could only partially compensate for this decrease. Gluconeogenesis is a relatively slow process that usually cannot match the glucose uptake rate by the working muscles. This results in a significant decrease in blood glucose concentration shortly after the start of exercise performed following a CHO-poor diet. Mean glucose concentration decreased from 5.0 to 2.8 mmol·l⁻¹ after 1 hour of exercise, and at least one subject had to stop working due to dizziness induced by the effects of low blood glucose content (1.7 mmol·l⁻¹) on the central nervous system [4]. The corresponding mean blood glucose concentration after a CHO-rich diet was 4.4. mmol·l⁻¹ following 1 hour of exercise and 3.5 mmol·l⁻¹ at the end of exercise (~3 hours).

Conclusions

It appears that adequate or increased liver glycogen stores, maintained through proper dietary intake of CHO, would be beneficial in most types of prolonged continuous or intermittent work, especially if the work is intense (75% of $\dot{V}o_2$max or greater). During exercise of several hours duration, a high liver glycogen content will delay the onset of hypoglycemia and the risk of impaired central nervous system function and exhaustion. A single day on a CHO-rich diet before competition is sufficient to produce high levels of glycogen in the liver. However, since liver glycogen stores become depleted in approximately 1 day, an overnight fast may decrease

stores by up to 50%. This is important to athletes engaging in early-morning exercise, which is necessary in the case of many endurance events that attempt to avoid environmental stresses such as heat. Under these circumstances, CHO should be consumed 2 to 4 hours before the event, as will be discussed later, to ensure adequate liver glycogen content.

CARBOHYDRATE INTAKE IMMEDIATELY PRIOR TO AND DURING EXERCISE

Proper dietary intake during the days and hours prior to exercise, ending with a CHO-rich meal no later than 2 to 4 hours before exercise, is important to ensure that the liver glycogen store is full. Clearly, an adequate diet in the days before exercise can ensure that the nutritional aspects of performance will be optimal. We now turn to the effects of CHO ingestion immediately prior to (0–60 minutes) or during exercise on muscle metabolism and exercise performance.

Rationale Behind Carbohydrate Feedings

Extended exercise can lead to hypoglycemia if the liver glycogen store becomes depleted. Central nervous system dysfunction in the form of nausea and dizziness will then cause fatigue. Muscle glycogen depletion also produces fatigue during prolonged exercise at 65 to 85% of $\dot{V}o_2$max. In an attempt to prevent these events from occurring, CHO supplements are routinely given to athletes prior to and during long- or ultra-long-distance events such as running, cross-country skiing, and cycling. Carbohydrate supplements appear to be indicated (a) during extended periods of exercise when the workload is light to moderate (30–70% of $\dot{V}o_2$max) and longer than 2 hours in duration and (b) during exercise lasting at least 1 hour at a heavy to intense workload (70–85% of $\dot{V}o_2$max).

Metabolic Responses to Glucose Ingestion

Two of the major metabolic effects of glucose ingestion are transient increases in plasma glucose and insulin concentrations. Elevation of the insulin level can produce a subsequent decrease in glucose concentration. This is especially true during exercise, when muscular activity and high insulin level act synergistically to increase muscle glucose uptake. Blood glucose concentrations below 3.5 mmol · 1^{-1} are routinely seen, and occasionally hypoglycemia occurs (glucose concentration <2.5 mmol · 1^{-1}). In addition, insulin is a potent inhibitor of adipose tissue lipolysis. As discussed earlier, plasma FFAs are an important energy source during prolonged work at submaximal workloads up to approximately 70% of $\dot{V}o_2$max. The elevated insulin concentration following glucose ingestion will impede fat mobilization, reduce oxidation of plasma FFAs and consequently place a greater dependence on CHO for the provision of energy during exercise. The initial elevation of glucose concentration may also inhibit FFA release by enhancing glucose uptake in adipose tissue and providing substrate for the production of α-glycerophosphate, a required precursor for the reesterification of triacylglycerol. However, with the onset of exercise and the lowering of blood glucose levels, this effect disappears.

In endurance-trained athletes, plasma FFAs are oxidized at a greater rate than in untrained subjects at both the same absolute and relative submaximal workloads. Plasma FFAs also contribute significantly to energy production at workloads as high as 80 to 85% of $\dot{V}o_2$max in well-trained athletes, since they often exercise at these high work intensities during endurance races. Therefore, glucose ingestion, which impedes FFA mobilization, may be expected to adversely affect the performance of trained subjects, because it places a greater dependence on plasma glucose uptake and muscle glycogen stores for energy provision.

From the foregoing discussion it is apparent that several factors will determine whether CHO ingestion is indicated in a given situation. These factors include the exercise intensity and duration and the nutritional and training status of the subject. We now present some of the experimental work examining the effectiveness of CHO ingestion in various exercise situations.

Glucose Ingestion Immediately Prior to Exercise

The feeding of a glucose solution 30 to 60 minutes prior to exercise appears to be of little benefit; in some studies it reportedly has reduced subsequent exercise performance. An example is the study of Costill and coworkers [13]. These investigators gave seven well-trained subjects 75 g of glucose 45 minutes prior to exercise. Immediately before exercise, insulin level was increased threefold and plasma glucose level was elevated 40%. Subsequent running for 30 minutes at 70% of $\dot{V}o_2$max reduced the plasma glucose level to below 3.5 mmol · 1^{-1} in most subjects. Glycogen utilization in the gastrocnemius muscle was increased 17% and total CHO utilization increased 13%, compared with values in a control trial. The authors concluded that the elevated insulin level was responsible for the hypoglycemia, thereby decreasing the availability of plasma glucose. Plasma FFA concentration was also slightly reduced. These findings suggest that the reduced availability of exogenous substrates places a greater dependence on muscle glycogen for providing energy substrate during exercise.

In a subsequent study from the same laboratory [25], cycling endurance time was reduced by 19% in trained subjects following preexercise glucose feedings. Eight men and eight women cycled to exhaustion at 84% of $\dot{V}o_2$max 30 minutes after ingestion of water or 75 g or glucose. During exercise, blood glucose concentration was lowest in those who had ingested glucose, R-values were highest, and FFA mobilization was impeded.

It appeared that an enhanced rate of muscle glycogen utilization following glucose ingestion led to earlier onset of glycogen depletion and reduced exercise performance, compared with control values.

In a more recent study [31], however, these findings have not been duplicated. Six men were studied to compare the effects of preexercise feeding of glucose, fructose, or a placebo beverage on endurance performance and muscle glycogen utilization during cycling to exhaustion at 75% of $\dot{V}O_2$max. No differences were observed among the three treatments for oxygen uptake, R-values, exercise time to exhaustion, or utilization of muscle glycogen. Following glucose ingestion there was a transient increase in blood glucose and insulin concentrations, but these returned to normal within 30 minutes of onset of exercise and reactive hypoglycemia did not occur. Fructose ingestion did not increase blood glucose or insulin concentrations but did increase preexercise lactate concentrations.

Fructose Ingestion Immediately Prior to Exercise

Recently, investigators have attempted to circumvent the potential detrimental effects of glucose ingestion by giving fructose, which does not significantly increase plasma glucose or insulin concentrations. It has been known for several years that fructose is taken up by the liver [51] and also directly taken up by skeletal muscles without prior conversion to glucose in the liver [7]. The infusion of glucose or fructose into subjects after an overnight fast and without preceding exercise produced similar small increases in muscle glycogen, but fructose was taken up by the liver at a greater rate than glucose [51]. When muscle glycogen was depleted by exercise, the infusion of glucose was more effective than fructose infusion in replenishing glycogen stores [7]. Infusing large amounts of fructose was also associated with a significant increase in blood lactate concen-

tration [8]. When metabolized in the liver, fructose is phosphorylated to fructose-1-phosphate and then split into two triose molecules, dihydroxyacetone phosphate and glyceraldehyde. Glyceraldehyde is further metabolized to lactic acid, and dihydroxyacetone phosphate can be further metabolized upward in the glycolytic pathway to glucose and glycogen. For example, the infusion of 1.0 g of fructose per kilogram of body weight per hour for 3 hours (~210 g) increased blood lactate to a plateau of 5 to 6 $mmol \cdot l^{-1}$[8].

Studies examining the effect of fructose feedings have routinely compared the ingestion of 50 to 75 g of placebo, glucose, or fructose given 45 to 60 minutes prior to exercise on muscle glycogen utilization during submaximal exercise. Levine and colleagues [44] reported equal glycogen depletion in the gastrocnemius muscles of eight untrained subjects during 30 minutes of running at 75% of $\dot{V}O_2$max following control and glucose feedings. Significantly less glycogen was used following fructose ingestion. Total CHO utilization calculated from R-values was lowest in the control trial and was equal during the glucose and fructose conditions. This suggests that increased uptake of exogenous fructose spares muscle glycogen utilization, even though overall CHO utilization was increased compared with the control trial. It is also interesting to note that glucose feeding did not produce hypoglycemia during exercise, as is usually reported. This was probably due to the fact that most studies have used subjects fasted overnight, whereas the subjects in this study consumed both a CHO-rich diet for 3 days and a CHO-rich meal 4 hours prior to each trial.

Koivisto and coworkers [42] found no difference in the vastus lateralis muscle glycogen utilization of moderately active subjects during 2 hours of cycling at 50% of $\dot{V}O_2$max following placebo, glucose, or fructose ingestions. Muscle utilization of exogenous glucose was enhanced by both glucose and fructose feedings. During this prolonged exercise, plasma FFA concentration increased from 0.6 to 1.3 $mmol \cdot L^{-1}$ in the control condition but only from 0.5 to 0.7 or 0.8 $mmol \cdot L^{-1}$ after CHO ingestion.

Therefore, in work of moderate intensity, glucose and fructose ingestions prior to exercise increased uptake by the muscles but also decreased FFA uptake. This meant that the reliance on muscle glycogen as a substrate was not reduced, accounting for the lack of glycogen sparing. The findings of this study suggest that because subjects were fasted overnight, the major effect of the CHO feedings may have occurred in the liver, where the glycogen store would be less than full. Such a benefit may only show up during exercise lasting longer than 2 hours at this intensity. It should also be noted that resting blood lactate levels were slightly elevated after fructose ingestion, increasing from 0.7 to 1.5 $mmol \cdot L^{-1}$ in the 45 minutes prior to exercise. In the control and glucose conditions, no increases in lactate were seen. However, the elevated lactate concentration in the fructose trial disappeared during exercise.

In a similar study, glucose ingestion actually increased the utilization of muscle glycogen [32]. Thirty minutes of cycling at 75% of Vo_2max in eight untrained men decreased vastus lateralis muscle glycogen utilization by 43, 55, and 46 $mmol \cdot kg^{-1}$ in control, glucose, and fructose trials, respectively. Corresponding estimates of oxidized CHO were 64, 79, and 65 g. The authors concluded that fructose ingestion before exercise prevented the extra CHO oxidation and glycogen usage found after glucose ingestion. Also, if fructose ingestion had any benefit it would be in preserving liver glycogen stores during prolonged exercise at this workload.

In the most recent study from this group [31], ingestion of 75 g of fructose 45 minutes prior to cycle exercise at 75% or Vo_2max, when compared with ingestion of 75 g of glucose or a placebo, had no effect on substrate utilization during exercise, vastus lateralis muscle glycogen depletion, or exercise time to exhaustion. In a similar study, Devlin, Calles-Escandon, and Horton [19] found that eating a candy bar 30 minutes before cycle exercise at 70% of Vo_2max did not affect substrate utilization during exercise, endurance time to exhaustion, or muscle glycogen depletion. Blood glucose concentration was maintained better and post exercise ketosis was less after snack feeding than after placebo.

Conclusions

The ingestion of glucose or sucrose immediately prior to exercise is associated with a transient increase in plasma insulin concentration, which may increase the tendency to hypoglycemia during exercise. In addition, plasma FFA concentration may be reduced, and in some studies muscle glycogen utilization has been found to be enhanced and exercise performance reduced.

Other studies, however, have not found this deleterious effect of preexercise feeding of carbohydrates. If fructose is given, major fluctuations in plasma insulin and glucose concentrations are not seen, hypoglycemia is not a problem, and glycogen sparing may occur under certain conditions. However, during extended exercise at workloads up to 70% of Vo_2max, plasma FFAs represent a major energy source, and both glucose and fructose severely inhibit the mobilization of this important substrate [42]. Clearly, more work needs to be done to determine the effects of feeding in the immediate preexercise period on substrate utilization and performance during exercise of different intensities and durations.

Proper diet in the days before exercise maximizes muscles glycogen stores, and a CHO-rich meal 2 to 4 hours before exercise does the same for liver stores. A recent study [40] has shown that 68% of a 100-g glucose load taken 3 hours prior to exercise was metabolized during 4 hours of exercise at 45% of Vo_2max. During extended exercise when CHO supplements are required to prevent hypoglycemia, the CHO can be given in frequent small amounts of low-concentration solutions, as discussed in the following section. If CHO is taken immediately before exercise, it should be in the form of fructose and should be administered prior to athletic events only after testing in training sessions, due to the variability of beneficial effects and fructose tolerance among subjects.

CARBOHYDRATE INGESTION DURING EXERCISE

Christensen and Hansen [11] recognized the potential benefits of supplemental CHO and gave 200 g of glucose to an exhausted man who then worked for an extra hour. Bergström and Hultman [6] infused 170 to 210 g of glucose into untrained subjects during 70 minutes of cycling exercise at 70% of $\dot{V}O_2max$. The infusion increased mean blood glucose concentration from 4.6 $mmol \cdot L^{-1}$ in the control trial to 21.5 $mmol \cdot L^{-1}$, and produced a 25% reduction in muscle glycogen utilization. The authors concluded that the sparing of glycogen was small given the drastically increased blood glucose concentration and that muscle glycogen was the most important fuel during this intensity.

We must then ask whether oral ingestions of smaller amounts of CHO, which transiently increase glucose or fructose concentrations by only 2 to 3 $mmol \cdot l^{-1}$, are sufficient to spare muscle glycogen and enhance endurance performance. During work at 70% of $\dot{V}O_2max$, muscle uptake of exogenous glucose contributed 12% of the total energy required [12]. During exercise at lower workloads, such as walking at 45% of $\dot{V}O_2max$ for 2 hours, exogenous glucose provided up to 55% of the CHO metabolized and 24% of the total energy expenditure [52]. Plasma FFAs are also more important as an energy source at low to moderate workloads and less important at intense workloads [29, 33]. Carbohydrate feedings increase overall CHO metabolism but adversely affect the rate of FFA mobilization and oxidation in muscle at both moderate and intense workloads. Therefore, for CHO

feedings to spare muscle glycogen and enhance endurance performance at any exercise intensity, the increase in exogenous glucose uptake and oxidation by muscle must provide more energy than is lost by decreased FFA oxidation. If the muscle glycogen utilization rate is not reduced during extended exercise, endurance may still be enhanced, since CHO feedings may postpone liver glycogen depletion and delay the onset of hypoglycemia.

Some investigations employing glucose feedings during prolonged exercise have reported no clear increase in performance even when hypoglycemia is prevented [23]. However, a recent study [30] reported enhanced exercise performance and less glycogen utilization following periodic ingestions of a total of 170 g of glucose during 4 hours of cycling at 50% of $\dot{V}O_2max$. Total glycogen utilization in the glucose and control trials were 101 and 126 $mmol \cdot kg^{-1}$, respectively. Enhanced performance was measured during a sprint bout to exhaustion at 100% of $\dot{V}O_2max$ following the submaximal cycling. During the glucose trial, blood glucose concentrations were maintained at a higher level, R-values were elevated, and increases in plasma FFA levels were severely blunted [30].

In another study, endurance was increased from 134 to 157 minutes during intense cycling at 74% of $\dot{V}O_2max$ when repeated glucose feedings totaling 105 to 120 g were given [18]. Fatigue was postponed in 7 of the 10 trained cyclists. Plasma glucose concentration decreased in these seven subjects during the control trial, but only two were severely hypoglycemic, suggesting that slower muscle glycogen depletion accounted for the greater endurance in the other five. Increases in plasma FFA levels in the control trial were about half those reported at lower workloads, and were only slightly reduced in the glucose trial because R-values were unchanged. In conclusion, glucose feeding left three subjects totally unaffected, delayed fatigue in two others by postponing hypoglycemia, and delayed fatigue in the remaining five presumably by slowing muscle glycogen depletion. In a similar study, nine trained cyclists were asked to do as much work as possible in 2 hours on an isokinetic bicycle with and without glucose feedings [39]. The average work rate was 71% of $\dot{V}O_2$max, and performance was not enhanced during the initial 90 minutes in the glucose trial. In the final 30 minutes, the glucose feedings maintained plasma glucose levels significantly above the control trial concentrations and increased the total work output during this period. Both of these studies also demonstrated that the large fluctuations in glucose and insulin concentrations that occur following preexercise glucose feedings are largely reduced by feeding during exercise.

Conclusions

Scientific work has confirmed the practical observation that carbohydrate ingestion during extended work is associated with increased performance. Fatigue is delayed in some individuals by postponing the onset of hypoglycemia and in others by decreasing the rate of muscle glycogen utilization. However, the success of delaying fatigue is highly dependent on the manner in which carbohydrate supplements are given during exercise. Since fluid loss can be as high as 2 L/hour during marathon running, fluid supplements are usually required, especially during exercise in the heat. Carbohydrate is therefore normally given dissolved in water at concentrations of 140 to 280 mmol $\cdot L^{-1}$ (25–50 g $\cdot L^{-1}$). The glucose concentration of the ingested fluid must be maintained this low because research has demonstrated that hypertonic solutions exert an osmotic effect forcing water into the stomach, since gastric emptying occurs only when fluids are isotonic [16]. Approximately 800 ml of water and 200 mmol of glucose can be absorbed from the gastrointestinal tract every hour during prolonged severe exercise [16, 24]. To avoid the risk of gastric overfilling and

discomfort to the athlete, no more than 1L/hour should be taken, preferably in small amounts (150–250 ml) at 10 to 20 minute intervals. Often sodium chloride is added to the solution in low concentration (20–30 mmol $\cdot L^{-1}$) to replace lost electrolytes. Potassium supplement is usually not needed during exercise, due to the release of potassium when glycogen is utilized, although it is added in low concentration in some commercially available sport drinks. During exercise in the heat, this amount of water absorption, together with the water release from glycogen metabolism, may still fall short of the rate at which water is lost, leading to dehydration and reduced work output. Finally, in hot situations, dilute glucose solutions may be chilled to 6 to 10°C to enhance gastric emptying [16] and assist in lowering core body temperatures to prevent overheating.

ELEVATED PLASMA FFAs, MUSCLE METABOLISM, AND EXERCISE PERFORMANCE

Plasma FFAs represent a significant energy source during prolonged exercise at workloads up to 70% of $\dot{V}O_2$max in untrained or moderately active subjects. Well-trained athletes metabolize FFAs at higher rates than untrained subjects at relative submaximal workloads, and fat continues to contribute to energy production up to 80 to 85% of $\dot{V}O_2$max in these subjects. The mobilization of fat from adipose tissue and subsequent elevations in plasma FFA levels occur rather slowly during prolonged exercise. Since muscle FFA oxidation is linearly related to the concentration of plasma FFAs, reliance on fat as a substrate slowly increases with time while CHO dependence decreases. Consequently, researchers have attempted to enhance FFA utilization early in exercise by artificially elevating plasma FFA levels prior to exercise. If this is successful, CHO stores may be metabolized more slowly and endurance time prolonged, since muscle glycogen depletion is delayed. Second, if the

CHO utilization rate is unchanged but FFA utilization increases, a higher intensity of work may be sustained leading to a shorter time to complete a race.

Costill and colleagues [13] had trained subjects eat a fatty meal 4 to 5 hours prior to exercise, and followed this with the infusion of 2000 units of heparin 30 minutes prior to exercise. This procedure increased the preexercise FFA concentration from 0.21 $mmol \cdot L^{-1}$ in the control trial to 1.01 $mmol \cdot L^{-1}$. Heparin directly stimulates plasma lipoprotein lipase, the enzyme responsible for hydrolyzing circulating triacylglycerol. Glycogen utilization was reduced by 40% in the heparin trial during 30 minutes of running at 70% of $\dot{V}O_2max$. Plasma glucose concentration was unaffected and R-values were significantly lower following heparin infusion compared with the control values. This study suggests that increasing the availability of plasma FFAs prior to or early in exercise reduces the rate of CHO utilization in human skeletal muscle.

Later studies [9, 14, 21, 39] examined the effects of caffeine ingestion on muscle metabolism and exercise performance. Caffeine is known to directly increase the mobilization of FFAs from adipose tissue by inhibiting the breakdown of the enzyme responsible for the degradation of cyclic adenosine monophosphate. Work from Costill's laboratory has demonstrated that 250 to 400 mg of caffeine ingested in the final hour prior to exercise enhances cycling endurance performance [14, 39]. This was true for trained cyclists and active noncyclists. The amount of caffeine ingested was the equivalent of two to four cups of percolated coffee. Caffeine also enhanced FFA mobilization, increased muscle fat oxidation, and reduced muscle glycogen utilization [21]. However, when caffeine was administered to trained or untrained runners, FFA mobilization was only marginally increased and no changes in substrate utilization were noted [9]. The ineffectiveness of caffeine ingestion during running may be linked to the amount of muscle mass involved. In cycling, a smaller muscle mass is required, and any increase in FFA concentration is distributed to these working muscles. In running, the increase in circulating FFAs would be distributed over a larger muscle mass, and a significant increase in fat oxidation may not be seen.

If caffeine is ingested prior to exercise in an attempt to enhance performance, it should be remembered that it has been proved beneficial only in cycling exercise. Additionally, large individual variations exist among individuals in their normal FFA response to prolonged exercise, and therefore the success of caffeine ingestion will also vary markedly among individuals. Also unknown is the effect the amount of caffeine normally consumed on a daily basis will have on the success of acute caffeine ingestion.

Last, we must emphasize that large fatty meals prior to competition are of no benefit and are not recommended, because they may cause gastrointestinal discomfort and because consumption of excess amounts of fat is linked to cardiovascular disease. Heparin involvement is also not advised, because heparin must be injected.

SUMMARY

Skeletal muscles metabolize dietary fuels or foodstuffs to produce energy for mechanical work. Fat and carbohydrate (CHO) are the major fuels utilized during exercise; protein is not a significant fuel during activity in healthy well-fed individuals. Fat is stored in extremely large amounts in adipose tissue, and the rate of fat mobilization is the factor limiting free fatty acid oxidation in exercising muscles. Carbohydrate is the major fuel at workloads above 50% of maximal oxygen uptake ($\dot{V}O_2max$), because it can be metabolized both aerobically and anaerobically. However, the limited glycogen stores present in muscle and liver can be depleted during prolonged exercise. For these reasons, proper CHO intake in the days and hours prior to and the hours during prolonged exercise is of paramount importance for optimal exercise performance.

The depletion of muscle glycogen stores during prolonged exercise at 65 to 85% of $\dot{V}O_2$max results in fatigue. If liver glycogen stores are depleted, the onset of hypoglycemia can also limit endurance performance. When muscle glycogen stores are significantly increased prior to exercise through dietary CHO "supercompensation" regimens, exercise endurance is enhanced. A CHO-rich meal 2 to 4 hours before exercise will ensure that the labile liver glycogen store is replenished. However, CHO ingestion in the final hour preceding exercise is not recommended, since it may induce hypoglycemia early in the exercise, place greater demands on muscle glycogen stores, and reduce endurance performance. The ingestion of CHO during exercise is recommended only during extended activity at moderate to heavy workloads. Endurance performance may be enhanced by delaying muscle glycogen depletion and/or the onset of hypoglycemia.

The proper management of CHO intake prior to and during exercise ensures that the nutritional aspects of exercise endurance performance are optimal.

REFERENCES

1. Ahlborg, G., P. Felig, L. Hagenfeldt, R. Hendler, and J. Wahren. Substrate turnover during prolonged exercise in man. *J. Clin. Invest.* 53:1080–1090, 1974.
2. Asmussen, E. Muscle metabolism during exercise in man: A historical survey. In Pernow, B., and B. Saltin (eds.). *Muscle Metabolism During Exercise.* New York: Plenum Press, 1971, pp. 1–12.
3. Bergström, J. Muscle electrolytes in man, determined by neutron activation analysis on needle biopsy specimens: A study on normal subjects, kidney patients, and patients with chronic diarrhea. *Scand. J. Clin. Lab. Invest.* (Suppl.) 68:1–110, 1962.
4. Bergström, J., L. Hermansen, E. Hultman, and B. Saltin. Diet, muscle glycogen and physical performance. *Acta Physiol. Scand.* 71:140–150, 1967.
5. Bergström, J., and E. Hultman. Muscle glycogen synthesis after exercise: An enhancing factor localized to the muscle cells in man. *Nature* 210:309–310, 1966.
6. Bergström, J., and E. Hultman. A study of the glycogen metabolism during exercise in man. *Scand. J. Clin. Lab. Invest.* 19:218–228, 1967.
7. Bergström, J., and E. Hultman. Synthesis of muscle glycogen in man after glucose and fructose ingestion. *Acta Med. Scand.* 182:93–107, 1967.
8. Bergström, J., E. Hultman, and A.E. Roch-Norlund. Lactic acid accumulation in connection with fructose infusion. *Acta Med. Scand.* 184:359–364, 1968.
9. Casal, D.C., and A.S. Leon. Failure of caffeine to affect substrate utilization during prolonged running. *Med. Sci. Sports Exer.* 17:174–179, 1985.
10. Cheetham, M.E., L.H. Boobis, S. Brooks, and C. Williams. Human muscle metabolism during sprint running. *J. Appl. Physiol.* 61:54–60, 1986.
11. Christensen, E.H., and O. Hansen, I. Zur Mehodik der respiratorischen Quotient-Bestimmungen in Ruhe und Arbeit. II. Untersuchungen über die Verbrennungs-Vorgänge bei langdauernder, schwere Muskelarbeit. III. Arbeitsfähigkeit und Ernährung. *Skand. Arch. Physiol.* 81:137–171, 1939.
12. Costill, D.L., A. Bennett, G. Branam, and D. Eddy. Glucose ingestion at rest and during prolonged exercise. *J. Appl. Physiol.* 34:764–769, 1973.
13. Costill, D.L., E. Coyle, G. Dalsky, W. Evans, W. Fink, and D. Hoopes. Effects of elevated plasma FFA and insulin on muscle glycogen usage during exercise. *J. Appl. Physiol.* 43:695–699, 1977.
14. Costill, D.L., G.P. Dalsky, and W.J. Fink. Effects of caffeine ingestion on metabolism and exercise performance. *Med. Sci. Sports Exer.* 10:155–158, 1978.
15. Costill, D.L., P.D. Gollnick, E.D. Jansson, B. Saltin, and E.M. Stein. Glycogen depletion pattern in human muscle fibers during distance running. *Acta Physiol. Scand.* 89:374–383, 1973.
16. Costill, D.L., and B. Saltin. Factors limiting gastric emptying during rest and exercise. *J. Appl. Physiol.* 37:679–683, 1974.
17. Costill, D.L., K. Sparks, R. Gregor, and C. Turner. Muscle glycogen utilization during exhaustive running. *J. Appl. Physiol.* 31:353–356, 1971.
18. Coyle, E.F., J.M. Hagberg, B.F. Hurley, W.H. Martin, A.A. Ehsani, and J.O. Holloszy. Carbohydrate feeding during prolonged exercise can delay fatigue. *J. Appl. Physiol.* 55:230–235, 1983.
19. Devlin, J.T., J. Calles-Escandon, and E.S. Horton. Effects of preexercise snack feeding on endurance cycle exercise. *J. Appl. Physiol.* 60(3):980–985, 1986.
20. Essén, B. Studies on the regulation of metabolism in human skeletal muscle using intermittent exercise as an experimental model *Acta Physiol. Scand.* (Suppl.) 454:1–31, 1978.
21. Essig, D., D.L. Costill, and P.J. vanHandel. Effects of caffeine ingestion on utilization of muscle glycogen and lipid during leg ergometer cycling. *Int. J. Sports Med.* 1:86–90, 1980.
22. Felig, P. Amino acid metabolism in man. *Annu. Rev. Biochem.* 44:933–955, 1975.
23. Felig, P., A. Cherif, A. Minagawa, and J. Wahren. Hypoglycemia during prolonged exercise in normal men. *N. Engl. J. Med.* 306:895–900, 1982.

24. Fordtran, J.S., and B. Saltin. Gastric emptying and intestinal absorption during prolonged severe exercise. *J. Appl. Physiol.* 23:331–335, 1967.

25. Foster, C., D.L. Costill, and W.J. Fink. Effects of preexercise feedings on endurance performance. *Med. Sci. Sports Exer.* 11:1–5, 1979.

26. Fröberg, S.O., L.A. Carlson, and L.-G. Ekelund. Local lipid stores and exercise. In Pernow, B., and B. Saltin (eds.). *Muscle Metabolism During Exercise*. New York: Plenum Press, 1971, pp. 307–313.

27. Fröberg, S.O., and F. Mossfeldt. Effect of prolonged strenuous exercise on the concentration of triglycerides, phospholipids and glycogen in muscle of man. *Acta Physiol. Scand.* 82:167–171, 1971.

28. Green, H.J. Glycogen depletion patterns during continuous and intermittent ice skating. *Med. Sci. Sports* 10:183–187, 1978.

29. Hagenfeldt, L., and J. Wahren. Metabolism of free fatty acids and ketone bodies in skeletal muscle. In Pernow, B., and B. Saltin (eds.). *Muscle Metabolism During Exercise*. New York: Plenum Press, 1971, pp. 153–163.

30. Hargreaves, M., D.L. Costill, A. Coggan, W.J. Fink, and I. Nishibata. Effect of carbohydrate feedings on muscle utilization and exercise performance. *Med. Sci. Sports Exer.* 16:219–222, 1984.

31. Hargreaves, M., D.L. Costill, W.J. Fink, D.S. King, and R.A. Fielding. Effect of pre-exercise carbohydrate feedings on endurance cycling performance. *Med. Sci. Sports Exer.* 19:33–36, 1987.

32. Hargreaves, M., D.L. Costill, A. Katz, and W.J. Fink. Effect of fructose ingestion on muscle glycogen usage during exercise. *Med. Sci. Sports Exer.* 17:360–363, 1985.

33. Havel, R.J., A. Naimark, and C.F. Borchgrevink. Turnover rate and oxidation of free fatty acids of blood plasma in man during exercise: Studies during continuous infusion of palmitate-1-C^{14}. *J. Clin. Invest.* 42:1054–1063, 1963.

34. Hermansen, L., E. Hultman, and B. Saltin. Muscle glycogen during prolonged severe exercise. *Acta Physiol. Scand.* 71:129–139, 1967.

35. Holloszy, J.O., and E.F. Coyle. Adaptations of skeletal muscle to endurance exercise and their metabolic consequences. *J. Appl. Physiol.* 56:831–838, 1984.

36. Hultman, E. Studies on muscle metabolism of glycogen and active phosphate in man with special reference to exercise and diet. *Scand. J. Clin. Lab. Invest.* (Suppl.) 94:1–63, 1967.

37. Hultman, E., and J. Bergstöm. Muscle glycogen synthesis in relation to diet studied in normal subjects. *Acta Med. Scand.* 182:109–117, 1967.

38. Hultman, E., and L.H. Nilsson. Liver glycogen in man: Effect of different diets and muscular exercise. In Pernow, B., and B. Saltin (eds.). *Muscle Metabolism During Exercise*. New York: Plenum Press, 1971, pp. 143–151.

39. Ivy, J.L., D.L. Costill, W.J. Fink, and R.W. Lower. Influence of caffeine and carbohydrate feedings on endurance performance. *Med. Sci. Sports Exer.* 11:6–11, 1979.

40. Jandrain, B., G. Krzentowski, F. Pirnay, F. Mosora, M. Lacroix, A. Luyckx, and P. Lefebvre. Metabolic availability of glucose ingested 3 h before

prolonged exercise. *J. Appl. Physiol.* 56:1314–1319, 1984.

41. Karlsson, J., and B. Saltin. Diet, muscle glycogen, and endurance performance. *J. Appl. Physiol.* 31:203–206, 1971.

42. Koivisto, V.A., M. Härkönen, S.-L. Karonen, P.H. Groop, R. Elovaino, E. Ferrannini, L. Sacca, and R.A. Defronzo. Glycogen depletion during prolonged exercise: Influence of glucose, fructose, or placebo. *J. Appl. Physiol.* 58:731–737, 1985.

43. Krogh, A., and J. Lindhard. The relative value of fat and carbohydrate as sources of muscular energy (with appendices on the correlation between stanard metabolism and the respiratory quotient during rest and work). *Biochem. J.* 14:290–363, 1920.

44. Levine, L., W.J. Evans, B.S. Cadarette, E.C. Fisher, and B.A. Bullen. Fructose and glucose ingestion and muscle glycogen use during submaximal exercise. *J. Appl. Physiol.* 55:1767–1771, 1983.

45. McCartney, N., L.L. Spriet, G.J.F. Heigenhauser, J.M. Kowalchuk, J.R. Sutton, and N.L. Jones. Muscle power and metabolism in maximal intermittent exercise. *J. Appl. Physiol.* 60:1164–1169, 1986.

46. McGilvery, R.W. The use of fuels for muscular work. In Howald, H., and J.R. Poortmans (eds.). *Metabolic Adaptations to Prolonged Physical Exercise*. Basel: Birkhäuser Verlag, 1975, pp. 12–30.

47. Munro, H.N. Control of plasma amino acid concentrations. In Wolstenholme, G.E.W., and Sitzsimons, D.W. (eds.). *Aromatic Amino Acids in the Brain*. Ciba Foundation Symposium 22. New York: Elsevier, 1974, pp. 5–18.

48. Nilsson, L.H. Liver glycogen content in man in the post-absorptive state. *Scand. J. Clin. Lab. Invest.* 32:317–323, 1973.

49. Nilsson, L.H., P. Fürst, and E. Hultman. Carbohydrate metabolism of the liver in normal man under varying dietary conditions. *Scand. J. Clin. Lab. Invest.* 32:331–337, 1973.

50. Nilsson, L.H., and E. Hultman. Liver glycogen in man: The effect of total starvation or a carbohydrate-poor diet followed by carbohydrate refeeding. *Scan. J. Clin. Lab. Invest.* 32:325–330, 1973.

51. Nilsson, L.H., and E. Hultman. Liver and muscle glycogen in man after glucose and fructose infusion. *Scand. J. Clin. Lab. Invest.* 33:5–10, 1974.

52. Pirnay, F., M. Lacroix, F. Mosora, A. Luyckx, and P. Lefebvre. Glucose oxidation during prolonged exercise evaluated with naturally labelled ^{13}C glucose. *J. Appl. Physiol.* 43:258–261, 1977.

53. Rennie, M.J., R.H.T. Edwards, S. Krywawych, C.T.M. Davies, D. Halliday, J.C. Waterlow, and D.J. Millward. Effect of exercise on protein turnover in man. *Clin. Sci.* 61:627–639, 1981.

54. Saltin, B., and J. Karlsson. Muscle glycogen utilization during work of different intensities. In Pernow, B., and B. Saltin (eds.). *Muscle Metabolism During Exercise*. New York: Plenum Press, 1971, pp. 289–299.

55. Sherman, W.M., D.L. Costill, W.J. Fink, and J.M. Miller. Effect of exercise–diet manipulation on muscle glycogen and its subsequent utilization during performance. *Int. J. Sports Med.* 2:114–118, 1981.

Chapter 10

FLUID AND ELECTROLYTE BALANCE DURING PROLONGED EXERCISE

Bengt Saltin, M.D., and David Costill, Ph.D.

An individual's physical performance capacity in endurance events is primarily restricted by the ability of the oxygen transport system and the capacity of the muscle tissue to utilize oxygen. A number of secondary factors influence the tolerable intensity and duration of the exercise bout, including water and electrolyte losses produced by heavy sweating. This chapter will describe the influence of these factors on performance during prolonged exercise.

SWEATING: HEAT, WATER, AND MINERAL LOSSES

As a result of the increased rate of metabolic heat production during exercise, the body's core temperature (central nervous system, thorax, abdominal cavity) is significantly elevated. This is true over a wide range of workloads and ambient temperatures. In his notable experiments, Nielsen [21] demonstrated that after about 30 minutes of exercise, rectal temperature had adjusted to the new level, and this level was then maintained until the completion of exercise, returning to the normal resting level within a half hour. The steady-state temperature during exercise is related to exercise intensity [32]. However, there are situations (e.g., swimming, light work without heavy clothing in cold weather, and heavy work in

very warm surroundings) in which the mechanisms of body temperature regulation are incapable of maintaining heat balance.

The temperatures in the skin and the muscle are also of interest from the point of view of heat regulation (Figure 1). Muscle temperature at rest is usually less than core temperature, but rises very quickly when muscles are put to work [31]. With an ambient temperature of 20°C, temperature gradient between the warmest part of the muscle and the arterial blood or core temperature is about 0.6°C. Skin temperature is not affected significantly by work intensity, but ambient temperature has a direct influence on it. Irrespective of workload, skin temperature is approximately 28, 30.5, and 33°C when ambient temperature is 10, 20 and 30°C, respectively (Figure 2 [37]).

Heat exchange with the environment enables the body to maintain a constant temperature even at different levels of energy metabolism. When heat losses via convection, radiation, conduction, and respiratory channels (insensible water loss) are insufficient, water also evaporates from the skin as sweat (Figure 3). In windless conditions, about 7 kcal disappear per hour from each square meter of body surface area (8 W/m² through radiation and convection per degree of temperature gradient between skin and surroundings) [24]. In steady-state conditions, remaining heat is disposed of through sweat-

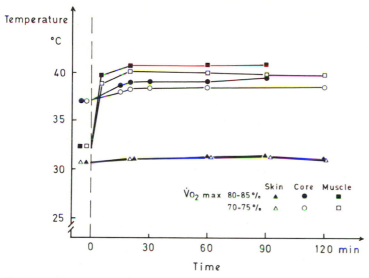

Figure 1. Temperatures in a leg muscle (vastus lateralis), temperatures in the core of the body (esophageal), and mean skin temperatures of a person during exercise at two intensities, one demanding approximately 70 to 75% and the other demanding 80 to 85% of maximal oxygen uptake, in an environmental temperature of 20°C (Data combined from 30, 32, and 37).

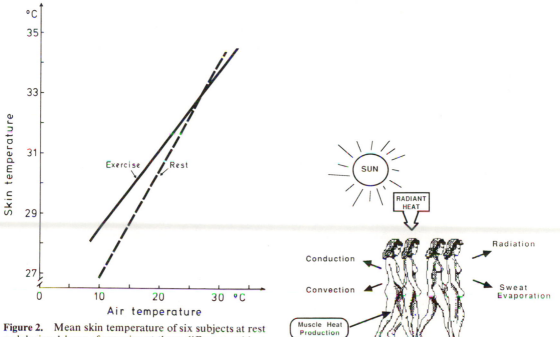

Figure 2. Mean skin temperature of six subjects at rest and during 1 hour of exercise at three different ambient temperatures with an oxygen uptake varying from 1.1 to 3.6 L/min. Of note is that the ambient temperature but not exercise has an influence on the skin temperature. (Data from 37).

Figure 3. Schematic illustration of heat exchange between an exercising woman and the surrounding environment.

ing, the magnitude of which can be calculated from the following equation:

$$\text{Sweat heat loss} = M \pm S \pm (R + C) - E$$

In this calculation, M stands for heat production through energy metabolism, S is heat stored in the body, B is radiation, C is convection, and E is heat consumed in the respiratory evaporation of water. When air temperature exceeds 32°C, the disposal of water via respiratory channels is limited [3].

Even with very heavy loads in warm surroundings, sweating does not start until work has gone on for 0.5 to 3 minutes; it then displays a linear increase until leveling off after 10 to 15 minutes of work [30]. The body's core temperature does not change in step with sweating when work is begun, but skin and muscle temperature, taken together, covary closely with sweating. In steady-state conditions, the correlation coefficient between skin, muscle, core temperature, and sweat rate approaches 1.0 [30, 31]. Thus, good covariation between temperature in different tissues and the magnitude of sweating can be demonstrated. However, it is not certain that these temperatures alone are active in the regulation of sweating. The existence of a factor unrelated to a tissue temperature in the body but related to, for example, the absolute magnitude of energy output may be required to provide a complete explanation of perspiration regulation during exercise [36].

A theoretical calculation of fluid loss through sweating is relatively easy with the aid of the equation given previously, at least in the case of cycling and running, in which the degree of mechanical efficiency is around 20% in these forms of exercise. This means that the remaining 80% of the energy metabolism is converted into heat. Current evidence indicates that fluid loss of 1 to 2 L/hr is quite common at around 20°C (Table 1). The observed values exceed the estimated values in Table 1 because part of the sweat produced did not evaporate from the skin, but fell to the ground in drops or remained in clothing. The calculations were made for windless conditions, and this causes a certain amount of error (e.g., in cycling), but the error is undoubtedly very small in other forms of exercise or at low ambient temperatures, when clothing counteracts any major increase in heat loss through convection. However, large amounts of heat can still be given off through convection during walking on a treadmill at a speed of 5 to 10 km/hr, 10 to 15 w/m²/°temperature gradient are lost [24]. Heat losses through convection are especially great from arms and legs.

DEHYDRATION: EFFECTS ON BODY FLUID VOLUMES

Traditional studies of the change in body water compartments during prolonged exer-

Table 1.   LOSS OF BODY FLUIDS DURING RUNNING
AT LOW OR HIGH SPEED

AMBIENT TEMPERATURE (NO WIND) °C	LOW SPEED CALCULATED* (L/HR)	HIGH SPEED, CALCULATED (L/HR)	HIGH SPEED, OBSERVED† (L/HR)
−5	0.3	1.1	1.1(0.6−1.4)
+10	0.6	1.5	1.6(1.2−1.5)
+20	0.9	1.8	2.0 (1.6−2.4)
+30	1.1	2.1	2.4 (2.0−2.8)

*Calculated values are based on subjects with a weight of 70 kg, working with 80% of their maximal oxygen uptake. Trained subjects have maximal oxygen uptake of 5.0 L/min; untrained have 3.0 L/min uptake. It is further assumed that clothing is adjusted to the ambient temperature.

†Observed values taken from unpublished investigations in different sports.

cise have been confined to measurements of constituents in plasma. Attempts to measure the distribution of water and ions between intracellular and extracellular spaces during muscular activity have been invalidated by the movement of proteins and isotope markers (e.g., ^{125}I-albumin, T-1824) between the various compartments. Since the mid-1960s, studies have been conducted using approaches such as an isolated leg muscle preparation in the cat [16] and the muscle biopsy procedure in humans [4, 7, 23], to determine the changes in water and electrolytes in muscle tissue during exercise. If we assume that the changes in plasma water and electrolytes during exertion are representative of changes in interstitial fluids, then it is possible to describe the influence of acute exercise and subsequent dehydration on various body fluid compartments.

On the basis of these methods, it has been shown that the water and electrolytes for production of sweat come initially from extracellular sources, though the losses are subsequently distributed evenly between the intracellular and extracellular compartments (Figure 4). The extracellular compartment includes both plasma and interstitial tissue water. There is rapid exchange of water between plasma and extravascular sources. When total body water declines during work, the level of plasma water is relatively well maintained [18]. Thus, water losses in absolute figures are, in large part, made up from intracellular water. The result is intracellular dehydration, which may impair cellular metabolism. Because perspiration is hypotonic, extracellular water tends to become hypertonic, a circumstance that contributes to intracellular dehydration. On the other hand, the osmolality in the exercising cell may be enhanced, which partly counteracts the flux of the water from the cell [19, 35].

DEHYDRATION: EFFECTS ON PERFORMANCE

Several studies have shown that a reduction in body water causes pronounced impairment of work ability with physical labor of long duration. Incomplete replacement of water losses also leads to increases in body temperature and pulse rate that are greater than normal [6, 28]. This occurs when fluid loss corresponds to about 2% or more of body weight. If the loss should amount to 4 to 5% of body weight, the capacity for very hard muscular work must be expected to decline by 20 to 30% (Figure 5). The risk of circulatory collapse is very great with work in a warm environment with dehydration amounting to 10% of body weight [1], though tolerance for exercise in the heat is markedly reduced with as little as 2% dehydration [6].

It has been shown that maximal oxygen uptake is unaffected by up to 4% dehydration [2, 29]. However, running performance is significantly impaired. Following the intake of a diuretic (40 mg of furosemide), subjects lost 1.2 to 1.6 kg of body water and experienced a reduction in plasma volume of 9.9 to 12.3% [2]. As a result, the runners' performance in test runs of 1500, 5000, and 10,000 m was reduced by 3.1, 6.7, and 6.3% respectively.

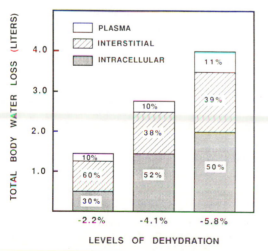

Figure 4. Distribution of water losses from intracellular, plasma, and interstitial compartments during varied levels of exercise-induced dehydration.

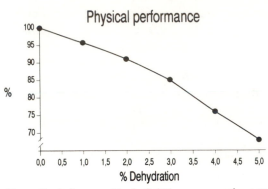

Figure 5. Influence of body fluid loss on exercise performance during intense endurance-type exercise. The decline in performance is based on measurements of power output and/or work done to exhaustion using an intense work load. This exercise was performed after various levels of dehydration and the performance was compared with measurements obtained during control conditions.

In a series of experiments, Nielsen et al. [22] have described in more detail the relative role of water losses, ion losses, elevated body heat, and reduction in availability of substrates in performance capacity. On separate days approximately a week apart, Nielsen let her subjects take diuretics ("pure" water loss), stay in a sauna (water and ion losses), submerge in hot water (elevated body temperature), and perform 2 hours of intense bicycle exercise (water and ion losses, elevated body temperature, and reduction in availability of substrates). Elevation of body temperature caused about the same reduction in work performance as did loss of water; a further small reduction was observed with water and ion losses after the sauna. The largest reduction in work performance occurred after the exercise challenge. Thus, all the treatment conditions appeared to play a role in the deterioration of work performance. If optimum performance at the end of prolonged effort is desired, efforts must be made to minimize water and ion losses as well as increase in body temperature, and ample substrates should be available.

The decline in work ability with dehydra-

tion cannot be accommodated through heat acclimatization, even though this leads to increased sweating with a lower salt content in the sweat [1]. Thus, the need for adequate water intake during exercise has been well documented. However, certain results suggest that trained persons more easily tolerate dehydration in exercise than do untrained persons [5, 6]. Unfortunately, humans cannot use thirst alone to gauge the amount of water that is lost through heavy sweating. This is particularly true during work. Only about 50% of the amount of water required is, in fact, voluntarily taken [1, 9, 13]. This phenomenon has been designated "voluntary dehydration during work." It is therefore necessary for people to take water beyond their subjective needs during work to prevent dehydration. Small-volume, frequent forced drinking is recommended before and during work efforts of long duration. Overhydration has never been described in persons with normal renal function, nor has increased water intake during exercise been found to lead to a pronounced increase in sweating beyond requirements. In fact, no negative effects of forced drinking have been documented.

ELECTROLYTE LOSSES

The exact content of sodium, chloride, potassium, and other ions in sweat has not been established. This is in part related to the difficulties of sampling sweat and ascertaining that the samples truly represent all parts of the body throughout the exercise. The problem has been considered by many researchers, and good critical reviews are available [27, 38]. Representative data, shown in Table 2, are taken from the work of Costill and coworkers [7]. Subjects experienced rather high sweat rates, were partly heat acclimatized, and had normal water and electrolyte stores at the start of the experiment. It should be noted that loss of sodium and chloride ions is substantially lower in heat acclimatized persons; it may be twice as

Table 2. ELECTROLYTE CONCENTRATIONS AND OS-MOLALITY IN SWEAT, PLASMA, AND MUSCLE OF MEN FOL-LOWING 2 HOURS OF EXERCISE IN THE HEAT

| | ELECTROLYTES (mEq/L) | | | | OSMOLALITY (mOsm/L) |
	Na^+	Cl^-	K^+	Mg^{++}	
Sweat	40–60	30–50	4–6	1.5–5	80–185
Plasma	140	101	4	1.5	302
Muscle	9	6	162	31	302

high in completely unacclimatized subjects who are sweating profusely.

Sodium and chloride are the dominant ions of the blood. Table 2 shows that the concentrations of sodium and chloride in sweat are roughly one-third those in plasma and five times those in muscle. The ionic concentration of sweat may vary markedly between individuals and, as mentioned earlier, is strongly influenced by the rate of sweating and the runner's state of heat acclimatization.

At the high rates of sweating reported during exercise in the heat, sweat contains relatively high levels of sodium and chloride, but little potassium, calcium, and magnesium. A sweat loss of nearly 4 L, representing a 5.8% reduction in body weight, resulted in sodium, potassium, chloride, and magnesium losses of 155, 16, 137, and 13 mEQ, respectively [7]. On the basis of estimates of the runner's body mineral content, these losses would lower the body's sodium and chloride content by roughly 5 to 7% At the same time, total body levels of potassium and magnesium, two ions principally confined to the inside of the cells, would decrease by less than 1.2% .

At the same time that electrolytes are lost from the body in sweat, there is a redistribution of the remaining ions among various tissues and organs. One such example is K^+. K^+ leaves contracting muscle fibers and contributes to the plasma K^+ pool during exercise [34]. However, the elevation in extracellular K^+ content is less than the K^+ release from active muscles, because inactive muscles and other tissues take up K^+

(Figure 6) [33]. During recovery following exercise, normalization of intracellular K^+ appears to occur rather rapidly [20, 33]. This redistribution cycle for K^+ in exercise and recovery is an efficient mechanism to conserve K^+ in the body. However, it does not eliminate the possibility that loss of K^+ from active muscles during prolonged exercise may be one factor that can contribute to impaired muscular function during exercise [34]. Endurance training appears to reduce the rate of K^+ loss from contracting skeletal muscle [14]. This may be related to the elevated number of $Na^+ - K^+$ pump sites

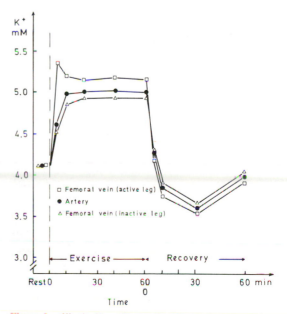

Figure 6. Illustration of potassium fluxes in an exercising and an inactive limb. [Data from 20 and 33].

[15] and greater $Na^+ - K^+$-activated ATPase [17] in skeletal muscle with training.

The other major source of electrolyte loss is via urine production. Under normal conditions, kidneys excrete about 50 ml of water per hour. During exercise, however, blood flow to the kidneys decreases, and urine production drops to near zero. Consequently, electrolyte losses by this avenue are quite diminished during exercise. There is another interesting facet of the renal management of electrolytes that is worthy of note. If an individual consumer eats 250 mEq of Na^+ and Cl^- per day, the kidneys will normally excrete an equal amount of these electrolytes to keep the body levels constant. Heavy sweating and dehydration, however, cause the release of aldosterone from the adrenal gland, a hormone that stimulates the kidneys to reabsorb Na^+ and CL^- As a result, after recovery the body's total Na^+ content is increased. This, of course, is accompanied by expansion of the extracellular fluid compartment. Repeated days of exercise in the heat, for example, have been shown to produce a 10 to 15% increase in plasma volume [11]. This expansion of the extracellular compartment appears to be only temporary, the compartment returning to normal within 48 to 72 hours after the cessation of exercise and heat exposure.

WATER AND ELECTROLYTE REPLACEMENT

Since the body loses more water than electrolytes during heavy sweating, the concentration of these minerals rises in the body fluids. Thus, even though there is a net loss of electrolytes from the body, the plasma electrolyte concentrations actually increase. Although this may seem confusing, it simply illustrates that during periods of heavy sweating, the need to replace body water is greater than the need to replace electrolytes.

There are obvious benefits to drinking fluids during prolonged exercise, especially during hot weather. Drinking will minimize

dehydration, lessen the rise in internal body temperature, and reduce the stress placed on the circulatory system [26]. It appears that the composition of fluids ingested during exercise has an effect on the rate that the fluid empties from the stomach [10]. Since little absorption of water occurs directly from the stomach, the fluids must pass into the intestine before entering the blood. In the intestine, absorption is rapid and unaffected by exercise, provided that the activity does not exceed 75% of the runner's $\dot{V}O_2$max [10, 12]. Many factors affect the rate at which the stomach empties including its volume, temperature, acidity, and the concentration of solutes (osmolality) [10].

Although large volumes of up to 600 ml empty faster from the stomach than do small portions, runners generally find it uncomfortable to run with a nearly full stomach, as this interferes with breathing. Drinking 100 to 200 ml at 10- to 15-minute intervals tends to minimize this effect.

Cold drinks have been found to empty more rapidly from the stomach than warm fluids. Although fluids at refrigerator temperatures of from 3 to 4°C may reduce the temperature of the stomach from 37 to 9 or 10°C, they do not appear to cause stomach cramps. Such stomach distress occurs more often when the volume of the drink is unusually large. It has been suggested that intake of very cold fluids may affect the normal electrical activity of the heart. Although some electrocardiographic changes have been reported in a few individuals following the ingestion of very cold drinks (4°C), the medical significance of these changes has not been established. It seems that drinking cold fluids during prolonged exercise in the heat seems to pose no threat to a normal heart.

Another factor known to regulate the rate at which the stomach empties is the osmolality of the fluid. Drink osmolalities above 200 mOsm/L tend to move out of the stomach more slowly than those below that level [10]. Thus, the addition of electrolytes and/or other ingredients that raise the osmolality can actually slow the rate of fluid replacement. However, solutions having high osmolalities may not have so marked a retarding effect on gastric emptying during running, as more recent studies have revealed that carbohydrate-rich solutions can be emptied rather quickly from the stomach [25; Mitchel et al. personal communication]. Since dehydration is the primary concern during hot-weather exercise, water seems to be the preferred fluid. Under less stressful conditions, where overheating and large sweat losses are not as threatening, runners might use liquid feedings to supplement their carbohydrate supplies.

A number of commercially available water—electrolyte solutions are available for use during exercise and work in the heat. Unfortunately, many of the claims used to sell these drinks are based on misinterpreted and often inaccurate information. Electrolytes, for example, have long been listed as important ingredients in sports drinks. But research shows that such claims are unfounded. A single meal adequately replaces the electrolytes lost during exercise. The body needs water to bring its concentration of the electrolytes back into balance. While the importance of minerals such as sodium, potassium, and magnesium should not be underestimated, blood and muscle biopsy studies have shown that heavy sweating has little or no sustained effect on water and electrolyte concentrations in body fluids [7, 23].

The control processes that regulate fluid volumes and electrolyte concentrations are quite effective. For example, it is normally difficult to consume too much water and dilute plasma electrolytes. Even marathoners who lose 3 to 5 L of sweat and drink 2 to 3 L of water retain normal plasma sodium, chloride, and potassium concentrations. Distance runners who run 25 to 40 km/day in warm weather and do not season their food, do not develop electrolyte deficiencies. Even subjects fed only 30% as much potassium as they normally consume and made to dehydrate by losing 3 to 4 L of sweat every day for 8 days, retain normal electrolyte levels [8].

It has been suggested, however, that during ultramarathon (80 km or more) running, some individuals may become hyponatremic. A case study of two runners who collapsed after an ultramarathon race in 1983 revealed that they had blood sodium values of 123 and 118 mEq/L (Costill, unpublished observations). One of the runners experienced a grand mal seizure; the other man became disoriented and confused. An examination of the runners fluid intake (21 to 24 L) and estimates of their sodium intake (224 to 145 mEq) during the run suggested that they diluted their body sodium levels by consuming fluids that contained little sodium. Thus, in ultra-long-duration exercise with large sweat losses, the fluid replacement should include not only carbohydrate but also ample amounts of electrolytes.

SUMMARY

It is apparent that adequate fluid balance is critical for optimal endurance performance. Electrolytes excreted in sweat are relatively small compared with total body stores. In fact, sweating results in a larger loss of body water than minerals, thereby concentrating the ions in body fluids. The consumption of fluids, primarily water, to minimize dehydration has a significant impact on heat tolerance and exercise performance. It is beneficial to replace the body water lost during exercise periods lasting more than 1 hour by ingesting water or very dilute solutions. In more prolonged exercise, the addition of carbohydrate can be essential, whereas in ultralong performance (greater than 4 hours), fluid replacement should also contain ions.

REFERENCES

1. Adolph, E.E. *Physiology of Man in the Desert*. New York: John Wiley, 1947.
2. Armstrong, L.E., D.L. Costill, and W.J. Fink. Influence of diuretic-induced dehydration on competitive running performance. *Med. Sci. Sports. Exer.* 17:456–461, 1985.
3. Barr, P.-O., G. Birke, S.-O. Liljedahl, and L.-O. Plantin. Oxygen consumption and water loss during

treatment of burns with warm air. *Lancet* 1:164, 1968.

4. Bergstrom, J. Muscle electrolytes in man. *Scand. J. Clin. Lab. Invest.* 14 (Suppl.) 68:1–100, 1962.

5. Buskirk, E.R., P.F. Iampietro, and D.E. Bass. Work performance after dehydration: Effects of physical training and heat acclimatization. *J. Appl. Physiol.* 12:189–194, 1958.

6. Claremont, A.D., D.L. Costill, W. Fink, and P. Van Handel. Heat tolerance following diuretic-induced dehydration. *Med. Sci. Sports Exer.* 8:239–243, 1976.

7. Costill, D.L., R. Cote, and W. Fink. Muscle water and electrolytes following varied levels of dehydration in man. *J. Appl. Physiol.* 40:6–11, 1976.

8. Costill, D.L., R. Cote, and W. Fink. Dietary potassium and heavy exercise: Effects on muscle water and electrolytes. *Am. J. Clin. Nutr.* 36:266–275, 1982.

9. Costill, D.L., W.F. Kammer, and A. Fisher. Fluid ingestion during distance running. *Arch. Environ. Health* 21:520–525, 1970.

10. Costill, D.L., and B. Saltin. Factors limiting gastric emptying during rest and exercise. *J. Appl. Physiol.* 37:679–683, 1974.

11. Costill, D.L. Sweating: Its composition and effects on body fluids. In P. Milvy (ed.). *The Marathon: Physiological, Medical, Epidemiological, and Psychological Studies.* N.Y. Acad. Sci. 301:160–174, 1977.

12. Fordtran, J.S., and B. Saltin. Gastric emptying and intestinal absorption during prolonged severe exercise. *J. Appl. Physiol.* 23:331–335, 1967.

13. Greenleaf, J., and F. Sargent II. Voluntary dehydration in man. *J. Appl. Physiol.* 20:719–724, 1965.

14. Kiens, B., and B. Saltin. Endurance training of man decreases muscle potassium loss during exercise. *Acta Physiol. Scand.* 126:P5, 1986.

15. Kjeldsen, K., E.A. Richter, H. Galbo, G. Lortie, and T. Clausen. Training increases the concentration of ^{3}H-ouabain binding sites in rat skeletal muscle. *Biochim. Biophys. Acta* 860:708–712, 1986.

16. Kjellmer, I. The effect of exercise on the vascular bed of skeletal muscle. *Acta Physiol. Scand.* 62:18–30, 1964.

17. Knochel, J.P., J.D. Blachley, J.H. Johnson, and N.W. Carter. Muscle cell electrical hyperpolarization and reduced exercise hyperkalemia in physically conditioned dogs. *J. Clin. Invest.* 75:740–745, 1985.

18. Kozlowski, S., and B. Saltin. Effect of sweat loss on body fluids. *J. Appl. Physiol.* 19:1119–1124, 1964.

19. Lundvall, J. Tissue hyperosmolality as a mediator of vasodilatation and transcapillary fluid flux in exercising skeletal muscle. *Acta Physiol. Scand.* 86(Suppl 379):1–142, 1972.

20. Medbø, J.I., and O.M. Sejersted. Acid-base and electrolyte balance after exhausting exercise in endurance-trained and sprint-trained subjects. *Acta Physiol. Scand.* 125:97–109, 1985.

21. Nielsen, M. Die Regulation der Korpertemperature bei Muskelarbeit. *Scand. Arch. Physiol.* 79:193–230, 1938.

22. Nielsen, B., R. Kubica, A. Bonnesen, I.B. Rasmussen, J. Stoklosa, and B. Wilk. Physical work capacity after dehydration and hyperthermia. *Scand. J. Sports Sci.* 3:2–10, 1981.

23. Nielsen, B., G. Sjøgaard, J. Ugelvig, B. Knudsen, and B. Dohlmann. Fluid balance in exercise dehydration and rehydration with different glucose-electrolyte drinks. *Eur. J. Appl. Physiol.* 55:318–325, 1986.

24. Nishi, Y., and A.P. Gagge. Direct evaluation of convective heat transfer coefficient by naphthalene sublimation. *J. Appl. Physiol.* 29:830, 1970.

25. Owen, M.D., K.C. Kregel, P.T. Wall, and C.V. Gisolfi. Effects of carbohydrate ingestion on thermoregulation, gastric emptying and plasma volume during exercise in the heat. (Abstract) *Med. Sci. Sports Exer.* 17:185, 1985.

26. Pitts, R.F. *Physiology of the Kidney and Body Fluids.* New York: Year Book, 1965.

27. Robinson, S., and A.H. Robinson. Chemical composition of sweat. *Physiol. Rev.* 34:202–206, 1954.

28. Saltin, B. Aerobic and anaerobic work capacity after dehydration. *J. Appl. Physiol.* 19:1114–1118, 1964.

29. Saltin, B. Aerobic work capacity and circulation at exercise in man. *Acta Physiol. Scand.* 62 (Suppl):230, 1964, (Thesis).

30. Saltin, B., A.P. Gagge, and J.A.J. Stolwijk. Muscle temperature during submaximal exercise in man. *J. Appl. Physiol.* 25:679–688, 1968.

31. Saltin, B., A.P. Gagge, and J.A.J. Stolwijk. Body temperature and sweating during thermal transients caused by exercise. *J. Appl. Physiol.* 28:318–327, 1970.

32. Saltin, B., and L. Hermansen. Esophageal, rectal and muscle temperature during exercise. *J. Appl. Physiol.* 21:1757–1762, 1966.

33. Saltin, B., G. Sjøgaard, S. Strange, and C. Juel. K$^+$ homeostasis during muscular exercise in man. In K. Shiraki (ed.). *Physiology of Stressful Environments.* Springfield, Mass.: C.C. Thomas, 1987.

34. Sjøgaard, G. Water and electrolyte fluxes during exercise and their relation to muscle fatigue. *Acta Physiol. Scand,* in press.

35. Sjøgaard, G., R.P. Adams, and B. Saltin. Water and ion shifts in skeletal muscle of humans with intense dynamic knee extension. *Am. J. Physiol.* 248:R190–R196, 1985.

36. Snellen, J.W. Mean body temperature and the control of thermal sweating. *Acta Physiol. Pharmacol. Neerl.* 14:99, 1966.

37. Stolwijk, J.A.J., B. Saltin, and A.P. Gagge. Physiological factors associated with sweating during exercise. *J. Aero. Med.* 39:101, 1968.

38. Vellar,. O.D. Studies on sweat losses of nutrients. I. Iron content of whole body sweat and its association with other sweat constituents, serum iron levels, hematological indices, body surface area and sweat rate. *Scand. J. Clin. Lab. Invest.* 21:157–167, 1968.

Chapter 11

INFLUENCE OF EXERCISE ON GASTROINTESTINAL FUNCTION

Alexander Bortoff, Ph.D.

INTRODUCTION

During the past few years, a number of reports have documented some of the apparent effects of strenuous or prolonged exercise on gastrointestinal activity [4, 13, 24, 29, 34, 35, 45, 50–52]. Most of these have been case reports or the results of surveys conducted on long-distance runners. The most striking aspect of survey results is the relatively high incidence of gastrointestinal disturbances reported to occur in association with long-distance running. In two surveys of distance runners [24, 51], the most common symptom experienced by the participants (approximately one-third of those responding) was the urge to defecate, either during or immediately after running. A bowel movement occurred relatively frequently after running, and diarrhea occurred immediately after a hard run in approximately 20% of those interviewed. A common complaint made by 10 to 20% of the runners was the occurrence of abdominal cramps either during or immediately after a run. One of the surveys differentiated between men and women, and revealed that all symptoms were significantly more common in women than in men.

Although no hard physiological data support the concept that exercise, especially running exercise, stimulates bowel movements, there is much anecdotal evidence to support it. Most dog owners will attest to a positive correlation between the pet's morning walk or run and the act of defecation. On the other hand, physicians for years have suggested that a similar correlation may exist between constipation and chronic lack of physical activity, constipation often occurring in elderly persons or immobilized patients. In the survey conducted by Keeffe and colleagues [24] involving 707 participants of a marathon, several runners commented that running alleviated their chronic constipation. In a preliminary study involving 14 distance runners, Sullivan [52] found that the weekly frequency of defecation was 16, compared with 7 in a group of healthy medical students. Thus, even though it has not been definitively established, there appears to be a positive correlation between running and the frequency of bowel movements. Possible physiological mechanisms that could be responsible for this correlation will be discussed.

Among the gastrointestinal consequences of running that have recently been reported, the most extreme is bleeding into the gut. Of the 707 marathoners interviewed by Keeffe and coworkers [24], 2.4% reported experiencing bloody stools associated with running. Again, the disturbance was reported more frequently by women than by men. In another study conducted after a marathon, 3 of 39 runners passed stools that tested positive for the presence of blood [35]. An even higher frequency of gastrointestinal blood loss during long-distance races was found in each of two other studies [29, 50]. In one, conducted on 32 runners who participated in the 1983 Boston Marathon, 7 or 22%, had blood-positive stools within 72 hours after the race [29]. In the other, stool samples were analyzed from 24 runners who participated in races of from 10 to 42.4 km. Fecal hemoglobin levels were found to increase in 20 of the 24 runners after a race [50]. Such blood loss has been implicated as a contributing factor in the iron-deficiency anemia that reportedly occurs in some long-distance runners. Although the basis for running-associated gastrointestinal bleeding has not been established, a number of authors have suggested that it may be due to relative gut ischemia resulting from increased splanchnic sympathetic tone [13, 45]. Experimental support for such a mechanism will be explored in some detail in this chapter.

THE SPLANCHNIC CIRCULATION

The splanchnic circulation supplies blood to most of the gastrointestinal tract and to the pancreas, liver, and spleen. Three major arteries, the celiac and the superior and inferior mesenterics, carry blood to the splanchnic bed, while a single vein, the hepatic, drains the bed. Within the wall of the gut, the arterial vessels supply two parallel capillary networks in the mucosa, one located around the crypts, the other in the intestinal villi [54]. Separate arterial vessels run from the submucosa to these capillary networks, thus providing the basic conditions for individual control of blood flow to the villi and to the crypts. This could also provide, in part, a basis for the differential blood flow response during exercise and could contribute to the occasional presence of blood in the stool following prolonged strenuous exercise.

The tissue around the crypts is provided by a dense capillary network supplied by numerous small arteries. Each villus is supplied with a single arterial vessel, which loses its smooth-muscle coat near the villus base. At the tip of the villus, the arteriole empties into a descending, monolayered capillary network that is in close contact with the epithelial cells. Drainage of these capillaries occurs by way of a vein or group of veins that conveys the blood back to the submucosa. Hence, the villus blood vessels are anatomically arranged in the form of a countercurrent exchanger [54].

The blood flow through the splanchnic circulation accounts for approximately 25% of the cardiac output at rest; in an individual whose resting cardiac output is 6 L/min, this amounts to 1.5 L/min. Under conditions of maximal work output, splanchnic blood flow can be reduced to 20% of its resting value [39, 40], which diverts more than 1 L/min to working muscle. Although this amount of blood contributes a relatively small fraction to the increase in cardiac output resulting from high-intensity exercise, it constitutes a large fraction of the splanchnic blood flow.

During graded exercise, splanchnic blood flow, as measured by hepatic clearance of indocyanine green (ICG), is inversely related to heart rate or percent of maximum oxygen consumption [5, 39, 40]. Furthermore, following a 5-week period of programmed physical training in humans, the reduction in heart rate for a given intensity of exercise was found to parallel an increase in ICG clearance [5]. However, no difference was found in ICG clearance with the body at rest, even though resting heart rate was lower after training than before. These findings indicate that the degree of splanchnic vasoconstriction is less for a given intensity of exercise following a period of training. They also have been interpreted as indicating that a common mechanism may mediate the increase in heart rate and reduction of splanchnic blood flow during exercise.

Exercise-induced changes occurring in the splanchnic circulation have been attributed primarily to increased sympathetic nervous activity. This concept was expressed by Rowell when, in describing the observed relationship between splanchnic blood flow and heart rate during exercise, he stated that "the increase in sympathetic nervous outflow to the heart to increase rate is directly proportional to the increase in sympathetic vasomotor outflow to vasoconstrict visceral organs" [39]. In several recent reports, relative gut ischemia resulting from sympathetic vasoconstriction of visceral organs has been suggested as the cause of the gastrointestinal blood loss that occurs in some long-distance runners [13, 29, 34]. The reduction in visceral blood flow has been compared to that occurring during hypovolemic shock [13, 45]. It is appropriate, therefore, to examine some of the results obtained from more direct studies dealing with the effects of sympathetic stimulation on splanchnic blood flow and related phenomena.

Svanvik [54] used an indicator-dilution method, which employs radiolabeled, beta-emitting tracers and is unaffected by the mucosal countercurrent exchanger, to study the effect of sympathetic stimulation on the villus circulation and total mucosal blood flow in isolated segments of cat intestine. In addition to blood flow, both blood volume and linear flow rate could be measured by this method. During regional sympathetic nerve stimulation, blood flow was monitored through an isolated segment of cat jejunum. After a transient reduction lasting 1 to 2 minutes, the blood flow returned toward normal levels ("autoregulatory escape") and stabilized somewhat below the prestimulatory control level (steady state). During the steady-state phase, mucosal blood flow returned toward its control level, while villus flow exceeded control and overall intestinal flow was reduced. Thus, a redistribution of blood flow occurred during the steady state, so that villus blood flow and oxygen supply actually increased while flow in deeper areas, probably through the parallel crypt circuit, decreased. Linear flow rate through the villus circulation was unchanged.

In a later study, Shepherd [46] showed that during intense (8–10 Hz) stimulation of perivascular sympathetic nerves innervating isolated loops of dog intestine, there was again an initially large but transient reduction in blood flow, followed by an increase to a new steady-state level. The steady-state blood flow at constant perfusion pressure was reduced below the prestimulatory control level by an average of 32%. Similar results were obtained by Granger and colleagues [16], who showed that under constant perfusion pressure conditions, steady-state blood flow through isolated segments of cat ileum was reduced an average of 26% during periarterial sympathetic nerve stimulation (4 Hz). In yet another study, Sjovall et al. [49], using a technique substantially different from that used by Svanvik [54], were able to study the effect of splanchnic nerve stimulation on the distribution of blood flow in an isolated segment of cat jejunum. Under constant pressure conditions, sympathetic stimulation at 4 Hz reduced steady-state blood flow through the intestinal segment by an average of about 40%. The reduction in flow was limited to the muscle layers (26% reduction) and to the nonabsorptive portion of the mucosa–submucosa (67% reduction). Villus blood flow was not affected by sympathetic stimulation.

In all of these studies the maximal reduction in blood flow to the gut resulting from sympathetic nerve stimulation was between 25 and 40%. This compares with a maximum reduction of 80% reported to occur in human subjects exercising at maximal oxygen uptake ($\dot{V}O_2$max). Thus, the larger reduction of splanchnic blood flow occurring in humans at $\dot{V}O_2$max is probably not due simply to increased sympathetic tone. Other factors must also be involved, such as vasopressin and the renin–angiotensin system.

A number of studies indicate that the redistribution of blood flow in the gut wall due to sympathetic stimulation is associated with complete closure of capillary beds, presumably in the tissue surrounding the crypts. In Shepherd's studies [46], it was found that under conditions of either constant perfusion pressure or constant flow, sympathetic stimulation resulted in a decrease in oxygen consumption of 28% and 38%, respectively. On the other hand, when blood flow was reduced by mechanical occlusion to the same level that was achieved during sympathetic stimulation at constant pressure, oxygen consumption was essentially normal due to an increased arteriovenous O_2 difference. This was interpreted as indicating that in addition to constricting resistance vessels, sympathetic stimulation closes precapillary sphincters, thereby reducing the density of the perfused capillary bed. Under these conditions the flux of oxygen from the capillary to the cell would become diffusion limited. In the studies of Granger et al. [16], capillary hydrostatic pressure (P_c) was measured with the venous occlusion method, making possible calculation of both precapillary and postcapillary resistances. The increase in total vascular resistance was found to be due almost entirely to increased precapillary resistance. The capillary filtration coefficient (K_f), determined by suddenly increasing the venous pressure and measuring the volume change of the intestinal segment, was found to decrease during sympathetic stimulation, probably due to a decreased capillary surface area (i.e., functional capillary density). As a result of a decrease in both P_c and K_f, capillary filtration rate is decreased during sympathetic stimulation.

A proposed mechanism of flow redistribution is based on anatomical studies of the mucosal vasculature and its innervation. It had been shown [47] that the major part of the adrenergic nerve endings in the mucosa are situated in the crypt region, becoming very sparse toward the villus tips. Svanvik [54] proposed that autoregulatory escape and redistribution of blood flow during sympathetic stimulation can be explained as follows. Initially, both villus and crypt arterioles constrict. However, accumulation of local metabolites causes vasodilation of the

villus arterioles, leaving the crypt vasculature constricted. This hypothesis is based on the supposition that either the villus arterioles are more sensitive to metabolic control or they are less densely innervated by sympathetic vasoconstrictor nerves.

A number of studies have shown that in addition to causing intestinal vasoconstriction and reduced blood flow, sympathetic nerve stimulation increases net fluid absorption [2, 48]. Recent evidence suggests that these two phenomena are regulated by sympathetic fibers that are functionally distinct from one another. Sjovall [48] studied the effects of splanchnic nerve stimulation on fluid transport and blood flow in segments of cat jejunum, prior to and after treating the animals with a ganglionic blocker, hexamethonium. He found that fluid absorption was essentially unaffected by hexamethonium at a concentration that totally eliminated the intestinal vasoconstrictor response. Since the absorptive response was eliminated by mesenteric denervation of the segment, the response did not involve an indirect mechanism such as the release of a humoral agent. Stimulation of the mesenteric nerves directly resulted in a 39% decrease in intestinal blood flow and a 158% increase in net fluid absorption. Thus, it is possible that the nerve fibers in the splanchnic nerve that regulate fluid absorption are postganglionic, while those regulating blood flow are, like the majority of efferent splanchnic fibers, preganglionic. The postganglionic fibers originate in one of the prevertebral ganglia. If, as this study indicates, intestinal fluid absorption and blood flow are regulated by functionally distinct sympathetic fibers, they may operate either independently or in concert under different physiological conditions. In view of the complexities surrounding the sympathetic control of intestinal fluid absorption and blood flow, it is not surprising that in an early study involving five human subjects, Fordtran and Saltin [14] found no consistent effect of exercise on intestinal fluid absorption. The more recent studies, such as those of Sjovall [48], should stimulate further work involving the effect of exercise on intestinal fluid transport and blood flow.

Intestinal blood flow during reduced perfusion pressure may differ in one important respect from that occurring during sympathetic stimulation alone. In a series of experiments designed to study mucosal hemodynamics during reduced perfusion pressure, Lundgren and Svanvik [28] found that villus blood flow was virtually unchanged when the perfusion pressure was reduced from 100 to 30 mmHg, while total venous outflow was reduced by approximately one-third. As is the case during sympathetic nervous stimulation, blood flow was shunted from the muscle layers and the nonabsorbing mucosa to the villi. However, the villus plasma volume also increased, resulting in a decreased linear velocity of flow. The decreased velocity of flow increases the efficiency of the countercurrent exchanger, thereby decreasing oxygen delivery to the tips of the villi. This condition is exacerbated during sympathetic nervous stimulation when superimposed on a reduction of perfusion pressure, resulting in a damaging level of hypoxia that is first evident at the tips of the villi [1]. This is evident macroscopically as petechial bleeding and microscopically as histological damage and even denudation of the villus tips. Such hemorrhagic lesions have been reported in a number of different animal species, including humans, during hypovolemic shock.

It has not been demonstrated whether the hemorrhagic lesions that sometimes occur in association with intensive and prolonged exercise, such as marathon running, are of the same type. Since perfusion pressure is not normally reduced under such conditions, it appears that villus blood flow and oxygen supply should not be adversely affected. On the other hand, blood flow to the crypts may be severely curtailed. It is apparent that the effects of severe, prolonged exercise on the regional redistribution of blood to the gut

wall is an area of physiology that is virtually devoid of substantive physiological data.

GASTROINTESTINAL MOTILITY DURING EXERCISE

Despite some early studies on the effects of exercise on gastric emptying [20] and colonic motility [7], surprisingly few laboratory studies have been conducted in this area of physiology. Hellebrandt and Tepper [20], in a fluoroscopic study of gastric emptying in young women, found that mild exercise tended to increase the rate of gastric emptying of a porridge–barium meal, while more severe exercise had the opposite effect. Forty years later, Ramsbottom and Hunt [37], using an aspiration method, studied the effect of exercise on gastric emptying of 750 ml of a glucose solution. The subjects were six male medical students who exercised on a bicycle ergometer for 20 minutes at work levels between 150 and 750 kpm (kilopond-meters)/min. The volume of the meal remaining in the stomach after 20 minutes of exercise did not change significantly from control values until work output exceeded 450 kpm/min, beyond which the rate of gastric emptying progressively decreased. Similar results had been reported earlier by Costill and Saltin [6], who observed no effect on gastric emptying until the work intensity exceeded 70% of V_{O_2}max. In a more recent study, Feldman and Nixon [11] found that exercise on a bicycle ergometer at 50 to 70% of maximum workload (210–475 kpm/min) for 45 minutes did not significantly affect the rate of gastric emptying over a 2-hour period in five untrained human volunteers (three women, two men). On the other hand, relatively low levels of exercise (100–150 kpm/min) have been reported to actually increase the rate of gastric emptying of a solid meal in six of seven subjects (six women, one man) studied by a radioactive-labeling technique [3]. A similar finding has recently been made in mice running on a treadmill at 0.5 mph [17]. Thus, it appears that under laboratory conditions, moderate levels of exercise have no significant effect on the rate of gastric emptying, but that more intense levels of exercise have an inhibitory effect and low levels of exercise may actually increase the rate of gastric emptying. The nature of the inhibitory mechanism operating at heavy workloads and of the excitatory mechanism working at light workloads is not known.

Moderate exercise does not appear to increase small-intestine transit time. With the breath hydrogen excretion method, transit time of a solid meal was measured in seven subjects during prolonged, intermittent exercise (equivalent to cycling of 35 miles over a 6-hour period). Small-bowel transit time during exercise was not significantly different from that during control periods [3]. In only one other comparable study, transit time of a liquid meal was found to actually decrease during mild exercise such as walking [24a].

Equally sparse are studies dealing with the effect of exercise on colonic motility. More than 50 years ago DeYoung et al. [7] recorded colonic motility, using intraluminal balloons, in a group of dogs surgically prepared with cecostomies while the animals ran on a treadmill. Control records were obtained prior to the onset of exercise, while the animals stood on the treadmill. Within minutes after the onset of exercise there was usually an abrupt rise in colonic tone (luminal pressure) and motility. The rise in motility was usually accompanied by defecation. The increased colonic motility was then followed by a prolonged period of inhibition, regardless of whether or not exercise was continued. On the basis of the effects of a variety of denervation procedures these investigators concluded that the rise in colonic motility was dependent on intact parasympathetic innervation from either the pelvic or vagal nerves. The subsequent decrease in colonic motility was attributed to "a non-nervous mechanism."

Although the mechanisms underlying the observed changes in colonic motility may be open to question, the observations themselves are significant, in light of the gastrointestinal symptoms experienced by long-distance runners described earlier in this chapter. Thus, the increase in colonic motility shortly after the onset of exercise may be related to the increased desire to defecate that is experienced by a substantial percentage of long-distance runners. The subsequent, protracted decrease in motility may be reflected by a reduction of colonic electrical spike activity recorded in dogs after exercise (Bortoff, unpublished observations). The mechanisms underlying these exercise-related changes in canine colonic motility and the relationship of the changes to gastrointestinal symptoms experienced by human runners remain to be elucidated.

A particular type of motility pattern occurs in humans and animals such as the dog only during the fasting state, beginning approximately 12 hours after ingestion of the last meal. It consists of a series of peristaltic contractions, often beginning in the stomach, that slowly migrate distally through the small intestine and possibly into the colon. These contractions are referred to as the *migrating motor complex* (MMC), the electrical counterpart of which is the *migrating myoelectric complex* (also MMC). MMCs occur at approximately 90-minute intervals and take about the same length of time to traverse the gut. The function of the MMC may be to periodically clear the intestinal lumen of accumulated debris (secretions, sloughed cells, bacteria, etc.) during the fasting state. Although it is not known exactly what triggers the MMC, both the hormone motilin and opioids such as morphine have been shown to elicit premature MMCs [41].

In one of the few studies designed to examine the effects of exercise on intestinal motility in humans, Evans, Foster, and Hardcastle [8] measured jejunal motility with a pressure-sensitive radiotelemetry capsule in 20 healthy volunteers. The subjects fasted overnight, for at least 12 hours prior to the study. The control group ($n=10$) sat quietly in the laboratory, while the experimental group ($n=10$) commenced a 12-mile walk over a 4-hour period. All 20 subjects had one MMC prior to the 4-hour test period. All subjects in the control group had at least one MMC during the test period, with a median number of 2. MMCs were recorded in 6 of 10 subjects in the exercise group during the test period, with a median number of 1. The difference between the two groups was significant. Of those subjects who had MMCs, the median interval in the control group was 100 minutes, that in the exercise group 150 minutes. Again the difference was significant. Thus, moderate exercise appears to reduce the incidence of MMCs in fasted subjects. However, the physiological significance of the exercise-related reduction in MMC frequency and the mechanism by which this occurs are not known.

EFFECTS OF EXERCISE ON GASTROINTESTINAL TRANSPORT

There is a paucity of studies dealing with the effects of exercise on gastrointestinal secretion and absorption, even though changes in these processes may be responsible for some of the symptoms associated with intense, prolonged exercise. In a study of six men who performed several levels of exercise on a bicycle ergometer, each for a 20-minute period, it was found that gastric acid secretion decreased up to a maximum work level of 750 kpm/min. Between 300 and 450 kpm/min, acid secretion appeared to increase, but the dominant effect over the entire work range was inhibition [37].

Similar results were obtained by Konturek, Tasler, and Obtulowicz [25], who studied the effects of exercise on gastric and pancreatic secretion in six dogs prepared with either a vagally innervated Pavlov gastric pouch ($n=3$) or a vagally denervated Heidenhain pouch ($n=3$). The dogs ran on a treadmill inclined at 8° for a period of 15 minutes at a speed of 10 km/hr. Mucosal

blood flow was measured by the aminopyrine clearance method. Gastric acid secretion and pancreatic secretion were measured in response to feeding and to intravenous infusion of pentagastrin and secretin. Exercise resulted in a decrease of acid secretion in both the Heidenhain and the Pavlov pouches in response to feeding and to pentagastrin. Gastric blood flow was also decreased during exercise, the percent decrease being even greater than that of the reduction in acid secretion. Exercise also decreased the pancreatic secretory response to feeding, to secretin, and to intraduodenal instillation of acid. The fact that acid output decreased in both the vagally innervated and vagally denervated pouches rules out an exercise-induced reduction of vagal tone as a possible mechanism. Inhibition seems to have occured at the level of the secretory cell, since exercise reduced pentagastrin-stimulated acid secretion and secretin-stimulated pancreatic secretion. The authors concluded that although all of the inhibitory mechanisms could not be determined, the measured decrease in blood flow could be an important contributing factor.

Fordtran and Saltin [14] studied the effect of 1 hour of moderately intense treadmill exercise (71% of maximum oxygen consumption) on acid secretion and intestinal absorption in four men and one woman. Before exercise each subject ingested 750 ml of an aqueous solution containing 100 g of glucose and 2.25 g of NaCl. Acid secretion was measured by an aspiration method and absorption by a constant perfusion technique. No effect of exercise was observed on acid secretion, nor was there any "consistent influence" on the rate of absorption of glucose, water, NaCl, potassium, or bicarbonate. It is interesting that the level of exercise in these studies was at about the level at which Ramsbottom and Hunt [37] noted a break in their regression lines of acid secretion plotted as a function of work.

When taken as a group, these studies suggest that moderate to intense exercise is associated with a reduction in gastric acid and pancreatic aqueous secretion, and that the effects of exercise on intestinal transport are, at best, equivocal.

EXERCISE AND GASTROINTESTINAL PEPTIDES

Improvements in radioimmunoassay techniques have led to a plethora of papers dealing with virtually every imaginable situation in which changes in circulating levels of gastroenteropancreatic (GEP) hormones might be involved. Exercise is but one example. Changes in circulating levels of GEP peptides during exercise have been measured in a number of animals, including humans [22, 53] and the horse [19].

In an extensive study, Hilsted and co-workers [22] measured plasma levels of GEP peptides in six normal men during a 3-hour period of exercise on a bicycle ergometer at 40% of $\dot{V}o_2$max. Significant increases were found in vasoactive intestinal polypeptide (VIP) (from 1.8 to 22.3 pmol/L), secretin (From 0.5 to 11.1 pmol/L), pancreatic polypeptide (PP) (from 4.0 to 46.3 pmol/L), somatostatin (SRIF) (from 12.8 to 17.7 pmol/L), and glucagon (from 5 to 23 pmol/L). Similar increases in VIP and pancreatic glucagon were found by Sullivan et al. [53], who measured plasma levels of GEP peptides in seven male marathon runners during a 30-km run. In addition, they found an increase in plasma levels of gastrin (from 7.5 to 25 pmol/L) and motilin (from 32 to 53 pmol/L). In an interesting study involving racehorses [19], it was found that after an 80-km ride or a 42-km race, significant increases had occurred in plasma levels of VIP, PP, and glucagon. Somatostatin increased only slightly. Secretin was not measured. Finally, a study involving 12 subjects who participated in a 90-km cross-country ski race showed significant increases in plasma concentrations of both VIP (5.5 to 33.7 pmol/L) and secretin (1.6 to 13.2 pmol/L) [33]. An interesting finding in this study was that plasma levels of these peptides remained

significantly above control levels for 2 hours after the race, even though both secretin and VIP have plasma half-lives of 2 to 4 minutes. In summary, these studies indicate that moderate to high intensity prolonged exercise of various types results in significantly elevated plasma levels of VIP, glucagon, and secretin, and probably also in elevated levels of PP, somatostatin, and motilin. Furthermore, the concentrations of VIP and secretin may remain higher than normal after termination of exercise for periods much longer than the half-lives of these peptides.

At least two major questions have yet to be satisfactorily resolved. What is the stimulus for release of these peptides during exercise? What function do they serve during exercise? Evidence regarding the stimulus for release of GEP peptides during exercise is contradictory. Increases in pancreatic glucagon levels are usually related to decreased plasma glucose levels. It has been shown, however, that plasma levels of glucagon are elevated during exercise regardless of whether glucose levels are above or below resting values [19]. Likewise, PP is thought to be released by activation of cholinergic reflexes, since its release during a meal or as a result of insulin hypoglycemia is blocked by atropine. Indeed, PP plasma levels have been proposed as an indicator of vagal tone [44], and increased levels during stress have been interpreted as indicating that stress may cause vagal hyperactivity [32]. However, exercise-induced increases in plasma levels of PP have been completely inhibited with propranolol, indicating that beta-receptors are involved in exercise-induced release of PP [12]. Furthermore, endurance training decreased both plasma catecholamine and PP concentration for a given level of exercise [15].

One of the most consistent findings in these studies is the large increase in plasma levels of VIP, the increases being a function of exercise duration [22, 53] and persisting long after termination of exercise [33]. VIP was originally classified as a gut candidate hormone, but has since been shown to be localized in gut neurons, especially those of myenteric and submucosal plexuses, as well as in neurons of the central nervous system and in peripheral nerves outside the gut [26]. Ingestion of a meal does not produce a significant increase in plasma levels of VIP [30], but vagal stimulation does [42]. The vagal effect is atropine resistant but is blocked by hexamethonium and by splanchnic nerve stimulation [9]. The response was enhanced by alpha-adrenergic blockade, indicating that splanchnic inhibition of VIP release is mediated by alpha-adrenergic fibers. Large quantities of VIP are released by the gut when the mucosa is mechanically stimulated [10], or following brief periods of ischemia [31].

The effect of intestinal ischemia on release of VIP from the intestine is intriguing, in light of the marked reduction (up to 80%) in blood flow that reportedly occurs during severe exercise [39]. Modlin and coworkers [31] found that intestinal ischemia, produced by clamping the superior mesenteric vascular pedicle for two periods of 15 minutes each, with rest periods of 30 minutes between, resulted in a fivefold increase in portal blood VIP concentration following the first ischemic period and a 10-fold increase following the second. Systemic VIP levels were not significantly affected, indicating rapid degradation of VIP by the liver. Although the gut certainly does not undergo total ischemia during exercise, even a 50% reduction in blood flow due to increased sympathetic tone to the gut may result in a much greater reduction to the nonabsorptive portion of the mucosa—submucosa. This is indicated by the study of Sjovall et al. [49], in which a 40% reduction in blood flow to the intestine at constant perfusion pressure resulted in a 67% reduction in flow to the nonabsorptive portion of the mucosa—submucosa. The nonabsorptive portion is the site of the submucosal plexus, a region rich in VIPergic neurons.

Although the physiological function of the GEP peptides during exercise is not known, some information is available regarding the effects of these peptides on certain gastrointestinal processes, such as transport and motility. Most transport studies have involved the use of segments of mucosa mounted in modified Ussing chambers. One such study evaluated the effect of VIP on sodium and chloride transport across the mucosal epithelium of rat colon under short-circuit conditions [37]. It was found that VIP at a concentration of 0.6 μM decreased sodium absorption and reversed chloride absorption to secretion. The changes produced by VIP were similar to those produced by theophylline, suggesting that the effect of VIP is mediated by cyclic adenosine monophosphate (cAMP). Similar results were obtained by Waldman and associates [55], who studied the effects of VIP and secretin on colonic transport and adenyl cyclase activity. Everted sacs of rat colonic mucosa were used. It was found that both VIP and secretin caused colonic secretion, by a mechanism involving the adenylate cyclase—AMP system. On a molar basis, VIP was found to be a thousand times more effective than secretin, with a threshold concentration of 10 pM. Pharmacokinetic studies indicated that VIP and secretin may produce their effects by acting on the same set of receptor sites. Inhibition of colonic absorption and stimulation of secretin by VIP have also been demonstrated in rat colon and ileum *in vivo* [58]. Thus, it appears that VIP, in concentrations found in blood plasma of human subjects undergoing prolonged high-intensity exercise (20–30 pM), can cause colonic secretion in *in vitro* preparations. In many cases, drug effects occur at even lower concentrations *in vivo* than they do *in vitro*. The concentrations of secretin occurring during exercise are probably not high enough to affect intestinal or colonic absorption, but it is interesting to note that they can exceed postprandial plasma levels, sufficient to stimulate aqueous pancreatic secretion when intravenously infused into human subjects [43]. Glucagon, administered by intravenous infusion, was found to reduce absorption of sodium chloride and water in the human jejunum [21]. Thus, it is possible that the diarrhea that sometimes afflicts long-distance runners during or after a long race may be attributable, at least in part, to the combined effects of VIP, glucagon, and possibly secretin on intestinal, colonic, and pancreatic secretion. This is an area of research that requires further attention.

The effects of glucagon, secretin, and VIP on motility are all inhibitory. Exogenously administered glucagon was found to inhibit motility in the upper small intestine of human subjects [see 56]. Secretin has been shown to inhibit upper small-intestine motility in humans [18], and to inhibit spike activity, the electrical counterpart of motility, in dogs [57]. The effect of exogenously administered secretin on MMCs has not been resolved, one group finding no effect [57], another than MMCs are inhibited in fasting dogs [27]. This may be a partial explanation for the reduction in MMCs found in human subjects during exercise (see previous section on motility). However, the effects of both secretin and glucagon are probably minor compared with the effect of VIP.

VIP is thought by many to be the major nonadrenergic inhibitory neurotransmitter in the gut. VIP has been shown to decrease lower esophageal sphincter pressure in the opposum (the experimental animal of choice for lower esophageal sphincter studies) [38], it inhibits antral motility, and it inhibits contractile activity of the small intestine [23]. As indicated by its name, VIP (vasoactive inhibitory polypeptide) is also an inhibitor of vascular smooth muscle, being, on a molar basis, one of the most potent vasodilators known. Its actions during exercise should, therefore, be predictable. It should inhibit gut motility and increase gastrointestinal blood flow, since it is probably present in the gut circulation in a significantly higher concentration than that found peripherally. Indeed, there are indications that gut motility, including lower esophageal sphincter (LES) pressure, is reduced during strenuous, prolonged exercise. Thus, approximately 10%

of runners complain of heartburn (due, most likely, to decreased LES pressure) [51], gastric emptying time is prolonged during severe exercise [36], and colonic motility is depressed, following an initial but transient increase [7]. On the other hand, in spite of the apparently large concentration of VIP in and around the splanchnic vasculature, blood flow to the gut can be markedly curtailed! The observed decrease in splanchnic blood flow (as much as 80%, [39]) becomes more and more puzzling.

The recent finding by Sullivan and coworkers [53] of an increase in plasma motilin levels is interesting, but its physiological significance is not known. Motilin stimulates gut motility, and it can, when administered exogenously, initiate an MMC. Indeed, some believe that motilin is responsible for normally triggering the MMC in fasting animals [see 41]. The physiological trigger for motilin release has not yet been determined. In view of the decreased gastrointestinal motility that occurs during prolonged, strenuous exercise and the apparent reduction in the number of MMCs generated during exercise, the finding that plasma motilin level increases during prolonged exercise adds but another piece to the puzzle.

CONCLUSIONS

Research in gastrointestinal physiology has produced more questions than answers. One of the more perplexing of these involves the marked reduction in splanchnic blood flow that reportedly occurs during periods of intense exercise. If, indeed, there can be a reduction of as much as 80% [39], how is this achieved? In experimental animals, maximal stimulation of the sympathetic nerves innervating the gut decreases blood flow no more than 40% [49]. Futhermore, blood concentrations of VIP, one of the most potent vasodilators known, rise to very high levels during intense, prolonged exercise [33, 53]. Supposedly, the VIP found in peripheral blood samples originates primarily in the gut, although this has not been definitely demonstrated. Recognizing that blood flow to the human gut does drop to very low levels during intense exercise, at least two explanations come to mind. First, human splanchnic resistance vessels may be more sensitive than those of laboratory animals. Second, other vasoconstrictors, such as vasopressin and angiotensin, may be involved. Clearly, more work is needed in this area. Further work is also required to determine the pattern of redistribution of blood flow that occurs within the gut wall during exercise. Both factors—reduction of blood flow and redistribution within the gut wall—may be involved in the gastrointestinal bleeding that sometimes occurs during intense, prolonged running exercise.

Our knowledge of motility changes occurring in the gut during exercise is also very limited. Gastric emptying seems to be unaffected until the intensity of exercise approaches very high levels. Experimental evidence regarding changes occurring in intestinal and colonic motility is virtually nonexistent. Colonic motility changes may be especially important because of the relationship they may have to the urge to defecate, which is experienced by many individuals either during or immediately after running.

Through the use of radioimmunoassay techniques, much information has been gathered regarding exercise-related changes in plasma levels of GEP peptides. However, because of our limited knowledge concerning the physiological function of these peptides, the fact that some of them show significant increases in plasma concentration during exercise does little to improve our understanding of the mechanisms underlying some of the gastrointestinal symptoms associated with exercise. Thus, PP concentration increases during exercise, but little is known about the physiological function of PP. Increases in glucagon, secretin, and VIP may affect gastrointestinal transport, es-

pecially in the colon where absorption may be decreased and net secretion increased. Does this actually occur, and is it a possible explanation for the diarrhea that sometimes occurs during or following a strenuous run? These are just a few of the questions raised by the studies in this area of physiology to date. It is indeed a fertile area for further research.

REFERENCES

1. Ahren, C., and U. Haglund. Mucosal lesions in the small intestine of the cat during low flow. *Acta Physiol. Scand.* 88:541–550, 1973.
2. Brunsson, I., S. Eklund, M. Jodal, O. Lundgren, and H. Sjovall. The effect of vasodilation and sympathetic nerve activation on net water absorption in the cat's small intestine. *Acta Physiol. Scand.* 106:61–68, 1979.
3. Cammack, J., N.W. Read, P.A. Cann, B. Greenwood, and A.M. Holgate. Effect of prolonged exercise on the passage of a solid meal through the stomach and small intestine. *Gut* 23:957–961, 1982.
4. Cantwell, J.D. Gastrointestinal disorders in runners. *JAMA* 246:1404–1405, 1981.
5. Clausen, J.P., K. Klausen, B. Rasmussen, and J. Trap-Jensen. Central and peripheral circulatory changes after training of the arms or legs. *Am. J. Physiol.* 225:675–682, 1973.
6. Costill, D.L., and B. Saltin. Factors limiting gastric emptying during rest and exercise. *J. Appl. Physiol.* 37:679–683, 1974.
7. DeYoung, V.R., H.A. Rice, and A.H. Steinhaus. Studies in the physiology of exercise. VII. The modification of colonic motility induced by exercise and some indications for a nervous mechanism. *Am. J. Physiol.* 99:52–63, 1931–32.
8. Evans, D.F., G.E. Foster, and J.D. Hardcastle. Does exercise affect the migrating motor complex in man? In Roman, C. (ed.). *Gastrointestinal Motility*. Boston: MTP Press, 1984, pp. 277–284.
9. Fahrenkrug, J., H. Galbo, J.J. Holst, and O.B. Schaffalitzky de Muckadell. Influence of the autonomic nervous system on the release of vasoactive intestinal polypeptide from the procine gastrointestinal tract. *J. Physiol. (London)* 280:405–422, 1978.
10. Fahrenkrug, J., U. Haglund, M. Jodal, O. Lundgren, L. Olbe, and O.B. Schaffalitzky de Muckadell. Nervous release of vasoactive intestinal polypeptide in the gastrointestinal tract of cats: Possible physiological implications. *J. Physiol. (London)* 284:291–305, 1978.
11. Feldman, M., and J.V. Nixon. Effect of exercise on postprandial gastric secretion and emptying in humans. *J. Appl. Physiol.* 53:851–854, 1982.
12. Feurle, G.E., A. Wirth, C. Diehm, M. Lorenzen, and G. Schlierf. Exercise-induced release of pan-

creatic polypeptide and its inhibition by propranolol; evidence for adrenergic stimulation. *Eur. J. Clin. Inves.* 10:249–251, 1980.

13. Fogoros, R.N. 'Runner's trots.' *JAMA* 243:1743–1744, 1980.

14. Fordtran, J.S., and B. Saltin. Gastric emptying and intestinal absorption during prolonged severe exercise. *J. Appl. Physiol.* 23:331–335, 1967.

15. Gingerich, R.L., R.C. Hickson, J.M. Hagberg, and W.W. Winder. Effect of endurance exercise training on plasma pancreatic polypeptide concentration during exercise. *Metabolism* 28:1179–1182, 1979.

16. Granger, D.N., J.A. Barrowman, S.L. Harper, P.R. Kvietys, and R.J. Korthuis. Sympathetic stimulation and intestinal capillary fluid exchange. *Am. J. Physiol.* 247:G279–G283, 1984.

17. Grunewald, K.K., and T.J. Tucker. Gastric emptying in exercised mice. *Comp. Biochem. Physiol.* 80A:173–175, 1985.

18. Gutierrez, J.G., W.Y. Chey, and V.P. Dinoso. Actions of cholecystokinin and secretin on the motor activity of the small intestine in man.

19. Hall, G.M., T.E. Adrian, S.R. Bloom, and J.N. Lucke. Changes in circulating gut hormones in the horse during long distance exercise. *Eq. Vet. J.* 14:209–222, 1982.

20. Hellebrandt, F.A., and R.H. Tepper. Studies on the influence of exercise on the digestive work of the stomach. II. Its effect on emptying time. *Am. J. Physiol.* 107:355–363, 1934.

21. Hicks, T., and L.A. Turnberg. Influence of glucagon on the human jejunum. *Gastroenterology* 67:1114–1118, 1974.

22. Hilsted, J., H. Galbo, B. Sonne, T. Schwartz, O.B. Schaffalitzky de Muckadell, K.B. Lauristen, and B. Tronier. Gastroenteropancreatic hormonal changes during exercise. *Am. J. Physiol.* 239 (*Gastrointes. Liver Physiol.* 2):G136–G140, 1980.

23. Kachelhoffer, J., C. Mendel, J. Dauchel, D. Hohmatter, and J.F. Grenier. The effects of VIP on intestinal motility: Study on ex vivo perfused isolated canine jejunal loops. *Am. J. Diges. Dis.* 21:957–962, 1976.

24. Keeffe, E.B., D.K. Lowe, J.R. Goss, and R. Wayne. Gastrointestinal symptoms of marathon runners. *W. J. Med.* 141:481–484, 1984.

24a. Keeling, W.F., and B.J. Martin. Gastrointestinal transit during mild exercise. *J. Appl. Physiol.* 63:978–981, 1987.

25. Konturek, S.J., J. Tasler, and W. Obtulowicz. Effect of exercise on gastrointestinal secretions. *J. Appl. Physiol.* 34:324–328, 1973.

26. Larsson, L., J. Fahrenkrug, O.B. Schaffalitzky de Muckadell, F. Sundler, R. Hakanson, and J.F. Rehfeld. Localization of vasoactive intestinal polypeptide (VIP) to central and peripheral neurons. *Proc. Nat. Acad. Sci. USA* 73:3197–3200, 1976.

27. Lee, K.Y., and W.Y. Chey. Effect of a meat meal and gut hormones on plasma immunoreactive motilin (PIM) concentrations and myoelectric activity of the duodenum in dogs. *Gastroenterology* 74:1131, 1978.

28. Lundgren, O., and J. Svanvik, Mucosal hemodynamics in the small intestine of the cat during reduced perfusion pressure. *Acta Physiol. Scand.* 88:551–563, 1973.

29. McMahon, L.F., M.J. Ryan, D. Larson, and R.L. Fisher. Occult gastrointestinal blood loss in marathon runners. *Ann. Intern. Med.* 100:846–847, 1984.

30. Mitchell, S.J., and S.R. Bloom. Measurement of fasting and postprandial plasma VIP in man. *Gut* 19:1043–1048, 1978.

31. Modlin, I.M., S.R. Bloom, and S. Mitchell. Plasma vasoactive intestinal polypeptide (VIP) levels and intestinal iscaemia. *Experientia* 34:535–536, 1978.

32. Oktedalen, O., I. Guldvog, P.K. Opstad, A. Berstad, D. Gedde-Dahl, and R. Jorde. The effect of physical stress on gastric secretion and pancreatic polypeptide levels in man. *Scand. J. Gastroenterol.* 19:770–778, 1984.

33. Oktedalen, O., P.K. Opstad, and O.B. Schaffalitzky de Muckadell. The plasma concentrations of secretin and vasoactive intestinal polypeptide (VIP) after long-term, strenuous exercise. *Eur. J. Appl. Physiol.* 52:5–8, 1983.

34. Papaioannides, D., Ch. Giotis, N. Karagiannis, and C. Voudouris. Acute upper gastrointestinal hemorrhage in long-distance runners. *Ann. Intern. Med.* 101:719, 1984.

35. Porter, A.M.W. Do some marathon runners bleed into the gut? *Br. Med. J.* 287:1427, 1983.

36. Racusen, L.C., and H.J. Binder. Alteration of large intestinal electrolyte transport by vasoactive intestinal polypeptide in the rat. *Gastroenterology* 73:790–796, 1977.

37. Ramsbottom, N., and J.N. Hunt. Effect of exercise on gastric emptying and gastric secretion. *Digestion* 10:1–10, 1974.

38. Rattan, S., S.I. Said, and R.K. Goyal. Effect of vasoactive intestinal polypeptide (VIP) on the lower esophageal sphincter pressure (LESP) (39740). *Proc. Soc. Exp. Biol. Med.* 155:40–43, 1977.

39. Rowell, L.B. Regulation of splanchnic blood flow in man. *Physiologist* 16:127–142, 1973.

40. Rowell, L.B., J.R. Blackmon, M.A. Kenny, and P. Escourrou. Splanchnic vasomotor and metabolic adjustments to hypoxia and exercise in humans. *Am. J. Physiol.* 247:H251–H258, 1984.

41. Sarna, S., P. Northcott, and L. Belbeck. Mechanism of cycling of migrating myoelectric complexes: Effect of morphine. *Am. J. Physiol.* 242: G588–G595, 1982.

42. Schaffalitzky de Muckadell, O.B., J. Fahrenkrug, and J.J. Holst. Release of vasoactive intestinal polypeptide (VIP) by electric stimulation of the vagal nerves. *Gastroenterology* 72:373–375, 1977.

43. Schaffalitzky de Muckadell, O.B., J. Fahrenkrug, S. Watt-Boolsen, and H. Worning. Pancreatic response and plasma secretin concentration during infusion of low dose secretin in man. *Scand. J. Gastroenterol.* 13:305–311, 1978.

44. Schwartz, T.W., B. Stenquist, L. Olbe, and F. Stadil. Synchronous oscillations in the basal secretion of pancreatic-polypeptide and gastric acid: Depression by cholinergic blockade of pancreatic-polypeptide concentrations in plasma. *Gastroenterology* 76:14–19, 1979.

45. Sharman, I.M. Gastrointestinal disturbances in runners. *Br. J. Sports Med.* 16:179, 1982.

46. Shepherd, A.P. Intestinal O_2 uptake during sympa-

thetic stimulation and partial arterial occlusion. *Am. J. Physiol.* 236:H731–H735, 1979.

47. Silva, D.G., G. Ross, and L.W. Osborne. Adrenergic innervation in the ileum of the cat. *Am. J. Physiol.* 220:347–352, 1971.

48. Sjovall, H. Evidence for separate sympathetic regulation of fluid absorption and blood flow in the feline jejunum. *Am. J. Physiol.* 247:G510–G514, 1984.

49. Sjovall, H., S. Redfors, D.-A. Hallback, S. Eklund, M. Jodal, and O. Lundgren. The effect of splanchnic nerve stimulation on blood flow distribution, villous tissue osmolality and fluid and electrolyte transport in the small intestine of the cat. *Acta Physiol. Scand.* 117:359–365, 1983.

50. Stewart, J.G., D.A. Ahlquist, D.B. McGill, D.M. Ilstrup, S.Schwartz, and R.A. Owen. Gastrointestinal blood loss and anemia in runners. *Ann. Intern. Med.* 100:843–845, 1984.

51. Sullivan, S.N. The gastrointestinal symptoms of running. *N. Engl. J. Med.* 304:915, 1981.

52. Sullivan, S.N. The effect of running on the gastrointestinal tract. *J. Clin. Gastroenterol.* 6:461–465, 1984.

53. Sullivan, S.N., M.C. Champion, N.D. Christofides, T.E. Adrian, and S.R. Bloom. Gastrointestinal regulatory peptide responses in long-distance runners. *Phys. Sportsmed.* 12(7):77–82, 1984.

54. Svanvik, J. Mucosal blood circulation and its influence on passive absorption in the small intestine. *Acta Physiol. Scand. (Suppl. 385)*, 1973.

55. Waldman, D.B., J.D. Gardner, A.M. Zfass, and G.M. Makhlouf. Effects of vasoactive intestinal peptide, secretin, and related peptides on rat colonic transport and adenylate cyclase activity. *Gastroenterology* 73:518–523, 1977.

56. Whalen, G.E. Glucagon and the small gut. (Editorial) *Gastroenterology* 67:1284–1286, 1974.

57. Wingate, D.L., E.A. Pierce, M. Hutton, A. Dand, H.H. Thompson, and E. Wunsch. Quantitative comparison of the effects of cholecystokinin, secretin, and pentagastrin on gastrointestinal myoelectric activity in the conscious fasted dog. *Gut* 19:593–601, 1978.

58. Wu, Z.C., T.M. O'Dorisio, S. Cataland, H.S. Mekhjian, and T.S. Gaginella. Effects of pancreatic polypeptide and vasoactive intestinal polypeptide on rat ileal and colonic water and electrolyte transport in vivo. *Diges. Dis. Sci.* 24:625–630, 1979.

Chapter 12

VITAMIN REQUIREMENTS FOR INCREASED PHYSICAL ACTIVITY

Daphne A. Roe, M.D.

The lay public has long been persuaded that it is possible to increase physical performance by taking vitamins. This belief in vitamins as the latter-day elixirs of life grew out of the old demonstration that in certain states of malnutrition, the ingestion of food sources of vitamins or vitamins themselves could bring about rapid recovery with remarkable improvement in ability to perform physical work.

Today it is still relevant and important to ask questions that have previously been asked but not always completely answered by our scientific forebears. For example, do vitamin deficiencies affect physical work performance? Does exercise increase vitamin needs? Can one improve exercise performance by taking vitamins? Answers to these questions are needed by physicians, exercise physiologists, athletic coaches, nutritionists who set guidelines on nutrient requirements, and people who take vitamins, often irrationally and sometimes dangerously, to improve their ability to perform in sports.

VITAMIN STATUS AND PHYSICAL WORK CAPACITY

Early observers of endemic nutritional deficiencies reported that inability to perform physical work was an outstanding feature of these states of malnutrition. Sailors with scurvy, prisoners with beriberi, and sharecroppers with pellagra were unable to work; their loss of physical strength was variously attributed to swelling of the limbs, cardiac insufficiency, and laziness. Lind (1716–1794), who demonstrated the efficacy of citrus fruit juices in curing scurvy, used as his end point the time taken for sailors to return to active duty [24, 26]. The early observation that beriberi was more common in men than in women was attributed to the greater metabolic rate, activity, and food consumption of men [7].

Whereas early observers were quick to recognize that a number of nutritional deficiencies were associated with impaired physical performance as well as with a more general state of unwellness and recognizable clinical signs, they were also astute enough to identify that a part of the impairment in physical performance was related to a certain disinclination for work. This disinclination for work could be related not only to loss of physical strength, but also to loss of motivation. Thus, in the late stages of pellagra patients have always shown a characteristic aversion to any form of activity [33].

In the forty years from 1915–1955, when major advances were made in our knowledge of vitamins and vitamin deficiencies in animals and humans, information transfer to the public was such that the laity came to believe that almost any vitamin deficiency could result in a marked decrease in physical strength and the capacity to perform muscular work. Indeed, people not only came to associate severe vitamin deficiencies with these functional deficits but also were of the opinion that minor degrees of depletion, such as that which might occur with a low intake of B vitamins, would also impair muscular strength. The comment by Herbert Evans [9], who did so much fundamental work in relation to vitamin E, "... that lack of vitamin E affected the body deleteriously in a more general way than merely by injury to the reproductive system ... could be interpreted to indicate that a deficiency or a depletion of this vitamin could undermine ability to carry out physical work or engage in exercise" is an expression of the same philosophy.

In another context, Kruse [20] introduced the idea of maladaptation to chronic marginal malnutrition. Such maladaptation would be associated with inactivity as well as poor appetite, and Kruse proposed that both the inactivity and the poor appetite could be protective mechanisms that helped the depleted person survive the ordeal.

INVESTIGATION OF THE RELATIONSHIPS BETWEEN VITAMIN STATUS AND PHYSICAL PERFORMANCE

In 1941, a study was carried out at the Rochester State Hospital on patients who had previously received an ample diet with daily supplements of 2 mg of thiamin, 2 mg of riboflavin, 2 mg of pyridoxine, 5 mg of calcium pantothenate, and 40 mg of nicotinamide for several weeks or months. It was assumed by the investigators that these patients would have optimal stores of B vitamins, particularly riboflavin, which was the vitamin of special concern. Subjects or patients were investigated apparently with their informed consent. They were divided into four groups. Group 1 consisted of four subjects studied for the effects of isolated restriction of

riboflavin. Group 2, consisting of two subjects, was studied for the effects of simultaneous deprivation of thiamin, pyridoxine, pantothenic acid, and niacin after development of riboflavin deficiency. Group 3, with only two subjects, served as a control for groups 1 and 2. These subjects received supplements of thiamin, pyridoxine, pantothenic acid, and niacin, and in addition received supplements of riboflavin. By varying the amount of the supplement it was possible to determine the approximate amount of riboflavin that would be required for maintenance of satisfactory tissue stores of this vitamin. Group 4 consisted of five subjects who were maintained on 0.5 mg riboflavin/1000 kcal because of another study that was going on at that time. The period of restriction of riboflavin (group 1) began on August 18, 1941, and extended to June 2, 1942 (288 days). The subjects had good appetites and felt well until the end of the period of investigation and depletion. Physical examinations gave consistently negative results. The concentrations of pyruvic acid and lactic acid in the blood were never abnormally elevated. Apparently there were no complaints or observations of muscle weakness. However, since these were patients in the State Hospital, one wonders whether this was an appropriate population to assess subjective responses. In the group that was restricted with respect to both riboflavin and other members of the B-complex vitamins, signs and symptoms of thiamin deficiency developed within 100 days, and the syndrome that was observed was not essentially different from the syndrome of chronic moderate restriction of thiamin that had previously been reported to cause weakness and prostration [31].

In another study by the same group of investigators, experimental thiamin deficiency was produced in 11 women patients aged 23 to 46 years at the Rochester State Hospital. Subjects received less than 0.45 mg daily for 132 days. There was no caloric restriction. Symptoms among the subjects included irritability, moodiness, and variable restriction of physical activity. According to the report, their sense of well-being and their physical and mental efficiency greatly improved when they were provided with 0.5 mg thiamin/1000 kcal after the period of restriction [32].

On the other hand, Keys et al. [18] studied eight normal young men who were maintained on a rigidly controlled regime of diet, physical work, and endurance testing for 40 days. During the first 21 days of the study, the subjects received an average intake of B vitamins that approximated the (then) recommended dietary allowances (RDAs). For the next 14 days the basal diet of five of the men provided an average of 0.16 mg of thiamin, 0.15 mg of riboflavin, and 1.8 mg of niacin per 1000 kcal. The three other men were studied as controls and received abundant daily supplements of a yeast concentrate as well as synthetic B vitamins. During the last 5 days of the study, all subjects received the same basal diet and these two supplements. A fixed schedule of standardized tests was maintained throughout the study, including tests of physical endurance, of anaerobic work, and of coordination and muscle strength. Blood lactate and pyruvate levels were repeatedly measured at rest and at fixed intervals after standard exhausting anaerobic work. Urinary excretion of thiamin and riboflavin was measured every few days. Psychometric tests were filled out by each subject on alternate days. The limitation in vitamin intake was found to have no effect on the functions that were measured. Neither blood lactate nor pyruvate findings could be interpreted as showing any relationship to the level of vitamin intake. Urinary excretion of thiamin and riboflavin over 24 hours showed marked group differences during the period of vitamin restriction.

In a 1948 review of investigations carried out on relationships between B-vitamin status and nutritional and performance parameters [16], statements are made that mild restriction of B vitamins over a long period can lead to physical and mental changes in chronically psychotic, sedentary old and young individuals. The predominant mental change observed was a decrease in motivation and dulling of attention. Physical changes included loss of appetite and, in older subjects, mild circulatory insufficiency. With severe restriction of B vitamins in similar subjects, mental changes were more severe and included paranoid trends as well as depression and confusion. Marked dependent edema, facial edema, and serous effusion were observed in some individuals, indicative of thiamin deficiency. It was noted that in older subjects, B-vitamin deficiency signs, particularly thiamin deficiency, was precipitated by exercise [16].

No specific adverse effect on physical work performance was found by Keys et al. [19] in a study of riboflavin restriction for 84 days. The intake of riboflavin was set at the level of 0.31 mg/1000 kcal.

MARGINAL MALNUTRITION AND PHYSICAL WORK CAPACITY OF CHILDREN, ADOLESCENTS, AND ADULTS

Studies carried out by Buzina et al. [6] in Yugoslavia have been interpreted as showing that nutritional status affects physical working capacity not only by causing changes in body mass, but also by affecting processes related to aerobic capacity.

The same investigators studied a population of school children, aged 12 to 15 years, in whom biochemical deficiencies of vitamin C, riboflavin, and pyridoxine were present in 30%, 33.9%, and 17.2%, respectively [5]. A small but statistically significant correlation was found between maximal oxygen uptake (Vo_2max) and vitamin C, riboflavin, vitamin A, and iron nutriture. The administration of tablets containing 70 mg of ascorbic acid, 2 mg of riboflavin, and 2 mg of pyridoxine for 3 months led to a small but statistically significant reduction in the prevalence of vitamin deficiency and to a small but statistically significant increase in Vo_2max. No such changes were observed in untreated control groups. The investigators commented that it would not be possible to conclude whether the increase in $\dot{V}o_2$max was a result of the correction of the vitamin deficiencies or was due to an effect of iron utilization.

Buzina [4] offered another possible interpretation of these studies in a review of the effects of marginal malnutrition on functional capacity. Since both ascorbic acid and riboflavin are involved in the absorption and utilization of iron, it is possible that the administration of vitamin pills to mildly hypovitaminemic subjects could result in improved physical work capacity because of a vitamin/mineral interaction; that is, both of these vitamins could have effects on iron nutriture. In this context it is important that both Viteri and Torun [30] and Gardner et al. [10] demonstrated that physical working capacity increases with hemoglobin level, even in nonanemic subjects.

DOES EXERCISE INCREASE VITAMIN REQUIREMENTS?

On the basis of the studies just discussed, it is possible to conclude that severe vitamin deficiencies, particularly B vitamin deficiencies, do indeed compromise ability to perform physical work. However, mild to marginal vitamin depletion/deficiency does not appear to have a uniform or large effect on physical performance, at least not as demonstrated by methods so far employed. In this context, however, it is important to note a study recently conducted in the Netherlands, that shows in a very convincing manner that concurrent restriction of pyridoxine, thiamin and riboflavin may have a modest effect on the aerobic threshold such that there is a slight reduction in physical endurance during the period of depletion (W. van Dokkum, personal communication, 1984.)

A separate but interrelated question is whether exercise or physical work increases vitamin requirements. In three studies we have examined the effect of exercise on riboflavin requirements of young women [1–3]. Execise was found to increase the riboflavin requirements of women of normal (desirable) body weight, as well as of overweight women. In the first of these studies [2], active women of normal body weight were found to require a mean riboflavin intake of 0.96 mg/1000 kcal during periods when they were not exercising, and an intake of 1.16 mg/1000 kcal during periods of prescribed exercise (jogging). The riboflavin requirement in this and the subsequent studies was defined as the intake of riboflavin needed to normalize the erythrocyte glutathione reductase activity coefficient (EGRAC) to within an acceptable range (< 1.25).

In the next study, that investigated moderately obese women [3], it was found that during weight reduction, women consuming a diet containing 0.8 mg riboflavin/1000 kcal became riboflavin depleted. However, it was the exercise, rather than the weight loss or the loss of lean body mass per se, that was associated with the decrease in riboflavin status.

A further study was designed to evaluate our earlier estimates of riboflavin requirements [1]. In this study of moderately obese women, an intake of 0.96 mg riboflavin/1000 kcal was not fully adequate during nonexercise or exercise to maintain an acceptable riboflavin status, as defined by the EGRAC, but a level of intake of 1.16 mg/1000 kcal was adequate. No evidence was obtained that the higher level of riboflavin in the diet increased physical performance or aerobic capacity. Both during periods when the subjects were relatively sedentary and during periods of exercise, riboflavin requirements, whether the subjects were maintaining or losing weight, were in excess of the 1980 RDAs.

One may ask why riboflavin requirements should be increased by exercise. It has been noted in rat studies that when the animals are exercised, they accumulate more riboflavin in their muscles [29]. Increased activity of certain flavoprotein dehydrogenases

(FADs), which has been observed during exercise, may indeed increase the requirement for riboflavin in working muscles. Two FAD-dependent enzymes that have been shown to increase in level with exercise endurance training are succinate dehydrogenase and palmityl coenzyme A (CoA) dehydrogenase. Increases in the activity of these dehydrogenase enzymes may be expected to increase flavin demand, which could result in decreased excretion of riboflavin. This indeed has been demonstrated in studies of the riboflavin requirements of exercising women [11, 12, 23].

Requirements for certain other B vitamins may possibly be increased by exercise. This is implied by results of studies of B_6 status of exercising men and women. Leklem, Munoz, and Walter [22] reported that during strenuous exercise plasma pyridoxal phosphate levels may increase, and suggested that a mobilization of pyridoxal phosphate is occurring, perhaps for pyridoxal phosphate to serve as a cofactor for gluconeogenesis. Though as yet there has been no follow-up, it is possible that the need for vitamin B_6 is modestly increased. We have monitored the folate status of normal women during exercise but have found no evidence of depletion when they were receiving 1980 RDA levels of folate (D.A. Roe and A.Z. Belko, unpublished).

DO VITAMIN SUPPLEMENTS IMPROVE EXERCISE PERFORMANCE OF INDIVIDUALS WITH NORMATIVE VITAMIN STATUS?

In our studies we have been unable to demonstrate any effect of riboflavin supplementation on aerobic capacity in exercising women. It is therefore of interest to note that Tremblay et al. [28], in studies of swimmers in training for 2 to 4 hours/day, showed that these athletes could undergo this amount of training and still maintain normative riboflavin status without supplementation. The swimmers' dietary intake of the vitamin,

however, was probably high, as the report stated that their intake of milk and other dairy products was in accordance with Canadian dietary recommendations. These swimmers submitted to a regimen in which they received 60 mg of riboflavin as a supplement during a 16 to 20 day period, but when they were compared with a control group, no differences were found in performance levels.

However, in another study of athletes, in which some subjects were found to have a biochemical deficiency of riboflavin, administration of 10 mg of riboflavin per day orally apparently resulted in a moderate lowering of neuromuscular irritability, particularly in leg muscles [14]. No evidence was presented to indicate whether overall physical performance was improved by this treatment.

In large doses, niacin can affect myocardial metabolism, both under resting conditions and during exercise. Niacin decreases the mobilization of fatty acids from adipose tissue in exercising individuals; as a result, the utilization of muscle glycogen stores may be increased. In summarizing human studies in which niacin has been given and the effects monitored under resting conditions and during exercise, Hankes [13] pointed out that niacin in pharmacological doses not only reduces the plasma free fatty acid turnover rate and concentration, but also reduces the myocardial extraction of free fatty acids and increases the extraction of blood carbohydrate substrates. In other words, the myocardial energy metabolism shifts from predominant utilization of lipids to predominant utilization of carbohydrate substrates. Information has also been obtained that large doses (200 mg) of niacin increase myocardial extraction of pyruvate and lactate. Hankes therefore concluded that niacin should not be given as a physiological requirement to exercisers. Indeed, it may be dangerous for athletes to take large doses of niacin before events [15]. Information is lacking suggesting that exercise confers a special requirement for niacin.

Vitamin E has been given to improve athletic performance on the basis of a finding that endurance is reduced in vitamin E-deficient rats. Trials of vitamin E have failed to demonstrate any significant improvement in athletic prowess [21, 25].

Vitamin C is taken by athletes to reduce physical stress and to lessen musculoskeletal symptoms. However, the taking of megadoses of this vitamin is not only not effective for these purposes, but is a well-known cause of runners' diarrhea. [17].

RESEARCH NEEDS AND PUBLIC INFORMATION GOALS

Scientific knowledge to date does not allow us to predict with certainty the vitamin requirements of exercisers or athletes. Systematic studies are therefore required in which the vitamin requirements of men, women, and children during sedentary conditions and with aerobic as well as anaerobic exercise are examined. Lest this endeavor be considered without practical merit, it is worth pointing out that people of different ages and at different levels of physiological stress are currently undertaking exercise when their vitamin status is marginal. This is particularly true in Third World countries were malnutrition is prevalent.

In a study of adolescent children of agricultural migrant workers in southern Brazil [8], Desai et al. found that marginal as well as severe malnutrition affected physical work capacity even at low levels of activity. The vitamin intake of these youngsters, particularly their intake of riboflavin, as well as their food energy intake was low. Their vitamin status was not measured, however, and therefore it is not possible to infer that they were vitamin depleted. It would be important to examine the question of whether, if they received adequate food energy intake without increase in vitamin intake, their physical work capacity would increase to that of well-nourished adolescents. We recognize that a confounding issue in such studies might be that better early nutrition

and higher socioeconomic status may be associated with better physical performance, in part because of the effects of training.

Another research question, as yet unanswered, is whether elderly individuals who undertake exercise have increased vitamin as well as food energy needs. It certainly would be of importance to learn whether, when such persons exercise to an extent to maintain or increase their lean body mass, their riboflavin requirement increases.

However, notwithstanding our lack of knowledge of the vitamin requirements of a variety of demographic groups, we do have enough information to know that megavitamin doses are not required by any who undertake physical work or specific forms of exercise. We see and have seen athletes who self-medicate with vitamins as well as those who take megadoses of vitamins on the advice of an athletic trainer or health professional, and we deplore these practices as unjustified and potentially dangerous. The public needs to be informed that neither vitamin A, vitamin E, B-complex vitamins, nor vitamin C should be taken in the hope that it will help win a contest, and that if they want to excel at sports, there are other helpful means that may be safer and more sure.

SUMMARY AND CONCLUSIONS

In this review of the relationships between vitamin nutriture and exercise or physical work performance, it has been shown that severe avitaminoses can significantly impair performance but that marginal deficiencies do not markedly affect ability to exercise efficiently. It has, however, been demonstrated that, at least with respect to riboflavin, a vitamin necessary for optimum energy utilization, requirements increase with exercise, and therefore if exercise is continued, a moderate increase in riboflavin intake is desirable.

It is clear from studies carried out in the past that marginal vitamin deficiencies can have different effects, depending on age, physiological stress, and activity level. Indeed, these conclusions were also reached by Thurnham [27] in his discussion on whether marginal vitamin deficiencies have any physiological significance.

Vitamin requirements of people of varying ages undertaking physical exercise under different physiological conditions, in relation to exercise levels, are of concern. However, we do not presently see nor do we foresee justification for prescription of or self-medication with megadoses of vitamins, since there is no physiological or pharmacological demonstration of need for such products. There is a need to discourage the intake of large doses of vitamins by athletes and other exercisers, because they risk hypervitaminoses. Not only is the practice of megadose vitamin intake ineffective in attaining a high level of physical performance, but with certain vitamins (vitamins A, B_6, and niacin), megadosage can be toxic.

REFERENCES

1. Belko, A.Z., Meredith, M.P., Kalkwarf, H.J., Obarzanek, E., Weinberg, S., Roach, R., McKeon, G., and Roe, D.A. Effects of exercise on riboflavin requirements: biological validation in weight reducing women. *Am. J. Clin. Nutr.* 41:270–277, 1985.
2. Belko, A.Z., Obarzanek, E., Kalkwarf, H.J., Rotter, M.A., Bogusz, S., Miller, D., Haas, J.D., and Roe, D.A. Effects of exercise on riboflavin requirements of young women, *Am. J. Clin. Nutr.* 37: 509—517, 1983.
3. Belko, A.Z., Obarzanek, E., Roach, R., Rotter, M., Urban, G., Weinberg, S. and Roe, D.A. Effects of aerobic exercise and weight loss on riboflavin requirements of moderately obese, marginally deficient young women. *Am. J. Clin. Nutr.* 40: 553–561, 1984.
4. Buzina, R. Marginal malnutrition and its functional consequences in industrial societies. In *Nutrition in Health and Disease and International Development.* Harper, A. E., and Davis, G. K. (Eds). New York: Alan R. Liss, 1981, pp. 285–303.
5. Buzina, R., C. Grgic, M. Jusic, R.J. Sapuna, N. Milanovic, and G. Brubacher. Nutritional status and physical working capacity. *Hum. Nutr. Clin. Nutr.* 36C:429–438, 1982.
6. Buzina, R., V. Horvat, D.J. Vukadinovic, K. Uemura, and H. Dixon. Growth and development of populations in different ecological settings. III.
Nutritional status and physical working capacity in adolescents. *Bibl. Nutr. Dieta.* 27:107–112, 1979.
7. Cowgill, G.R. Vitamin B_1 in relation to the clinic. In *The Vitamins. Symposium on the Present Status of Knowledge of Vitamins. JAMA,* 1932. Evansville, Ind.: Mead Johnson, 1933 (reprinted).
8. Desai, I.D., C. Waddell, S. Dutra, S. Dutra de Oliveira, E. Duarte, M.L. Robazzi, L.S. Cevallos Romero, M.I. Desai, F.L. Vichi, R.B. Bradfield, and J.E. Dutra de Oliveira. Marginal malnutrition and reduced physical work capacity of migrant adolescent boys in Southern Brazil. *Am. J. Clin. Nutr.* 40:135–145, 1984.
9. Evans, H.M. Relation of vitamin E to growth and vigor. *J. Nutr.* 1:23–28, 1928.
10. Gardner, G.W., V.R. Edgerton, B. Seniwiratne, R.J. Bernard, and Y. O'Hira. Physical work capacity and metabolic stress in subjects with iron deficiency anemia. *Am. J. Clin. Nutr.* 30:910–917, 1977.
11. Gollnick, P.D., G.W. Armstrong, C.W. Saubert, K. Piehl, and B. Saltin. Enzyme activity and fiber composition in skeletal muscle of untrained and trained men. *J. Appl. Physiol.* 33:312–319, 1972.
12. Gollnick, P.D., R.B. Armstrong, B. Saltin, C.W. Saubert, W.L. Sembrowich, and R.E. Shepard. Effect of training on enzyme activity and fiber composition of human skeletal muscle. *J. Appl. Physiol.* 34:107–111, 1973.
13. Hankes, L.V. Nicotinic acid and nicotinamide. In Machlin, L.J. (ed.). *Handbook of Vitamins. Nutritional, Biochemical and Clinical Aspects.* New York: Marcel Dekker, 1984, pp. 329–377.
14. Haralambie, G. Vitamin B_2 status in athletes and the influence of riboflavin administration on neuromuscular irritability. *Nutr. Metab.* 20:1–8, 1976.
15. Hegsted, M.D. Niacin and myocardial metabolism. *Nutr. Rev.* 31:80–81, 1973.
16. Horwitt, M.K., E. Liebert, O. Kreisler, and P. Wittman. Investigations of human requirements for B-complex vitamins. *Bull. Nat. Res. Coun.* 116:101–106, 1948.
17. Hoyt, C.J. Diarrhea from vitamin C ("runners' trots"). (Letter) *JAMA* 244:1674, 1980.
18. Keys, A., A. Henschel, H. Longstreet-Taylor, O. Mickelsen, and J. Brozek. Absence of rapid deterioration in men doing hard physical work on a restricted intake of vitamins of the B complex. *J. Nutr.* 27:485–496, 1944a.
19. Keys, A., A.F. Henschel, O. Mickelsen, J.M. Brozek, and J.H. Crawford. Physiological and biochemical functions in normal young men on a diet restricted in riboflavin. *J. Nutr.* 27:165–178, 1944b.
20. Kruse, H.D. A concept of the deficiency states. *Milbank Fund.* 20:245–261, 1942.
21. Lawrence, J.P., R.C. Bower, W.P. Reihl, and V.L. Smith. Effects of alpha-tocopherol acetate on the swimming endurance of trained swimmers. *Am. J. Clin. Nutr.* 28:205–208, 1975.
22. Leklem, J., K. Munoz, and C. Walter. Vitamin B_6 metabolism in men and women following a run or cycle exercise. *Fed. Proc.* 42:1066, 1983.
23. Mole, P.A., L.B. Oscai, and J.O. Holloszy. Adapta-

tion of muscle to exercise: Increases in levels of palmityl CoA synthetase, carnitine palmityl-trans-
ferase, and palmityl CoA dehydrogenase and in the
capacity to oxidize fatty acids. *J. Clin. Invest.*
50:2323–2330, 1971.

24. Rolleston, H. James Lind, Pioneer of Naval
Hygiene. *J. Roy. Nav. Med. Svc.* 1:181, 1915.

25. Sharman, I.M., M.G. Down, and M.G.J. Morgan.
The effect of vitamin E on physiological function
and athletic performance of trained swimmers.
Sport Med. Phys. Fit. 16:215, 1976.

26. Stockman, R. James Lind and scurvy. *Edin. Med. J.*
37:329–350, 1926.

27. Thurnham, D.I. Red cell enzyme tests of vitamin
status: Do marginal deficiencies have any physiological significance? *Proc. Nutri. Soc.* 40:155–162,
1981.

28. Tremblay, A., F. Boilard, M.-F- Bratton, H. Bes-
sette, and A.G. Roberge. The effects of a riboflavin
supplementation on the nutritional status and performance of elite swimmers. *Nutr. Res.* 4:201–208,
1984.

29. Turkki, P., and K. Lepisto Hunter. Effect of exercise on riboflavin status of the rat. *Fed. Proc.*
44:1282, 1985.

30. Viteri, F.E. and B. Torun. Anaemia and physiological work capacity. *Clin. Haematol.* 3:609–626,
1974.

31. Williams, R.D., H.L. Mason, P.L. Cusick, and
R.M. Wilder. Observations on induced riboflavin
deficiency and the riboflavin requirement of man. *J.
Nutr.* 25:361–377, 1943.

32. Williams, R.D., H.L. Mason, B.F. Smith, and R.M.
Wilder. Induced thiamine (vitamin B_1) deficiency
and the thiamine requirement of man. *Arch. Intern.
Med.* 69:721–738, 1942.

33. Wood, E.J. *A treatise on pellagra for the general
practitioner.* New York: Appleton-Century-Crofts,
1912, pp. 144–150.

Chapter 13

TRACE MINERALS AND EXERCISE

Richard A. Anderson, Ph.D., and Helene N. Guttman, Ph.D.

Since the early times of athletic competition, athletes have been searching for elusive dietary substances to improve performance, and numerous dietary modifications have been attempted. No evidence exists, however, that supplementation with any specific nutrient influences athletic performance more than the performance level obtained with a well-balanced diet [5]. The effects of trace elements on overall health and performance is an emerging field, and many of the studies involving the effects of strenuous exercise on short- and long-term health as well as on athletic performance have not been completed. The effects of exercise on trace element status and overall health are of particular importance for the following reasons:

1. Dietary intake of the trace elements zinc, copper, and chromium, even for sedentary individuals, is marginal.
2. Dietary intake of selenium appears to meet the suggested intake, but additional selenium may be involved in the prevention of certain forms of cancer.
3. Strenuous exercise stimulates trace element losses.
4. Chronic diseases such as maturity-onset diabetes, cancer and cardiovascular diseases are associated with suboptimal trace element status.

In this chapter we put into perspective current understanding and gaps in our knowledge concerning the effects of strenuous exercise on the nutrition and metabolic roles of four essential trace elements—zinc, copper, chromium, and selenium. The areas covered include (a) the nutritional role of each of these elements, (b) food sources and requirements, (c) exercise-induced changes in the blood, and (d) exercise-induced changes in excretion.

ZINC AND EXERCISE

Role of Zinc

Zinc is a multifunctional nutrient that is involved in numerous phases of growth and development, including protein and DNA synthesis and cell division. It is the most abundant trace mineral in tissues other than the blood and is widely distributed in the nuclear, mitochondrial, and supernatant fractions of the cell in every tissue of the body.

Zinc nutriture is of critical importance to the athlete for the following reasons: (a) Exercise and other forms of stress alter zinc metabolism and stimulate zinc losses; (b) dietary intake, even of sedentary individuals, is suboptimal compared with recommendations of the National Research Council; and (c) abnormal zinc metabolism, whether due to slight excess or deficiencies, will alter body function. Suboptimal intake of zinc in humans is associated with slow wound healing, skin lesions, anorexia, oligospermia, loss of taste and smell acuity, and decreased immune responses [56], while slight excesses of zinc may lead to lower levels of the high-density lipoprotein (HDL)-cholesterol, which is associated with increased risk of cardiovascular disease.

Sources of Zinc and Requirement

The recommended dietary allowance (RDA) of zinc for adults is 15 mg [42]. Dietary zinc intake for most individuals appears to be marginal [56], and the consequences of this may be exacerbated by exercise, as evidenced by the hypozincemia experienced in runners [14]. Dietary habits associated with strenuous exercise, such as carbohydrate loading by competitive athletes, may also exacerbate the consequences of suboptimal zinc intake, since high carbohydrate foods such as pasta, ice cream, pastry, and fruits are not good sources of zinc (Table 1). Furthermore, zinc obtained from vegetable sources is less available than zinc in meat, poultry, or seafood because of the presence of phytate and dietary fiber in foods derived from plants [56]. Foods high in zinc include oysters (which may contain over 1 mg of zinc per gram), beef, liver, and dark meat from turkey and chicken (Table 1). The poorest sources are white sugar, some citrus fruits, nonleafy vegetables, tubers, and vegetable oils (Table 1) [59].

Exercise-Induced Changes in Blood Zinc

Strenuous training leads to decreases in circulating levels of zinc. Mean serum zinc of 77 male runners was 76 ± 13 μg/100 ml compared with 94 ± 12 μg/100 ml for 21 male nonrunners. Serum zinc concentrations tended to decrease with greater training distance, but because of wide individual variations, the effects of weekly mileage were not statistically significant [14]. Of the males with an average weekly training distance of

only 22 miles, 23% displayed serum zinc levels in the hypozincemic range (less than 65 μg/dl). Haralambie [21] reported a similar incidence of hypozincemia in male runners who trained for 90 to 120 minutes four times per week and a higher incidence (43%) of abnormally low zinc values for female runners. Depressed blood zinc levels have also been observed by others [15, 19]. In a separate study, the plasma zinc levels of young college-age athletic participants and of nonparticipants were not significantly different. However, the mean maximal oxygen uptake ($\dot{V}O_2$max) of both the athletes and nonathletes was in the good or above range, indicating that the group classified as nonathletes was in good physical condition. Athletes were defined as representative members of the various college sport teams including football, basketball, wrestling, hockey, weight lifting, and track and field [39].

Following acute exercise, changes in serum zinc are time dependent. Anderson, Polansky, and Bryden [3] reported no change in serum zinc level immediately following a strenuous run but a significant decrease after 2 hours. The decrease may have been due to a redistribution of zinc. Hetland et al. [23] reported that serum zinc level was 19% higher immediately following a 70-km cross-country ski race compared with prerace values but returned to prerace values 1 day following the race; zinc values were insignificantly elevated on the second day following the race. Erythrocyte zinc concentration, which is approximately 10-fold that of the serum, was not altered by strenuous exercise. These authors postulated that the transitory increase in serum zinc in response to exercise may be caused by leakage of zinc from skeletal muscle to the extracellular fluid. Muscle breakdown and localized injury due to exercise could also explain the increase. Similarly, tissue breakdown due to fasting leads to elevated serum zinc concentration [58]. Oh et al. [44] reported that plasma zinc levels fell in rats after acute swimming and that the

Table 1. ZINC, COPPER, SELENIUM, AND CHROMIUM CONTENT OF SELECTED FOODS.

SELECTED FOOD ITEMS	SERVING SIZE	ZINC (MG)(15 mg*)†	
		Per 100 g	*Per serving*
Edam cheese	1 slice = (24 g)	3.75	0.90
Cottage cheese, 1%	1/2 cup = (72 g)	0.38	0.27
Whole milk	1 cup = (244 g)	0.38	0.92
Butter	1 pat = (5 g)	0.05	0.00
Margarine	1 pat = (5 g)	0.00	0.00
Hard-boiled egg	1 med = (50 g)	1.44	0.72
Chicken meat, dark	3 oz = (90 g)	2.80	2.52
Chicken meat, light	3 oz = (90 g)	1.23	1.11
Turkey meat, dark	3 oz = (90 g)	4.46	4.01
Turkey meat, light	3 oz = (90 g)	2.04	1.84
Pork, broiled	3 oz = (90 g)	2.23	2.01
Beef, round, broiled	3 oz = (90 g)	6.31	5.70
Liver, calf, fried	3 oz = (90 g)	5.13	4.61
Haddock, raw	3 oz = (90 g)	0.80	0.72
Oyster, raw	3 oz = (90 g)	74.70	67.23
Special K cereal	1 cup = (25 g)	13.20	3.30
Corn Flakes	1 cup = (25 g)	0.28	0.07
White bread	1 slice = (25 g)	0.62	0.16
Wholewheat bread	1 slice = (25 g)	1.89	0.47
Oatmeal, dry	1/3 cup = (27 g)	3.07	0.83
Wheat germ, toasted	1 Tb = (6 g)	16.67	1.00
Brown rice, raw	1/6 cup = (66 g)	1.60	1.06
White rice, raw	1/6 cup = (66 g)	1.30	0.86
Potato, raw	1 cup = (250 g)	0.39	0.98
Apple, raw, w/skin	1 med = (150 g)	0.04	0.06
Raisins, seedless	2 Tb = (20 g)	0.27	0.05
Broccoli, fresh	1/2 cup = (92 g)	0.15	0.14
Chickpeas	1 oz = (25 g)	2.94	0.74
Peanuts, roasted	1 Tb = (9 g)	1.27	0.11
Mushrooms, Shiitake, dried	4 = (15 g)	7.66	1.15
Mushrooms, white, new	1/2 c = (35 g)	0.73	0.26
Spaghetti, dry	1/2 cup = 52 g	0.97	0.50
Beer	12 oz = (360 g)	0.02	0.07
Brewer's yeast	1 Tb = (8 g)	—	—
Cocoa	1 Tb = (5 g)	6.700	0.34
Black pepper	1/8 t = 0.25 g	1.42	0.00
Wine, table	3 1/2 oz = (102 g)	0.08	0.08

*Data from Human Nutrition Information Service [27].
†Number(s) denotes recommended dietary allowance or suggested safe and adequate intake [42].
‡Data from Fachman, Souci, and Kravt [16].
◖Data from Schubert, Holden, and Wolf [54].
§Data from Koivistoinen [34] and unpublished data from our laboratory.

COPPER (MG) (2–3MG†)		SELENIUM (μG) (50–200 μG¶)†		CHROMIUM (μG) (50–200 μG§)†	
Per 100 g	Per serving	Per 100 g	Per serving	Per 100 g	Per serving
0.04	0.01	11	2.6	2.0	0.5
0.03	0.02	6.0	4.3	2.0	1.4
0.01	0.02	1.6	3.9	1.0	2.4
0.02	0.00	—	—	6.0	0.3
0.00	0.00	—	—	2.0	0.1
0.06	0.03	25	12.5	0.5	0.2
0.08	0.07	21	18.9	3.0	2.7
0.05	0.05	21	18.9	3.0	2.7
0.16	0.14	25	22.5	1.0	0.9
0.04	0.04	25	22.5	1.0	0.9
0.08	0.07	35	31.5	3.0	2.7
0.14	0.12	26	23.4	1.0	0.9
12.00	10.80	56	50.4	1.0	0.9
0.16	0.14	48	43.2	1.0	0.9
7.60	6.84	57	51.3	14.0	12.6
0.45	0.11	63	15.8	—	—
0.07	0.02	6.3	1.6	7.0	1.8
0.14	0.04	32	8.0	—	—
0.37	0.09	44	11.0	3.0	0.8
0.34	0.09	29	7.8	<2.0	<0.5
0.62	0.04	—	—	<2.0	<0.1
0.30	0.20	—	—	3.0	2.0
0.26	0.17	29	19.1	2.0	1.3
0.26	0.70	1.3	3.2	0.5	1.2
0.04	0.06	0.4	0.6	5.0	7.5
0.31	0.06	—	—	10.0	2.0
0.07	0.06	—	—	1.0	0.9
0.57	0.14	—	—	4.0	2.0
6.62	0.60	—	—	8.0	0.7
5.17	0.78	—	—	47.0	16.4
0.49	0.17	—	—	47.0	16.4
0.25	0.13	66	34.3	4.0	2.1
0.01	0.03	—	—	0.9	3.2
—	—	—	—	1.0	3.4
3.61	0.18	—	—	14.0	0.7
3.32	0.01	—	—	17.0	0.8
0.01	0.01	—	—	7.5	7.6

decline was related to the increased synthesis of hepatic metallothioneine, a metal-binding protein. A second zinc binding protein, α_2-macroglobulin, is also found in higher levels in athletes than in sedentary controls [38].

Leukocytic endogenous mediator, a hormone-like substance released by phagocytes in response to stress such as infection or exercise, leads to a redistribution of zinc from the blood to the liver. This may be responsible for the decreased level of serum or plasma zinc observed following exercise [47]. A stable messenger or factor seems to be present in the blood after exercise, since human plasma collected immediately or 3 hours after strenuous exercise depressed plasma zinc level when injected intraperitoneally into rats.

Zinc Excretion and Exercise

Zinc is excreted primarily in the feces, with lesser amounts occurring in urine and sweat. Fecal zinc consists mostly of unabsorbed dietary zinc, with small amounts being secreted via the bile into the cecum and colon. Urinary zinc excretion of healthy adults is normally 0.3 to 0.5 mg/day, compared with the 8 to 12 mg/day normally ingested. Exercise leads to increased urinary zinc losses [3, 9]. Two hours after a strenuous 6-mile run, urinary zinc concentration in nine male runners was elevated more than twofold; total urinary losses on the day of the run were more than 1.5-fold higher than on a nonrun day [3].

Significant quantities of zinc also can be lost in sweat, especially during strenuous exercise [10, 11]. Whereas normal sweat losses of zinc by sedentary subjects may account for 5% or less of the normal intake, sweat losses following extended strenuous exercise may be substantially higher. With prolonged heavy sweating, the amount of zinc lost could theoretically exceed 3 mg/day (20% of the RDA) [43].

Zinc Status and Exercise

There is no single reliable clinical index of zinc status in humans. However, fasting serum and plasma zinc levels have been used to assess status. While circulating zinc may in some instances reflect the body's zinc status, it also may reflect zinc from a body storage pool that is available as necessary for metabolically active tissues. Mobilization of this available zinc occurs under conditions of stress such as exercise, infection, or inflammation [49, 47]. Mobilization of zinc may be part of an initial defense mechanism, which would be consistent with the role of zinc in immune function. Functional tests including neuropsychological function, immune response, reproductive competence, and work capacity have been suggested as methods to assess zinc status more accurately [57]. Lukaski et al. [40] reported that postexercise changes in plasma zinc content are sensitive to changes in body zinc level, and thus may represent a suitable functional test to assess zinc status. Increases in plasma zinc concentration following exercise in subjects consuming zinc-adequate diets indicate that tissue pools, including muscle, contain adequate zinc. When subjects were placed on a low-zinc diet, postexercise changes in plasma zinc levels decreased, presumably due to depletion of muscle zinc stores. This postulate is confirmed by animal studies that show that zinc concentration of muscles containing slow-twitch fibers (e.g., the soleus) is sensitive to dietary zinc intake [46].

Exercise and Zinc Supplementation

Due to the apparent compromise of zinc status associated with strenuous exercise, zinc supplementation has been suggested as a means of improving not only zinc status but also physical performance. Zinc supplementation (135 mg/day) for 14 days resulted in a significant increase in isokinetic leg strength at high angular velocities and in isometric endurance [36]. Beneficial effects of zinc supplementation were postulated to be due to an effect of zinc either on lactate dehydrogenase activity or on glucose transport and metabolism in muscles. Zinc supplementation of rats also led to increased performance in that the gastrocnemius muscles of zinc-supplemented animals took longer to fatigue than did muscles taken from control animals [50].

While the human dietary zinc intake should be maintained near the daily RDA of 15 mg, excess dietary zinc should be avoided. High levels of dietary zinc compared with copper (zinc level 40-fold higher than copper level; control zinc level 5-fold higher) have been associated with hypercholesterolemia in rats and have been postulated to increase the risks of coronary artery disease [33]. Large supplemental doses of zinc (160 mg/day) in humans may decrease HDL cholesterol (the protective form of cholesterol) without changing total cholesterol, thus increasing the risks of coronary artery disease [26]; it can also lead to impaired copper metabolism. This effect is well documented in animal studies, and depressed copper levels in humans due to long-term (2 years) daily zinc supplementation of 150 mg has been reported [48]. Zinc supplementation (greater than 15 mg/day) of elderly subjects has been shown to inhibit the increase in HDL cholesterol normally associated with increased exercise [18]. With sex, alcohol intake, and body mass controlled there was a significant positive correlation between level of exercise and serum HDL cholesterol in the subjects over age 60 not taking supplemental zinc. Multiple regression analysis showed a significant interaction of zinc intake and activity level on HDL cholesterol concentration. In the 22 subjects who stopped taking supplemental zinc for 8 weeks, HDL cholesterol levels increased significantly (2 mg/dl; $P = 0.04$) and the change in HDL cholesterol was positively correlated with the level of exercise of the subjects [18]. Results of this study, however, should be treated with caution due to the small changes observed and the exercise

levels of the subjects. While there was a significant increase in HDL ($P = 0.04$) following supplemental zinc cessation in the 22 subjects, there was a more significant unexplained increase ($P = 0.0001$) in body mass index. In a separate study from the same laboratory, involving sedentary and endurance-trained men, zinc supplementation (zinc sulfate, 50 mg daily) did not alter HDL cholesterol levels [11]. These studies may also illustrate the need for balanced nutritional supplementation. Ingestion of a supplement consisting of a single nutrient or a small group of nutrients may upset the normal balance of nutrients and lead not to beneficial but to detrimental effects. Unless the subject is closely followed and there is irrefutable evidence of no detrimental effects, supplementation with single nutrients or small groups of nutrients should be avoided in healthy normal subjects.

COPPER AND EXERCISE

Role of Copper

Copper is involved in numerous essential physiological functions, including carbohydrate and lipid metabolism, integrity of the immune system, collagen and elastin formation, amino acid metabolism, hematopoiesis, and protection against cellular damage due to the accumulation of toxic free radicals. Copper is also an essential cofactor of numerous enzymes.

Clinical signs of copper deficiency have been associated with hypercholesterolemia, abnormal electrocardiogram, glucose intolerance, and ischemic heart disease. Copper deficiency in animals is characterized by weakening of arteries, lesions in blood vessels, hypercholesterolemia, cardiac hypertrophy, anemia, inflammation and fibrotic changes of the heart, and sudden death [31, 32].

The clinical significance of newer findings regarding the consequences of inadequate dietary copper, which have been published in experimental nutrition literature, has not been recognized by the medical community or the general public. This lack of awareness of the nutritional importance of copper and the risk factors associated with copper deficiency is dangerous, because typical diets in the United States and other westernized countries contain only about half of the daily lower limit of the recommended safe and adequate level of copper [17].

Sources of Copper and Requirement

The suggested safe and adequate intake of copper for adults is 2 to 3 mg/day [42]. However, some studies indicate that normal daily copper intake is in the region of only 1 mg [17, 33, 62]. Under certain circumstances this may lead to serious health problems. For example, electrocardiogram irregularities returned to normal following supplemental copper in a subject consuming a diet similar in copper content to that often consumed by "normal" free-living individuals [32]. In addition, 4 of 24 male subjects participating in a study to determine the effects of feeding diets low in copper (1.03 mg/2850 Cal) containing 20% fructose or starch exhibited heart-related abnormalities and the study had to be discontinued [49]. (The reader is reminded that 1 mg/day of copper is similar to the amount normally consumed in the United States.)

Good sources of dietary copper include liver, shiitake mushrooms, potatoes, and peanuts (Table 1). The poorest sources include white sugar, honey, and dairy products. Type of dietary carbohydrate, in addition to absolute copper concentration, also affects copper nutriture. For example, a diet containing fructose instead of starch as the source of carbohydrate, with the same copper concentration, has profound detrimental effects, including changes in numerous clinical parameters, heart morphology, and even survival [17].

Exercise-Induced Changes in Blood Copper Level

While long-term training leads to lower blood zinc levels, training usually leads to elevated serum copper concentrations. Ohla et al. [45] reported that runners had significantly higher mean resting serum copper concentrations compared with sedentary controls (116 vs. 108 μg/dl); similar results were reported by others [19, 20, 22]. Lukaski et al. [39] reported that varsity athletic participants had significantly higher plasma copper levels than did nonparticipants; plasma zinc levels of these subjects were not significantly different. However, Dressendorfer and Sockolov [14] studied the relationship between training mileage and serum copper levels; mean copper levels were similar for runners and controls (96 and 93 μg/dl, respectively) and there was no relationship between training mileage and serum copper, while an inverse relationship with serum zinc was observed. Dowdy and Burt [13] followed competitive swimmers during a 6-month training period and reported that serum copper level decreased with duration of training. The concentration of ceruloplasmin, the principal copper-binding protein, also decreased. Similar decreased ceruloplasmin activity was reported for adolescents during intense ski training. The combined stresses of training and growth also resulted in a 29% decrease in copper oxidase activity [51].

Reports on the effects of acute exercise on serum copper level are also somewhat conflicting. Some reports cite increases [20, 45], decreases [52], or no change [3] in blood copper level due to acute exercise. Haralambie [20] reported that serum copper concentration of untrained men increased initially during exercise and then decreased after 30 minutes. The decrease was accompanied by a decrease in ceruloplasmin; in the ensuing 90 minutes, both serum copper and ceruloplasmin levels increased. Degree of training may also alter serum copper values in response to acute exercise. Olha et al. [45]

reported a 35% increase in serum copper level in trained athletes compared with a 15% increase in untrained athletes following 90 minutes of intense exercise on an ergometer. Possible explanations for the above-mentioned inconsistencies include (a) duration and type of training, (b) copper status of subjects, and (c) type of exercise performed, for example, swimming versus running.

Copper Excretion and Exercise

In all species studied, a high proportion of ingested copper appears in the feces, most of which is unabsorbed copper; active excretion of some copper does occur via the bile. The major fraction of the absorbed copper binds to plasma albumin; a small fraction is chelated to histidine. Albumin copper is the most rapidly available source of copper for the tissues. While brain, heart, and kidney ultimately show relatively high tissue levels, most absorbed copper is preferentially taken up by the liver. The majority of this hepatic copper is excreted in the bile to maintain total body copper balance. A significant portion of the recently absorbed copper also is incorporated into ceruloplasmin, which then is secreted into the serum. The remainder of the copper is lost via the urine (1–2%), gastric secretions, and sweat [59].

The amount of copper lost via sweat, although significant, often is not reported in studies involving copper losses. Reported copper concentrations of sweat vary from 58 μg/L [41] to 550 μg/L [24]. The large differences reported, besides analytical problems and problems with contamination, may be related to copper intake and status of subjects, area of the body from which sweat was collected, and methods and conditions used to induce sweating. Sweat due to strenuous exercise is probably very different from that collected in a sauna or after nervous perspiration. The American Dietetic Association [1] has stated that some individuals may lose as much as 2 to 4 L of sweat per hour when competing in endurance events. If one assumes an average copper concentration in sweat of 304 μg/L (average of the two values listed previously) and a daily sweat loss of 3 L (average amount lost during 1 hour of strenuous exercise), this amounts to approximately 1 mg of copper lost in sweat per day. Normal whole-body surface losses of copper are approximately 33% of this value for sedentary subjects [28]. These increased copper losses via sweat become very significant, since recent values for dietary copper intake are less than 2 mg/day (see section on copper intake). This theoretical calculation for copper lost per day due to strenuous exercise is similar to the 1.04 mg of copper lost in sweat by three men exposed to 37.8°C, 50% relative humidity [10]. Therefore, sweat losses of individuals who exercise strenuously could lead to gradual depletion of body copper stores unless significant physiological adaptive changes occur. Increases of copper intake of two-fold or more may be required to offset sweat losses due to strenuous exercise.

Copper Status and Exercise

Assessment of copper status cannot be achieved simply by measuring blood copper level. While this measurement may be useful under certain circumstances, it should not be the only measurement; normal or even slightly elevated serum copper level has been observed in subjects consuming a low-copper diet (low copper intake was obvious from the red blood cell superoxide dismutase activity) [49]. Superoxide dismutase is widely distributed metalloenzyme containing both zinc and copper, with copper at the active site. Decreases in copper status in humans appear to be reflected in red-cell superoxide dismutase activity [49] and should be monitored in individuals who exercise strenuously over long duration.

The potential long-term effects of altered serum zinc and copper levels in response to exercise are not known. An issue that needs to be resolved is whether the increased copper output from the liver leads to depressed hepatic copper activity. If this is the case, trained athletes may have an increased copper requirement [29]. However, supplemental copper in excess of the suggested safe and adequate intake (2–3 mg for adults) should be avoided, since excess copper is quite toxic [59].

CHROMIUM AND EXERCISE

Role of Chromium

Chromium, an essential element for humans and animals, functions in normal carbohydrate, lipid, and nucleic acid metabolism. Chromium's role in carbohydrate and lipid metabolism is related to that of insulin, with chromium potentiating the action of insulin. Less insulin is required, both *in vivo* and *in vitro*, if sufficient chromium in a useable form is present [7]. Chromium's role in nucleic acid metabolism appears to be related to the structural integrity of the nuclear strands.

Clinical signs of chromium deficiency that are present in sedentary individuals include impaired glucose tolerance, decreased insulin receptor number, elevated serum cholesterol and triglyceride levels, decreased HDL cholesterol level, and increased incidence of aortic plaques. More severe chromium deficiency leads to disorders that are not normally observed except with special diets, for example, total parenteral nutrition. These more severe signs of chromium deficiency include peripheral neuropathy and brain disorders [7].

Sources of Chromium and Requirement

In 1980 the recommended or suggested safe and adequate adult intake of chromium was established at 50 to 200 μg [42]. Many earlier studies reported dietary chromium intakes in excess of the suggested intake [for review, see 2], but these higher values likely were due to chromium contamination in the collection, to homogenization, or to the analysis of the samples. Samples often were contaminated in the homogenization steps, since stainless-steel blades, which are approximately 18% chromium, were used in blending; apparent chromium content of the diet samples is then related to the duration of blending and does not reflect the endogenous chromium in the food as consumed [2]. Recent well-controlled studies from the United States, Canada, England, and Finland [for original references, see 2] all indicate that dietary chromium intake of normal free-living subjects is suboptimal. In a recent study involving 10 male and 22 female adult subjects, diets were collected for 7 consecutive days and analyzed for chromium [2]; the 7-day dietary chromium intake was below the minimum suggested intake for all of the subjects. Mean intake was 25 ± 1 (standard error of the mean) μg/day for the females and 33 ± 3 μg/day for the males. Mean chromium intake per thousand Calories was approximately 15 μg. In a separate study in which a constant diet designed by nutritionists to be well balanced was fed to trained and untrained runners, the chromium content per thousand Calories was only 9 μg [4]. Therefore, to obtain the minimum suggested intake for chromium would require consumption of between 3000 and 5500 Cal and to obtain the upper limit of the safe and adequate intake of 200 μg would require consumption of 13,000 to 22,000 Cal. Obviously care must be taken in the selection of foods by individuals who exercise regularly, since exercise also leads to increased chromium losses that need to be compensated for by some as-yet unknown means [3, 6].

Good dietary sources of chromium include mushrooms, oysters, apples with skins, wine, and beer (Table 1). Poor sources of chromium include highly processed or refined foods such as sugar and white flour. Carbohydrate loading by ingestion of pastries, pastas, and foods high in carbohydrate but low in chromium may lead to insufficient intake of chromium. Not only are these foods low in chromium, but highly refined-sugar foods also stimulate chromium losses [35]. Carbohydrate loading should include complex carbohydrates such as those present in potatoes and not simple carbohydrates such as table sugar (sucrose).

Exercise-Induced Changes in Blood Chromium

Circulating chromium does not appear to reflect chromium status; increases in serum chromium in response to a stress such as a glucose load may be a better reflection of status. Similarly, the stress of acute exercise may be an indicator of status similar to that for zinc (see section on zinc status and exercise). To our knowledge there is only one report of the effect of exercise on serum chromium [3]. Immediately following a strenuous 6-mile run, serum chromium level was elevated approximately 50% above preexercise levels and remained elevated 2 hours following exercise. In these same subjects, serum copper level was not altered by acute exercise and serum zinc level was significantly lower 2 hours following exercise and was unchanged immediately following running.

Chromium Excretion and Exercise

Urinary excretion is the primary route of excretion of absorbed chromium. Various stresses including glucose loading, infection, physical injury, and strenuous exercise all stimulate chromium loss. Urinary chromium concentrations of samples collected 2 hours following a strenuous run were approximately fivefold higher than basal levels [6]. Values were still more than threefold higher when expressed as a chromium/creatinine ratio, and the 24-hour chromium excretion

on a run day compared with a nonrun day was also more than double [3, 6].

Basal urinary chromium excretion of subjects with $\dot{V}o_2$max scores in the good or excellent range (trained subjects) was twofold less on nonrun days than that of subjects with $\dot{V}o_2$max values in the average or below range (untrained subjects) [2]. Even after subjects were placed on a constant diet, basal urinary chromium excretion of untrained subjects remained twofold higher than that of the trained subjects. While consuming the constant diet, subjects exercised on a treadmill at 90% of $\dot{V}o_2$max to exhaustion with 30-second exercise and 30-second rest periods. Trained subjects excreted significantly more chromium on the day of controlled exercise compared with nonexercise days. The amount of urinary chromium excretion of untrained subjects was not altered by the controlled exercise bout. Therefore, basal urinary chromium excretion and chromium excretion in response to exercise are related to maximal oxygen consumption and thus to degree of physical training [2].

Whether the decreased basal chromium excretion of trained runners is a sign of marginal deficiency or an adaptive defense mechanism to conserve chromium remains to be established. The body undergoes numerous changes in response to training, and conservation of body chromium may be yet another example. In studies involving rats, exercise-trained animals had higher tissue chromium levels than sedentary controls [60]. Similarly, trained subjects may have higher tissue chromium levels than untrained subjects, and some of the decreases in basal chromium excretion may be related to the possible increases in tissue chromium concentration.

Loss of chromium in sweat has not been determined with acceptable collection and analytical techniques. This area of research needs to be explored to ascertain not only the basal and exercise-induced sweat losses of chromium but also if the chromium content of sweat is altered by physical training.

Chromium Status and Exercise

Due to the increased losses of chromium associated with strenuous exercise, chromium status of exercising individuals may be compromised. There are no known parameters that can be used to assess chromium status in a single measurement, but changes in glucose tolerance in response to chromium supplementation can be used to assess status [7].

SELENIUM AND EXERCISE

Role of Selenium

Selenium is present in all cells of the body in concentrations dependent on the amount and form of selenium in the diet. The liver and kidney usually contain the highest selenium concentrations, with much lower levels in the muscles, bones, blood, and adipose tissues. Cardiac muscle contains higher concentrations of selenium than skeletal muscle [59]. Signs of selenium deficiency in animals include muscular dystrophy (white-muscle disease) in lambs, calves, and other species; resorption sterility; and liver necrosis [59]. In humans, selenium deficiency has been associated with severe muscular discomfort in the quadriceps and hamstring muscles in a patient receiving total parenteral nutrition [61]; all muscular symptoms disappeared within 7 days of selenium supplementation. Keshan disease, an endemic cardiomyopathy that primarily affects children (1 to 9 years of age) in certain areas of China is also associated with low selenium intake. Symptoms of Keshan disease include heart failure, cardiogenic shock, abnormal electrocardiograms, and heart enlargement [30]. Increasing evidence linking selenium deficiency with Keshan disease led to a large-scale selenium intervention study. (Dosage was 0.5 mg selenite/week for children 1 to 5 years of age and 1 mg for those aged 6 to 9 years). The effects of supplemental selenite was so positive in the first 2 years of the study (1 death due to Keshan disease vs. 53 deaths in the placebo group) that the placebo group was eliminated and all subjects were given supplemental selenium the following years.

Sources of Selenium and Requirement

The suggested safe and adequate daily intake of selenium for adults is 50 to 200 μg [42]. Dietary intake for most individuals appears to be in this range, but due to the variable nature of selenium bioavailability and content in foods, certain individuals may inadvertently select a low-selenium diet. An example of the extreme variation of the selenium content in the same food was reported by Schroeder, Frost, and Balassa [53], who found that the selenium content of wheat from different geographical regions ranged from 0.04 to 21.4 $\mu g/g$. Other factors such as milling, cooking, and processing also alter the selenium content of foods, but these effects are minor compared with variations due to geographical origin. Good sources of selenium, in decreasing order, usually include muscle meats, liver, cereal products, dairy products, vegetables, and fruits (Table 1). However, the selenium content of all of these foods would be altered due to the selenium content of the soils in the region of origin of the foods. Poor sources of selenium include sugar and many highly refined foods.

To our knowledge there are presently no comprehensive studies regarding the effects of acute exercise or chronic training on selenium levels in the blood, urine, or sweat. Therefore this section discusses the available studies together.

Selenium, as a component of glutathione peroxidase, in conjunction with vitamin E, functions in the removal of peroxide free radicals. Selenium and vitamin E interact critically; vitamin E has a definite sparing effect on selenium metabolism. Much lower levels of selenium are required to induce selenium deficiency symptoms in the presence of sufficient vitamin E than at suboptimal levels.

Since both selenium and vitamin E are involved in the removal of free radicals, this becomes important to the field of exercise physiology—strenuous exercise leads to increased production of free radicals [12]. In rats, exercise to exhaustion led not only to increased free radical production but also to increased levels of lipid peroxidation products. Thiobarbituric acid reactive substances, indicators of lipid peroxidation, increased in liver and muscle following swimming [9]. This increase was reduced in liver by dietary E supplementation but not by dietary selenium. Increased peroxidation in horses due to exercise also has been reported, and was not altered due to supplemental selenium intake [8]. However, selenium status, on the basis of plasma selenium, was normal in both groups of horses, and therefore additional selenium would not be expected to show beneficial effects. Increased lipid peroxidation appears to be a normal response to exercise regardless of the nutritional intake. Effects of a nutrient on experimental animals or people consuming sufficient amounts of nutrient in question are pharmacological effects, and these should not be confused with the beneficial nutritional effects observed in people or animals consuming suboptimal dietary amounts.

Symptoms of white-muscle disease, a disease in lambs that can be prevented by adequate dietary selenium, are exacerbated by exercise [63]. When one foreleg of lambs born to ewes fed a "dystrophy-producing" diet was restrained, lesions of white-muscle disease did not develop; lesions occurred only in the exercising limb. While this is an extreme case, it does point out potential problems associated with improper selenium intake and exercise. Problems of this nature are not likely to occur in humans consuming an average diet, but the risks of long-term problems of marginal selenium deficiency, for example, the incidence of cancer, need to be studied. There is no reported evidence that strenuous exercise leads to increased incidence of cancer in later life, but there is evidence that exercise enhances selenium deficiency, and low dietary selenium is associated with an increased incidence of certain forms of cancer [55].

Selenium Status and Exercise

No single technique for assessing selenium status is satisfactory, and different methods yield conflicting results. Extremely low selenium status, such as that observed in patients with Keshan disease, can be assessed by blood selenium levels. Glutathione peroxidase, a selenoenzyme, provides a convenient tool for assessing selenium status, but appears to reflect status only when blood selenium levels are low, a situation commonly found in New Zealand. Blood glutathione peroxidase activity is usually saturated at blood selenium levels present in individuals living in North America. Platelet glutathione peroxidase activity appears to be a better indicator of selenium status, since its activity is responsive to selenium intake in the range of most individuals [37].

GAPS IN OUR KNOWLEDGE AND FUTURE STUDIES REGARDING TRACE ELEMENTS AND EXERCISE

Longitudinal studies of the effects of strenuous exercise on trace element intake, excretion (including sweat), and trace element status are needed. The effects of trace elements on athletic performance, or parameters associated with performance such as muscle glycogen, are also needed. Documentation of increased requirement of trace elements for individuals who exercise strenuously is lacking. Are the increased losses of trace elements compensated for by unknown means, such as increased absorption or utilization? Are the increased needs in energy intake due to exercise sufficient to meet the increased needs for trace elements and other nutrients? What are the long-term effects of marginal intakes of trace elements coupled with increased losses on long-term health? These questions and many more regarding trace elements remain to be answered and serve to illustrate the importance of this emerging area of research.

SUMMARY

Zinc

- Zinc is the most abundant trace mineral in tissues other than blood and is involved in essentially all phases of growth and development.
- Dietary intake of zinc is suboptimal for most Americans. This situation is exacerbated by exercise, which increases zinc losses.
- Carbohydrate-loading diets, currently associated with athletic training programs, are often low in zinc.
- Supplementation with high doses of zinc is associated with an increased risk of cardiovascular disease.
- Bioavailability of zinc from different food sources is not uniform. Thus, the sum of all zinc ingested without regard to the source and without regard for dietary components that modulate zinc nutriture can yield a misleading impression of the quality of the dietary program.
- The foods with the highest amounts of zinc per serving include oysters, liver, beef, chicken, and turkey.

Copper

- Copper is an essential cofactor of numerous enzymes. It is involved in several essential physiological functions, including carbohydrate and lipid metabolism, immune system integrity, collagen and elastin formation, hematopoiesis, and protection against cellular damages due to toxic free-radical accumulation.
- Copper deficiency is associated with hypercholesterolemia, cardiovascular irregularities, and glucose intolerance.
- Dietary intake of copper for most Americans is only half to one-third the recommended intake of 2 to 3 mg/day for adults. This situation is exacerbated by megadosing with zinc and by high doses of dietary fructose (supplied as fructose itself, in sucrose, or in corn sweeteners) that increase copper requirements.
- Training and acute exercise alter copper metabolism and increase copper losses.
- Clinical indices of human copper status include erythrocyte superoxide dismutase activity and ceruloplasmin levels.
- The foods with the highest amounts of copper per serving include liver, oysters, potatoes, mushrooms, and peanuts.

Chromium

- Chromium functions by potentiating insulin action in carbohydrate and lipid metabolism. Chromium also helps maintain structural integrity of nuclear strands.
- Signs of chromium deficiency include impaired glucose tolerance, decreased number of insulin receptors, elevated levels of serum cholesterol and triglycerides, decreased HDL cholesterol levels, and increased incidence of aortic plaques.
- Normal dietary intake of chromium is approximately half the minimum suggested intake.
- Urinary chromium excretion is related to $\dot{V}O_2$max and therefore to degree of physical fitness.
- The foods with the highest amounts of chromium per serving are mushrooms, oysters, apples with skins, wine, and beer.
- There are no suitable methods to assess chromium status, but functional chromium status can be determined retrospectively by measuring glucose tolerance before and after chromium supplementation.

Selenium

- Selenium is present in all cells of the body in concentrations dependent on the amount and form of selenium in the diet.
- Selenium functions in removal of toxic free radicals, and low selenium intake is associated with skeletal and cardiac muscle degeneration.
- Dietary intake of selenium is usually within the recommended range; higher dietary intake is associated with a decreased risk of certain forms of cancer.
- In animals, exercise enhances signs of white-muscle disease due to insufficient intake of selenium.
- There are considerable gaps in our knowledge regarding selenium and exercise due to limited research in this area.

REFERENCES

1. American Dietetic Association. Nutrition and physical fitness. *J. Am. Diet. Assoc.* 76:437–443, 1980.
2. Anderson, R.A., and A.S. Kozlovsky. Chromium intake, absorption and excretion of subjects consuming self-selected diets. *Am. J. Clin. Nutr.* 41:1177–1183, 1985.
3. Anderson, R.A., M.M. Polansky, and N.A. Bryden. Strenuous running: Acute effects on chromium, copper, zinc and selected clinical variables in urine and serum of male runners. *Biol. Trace Element Res.* 6:327–336, 1984.
4. Anderson, R.A., M.M. Polansky, N.A. Bryden, and P.A. Deuster. Exercise effects on chromium excretion of trained and untrained runners consuming a constant diet. *J. Appl. Physiol.* (in press).
5. Anderson, R.A., M.M. Polansky, N.A. Bryden, and H. Guttman. Strenuous exercise may increase dietary needs for chromium and zinc. In F. I. Hatch (ed.). *Sport, Health, and Nutrition: Olympic Scientific Congress Proceedings.* Vol. 2. Champaign, Il. Human Kinetics, 1984, pp. 83–88.
6. Anderson, R.A., M.M. Polansky, N.A. Bryden, E.E. Roginski, K.Y. Patterson, and D.C. Reamer. Effect of exercise (running) on serum glucose, insulin, glucagon and chromium excretion. *Diabetes* 31:212–216, 1982.
7. Borel, J.S., and R.A. Anderson. Chromium. In Frieden, E. (ed.). *Biochemistry of the Essential Ultratrace Elements.* New York: Plenum Press, 1984, pp. 175–199.

8. Brady, P.S., P.K. Ku, and O. Ullrey. Lack of effect of selenium supplementation on the response of the equine erythrocyte glutathione system and plasma enzymes to exercise. *J. An. Sci.* 47:492–496, 1978.
9. Bray, J.T., A.M. Van Rij, M.T. Hall, and W.J. Pories. Analytical and sampling factors affecting urinary zinc analyses. In D.D. Hemphill (ed.). *Trace Substances in Environmental Health-XIII.* Columbia, Miss. Univ. of Missouri, 1979, pp. 163–171.
10. Consolazio, C.F., R.A. Nelson, L.R. Matoush, R.C. Hughes, and P. Urone. The trace element mineral losses in sweat. Denver, Colo. U.S. Army Medical Research and Nutrition Laboratory, 1964. Report No. 284.
11. Crouse, S.F., P.L. Hooper, H.A. Alterbom, and R.L. Papenfuss. Zinc ingestion and lipoprotein values in sedentary and endurance-trained men. *J. Am. Med. Assoc.* 252:785–787, 1984.
12. Davies, K.J.A., A.T. Quintanilha, G.A. Brooks, and L. Packer. Free radicals and tissue damage produced by exercise. *Biochem. Biophys. Res. Comm.* 107:1198–1205, 1982.
13. Dowdy, R.P., and J. Burt. Effect of intensive, long-term training on copper and iron nutriture in man. (Abstract) *Fed. Proc.* 39:786, 1980.
14. Dressendorfer, R.H., and R. Sockolov. Hypozincemia in runners. *Phys. Sports Med.* 8:97–100, 1980.
15. Dressendorfer, R.H., C.E. Wade, C.L. Keen, and J.H. Scoff. Plasma mineral levels in marathon runners during a 20-day road race. *Phys. Sports Med.* 10:113–118, 1982.
16. Fachman, W., S.W. Souci, and H. Kravt. *Food Composition and Nutrition Tables.* Stuttgart: Wissenschaftliche Verlagsgesellschaft, 1981.
17. Fields, M. Newer understanding of copper metabolism. *Inter. Med.* 6:91–98, 1985.
18. Goodwin, J.S., W.C. Hunt, P. Hooper, and P.J. Garry. Relationship between zinc intake, physical activity, and blood levels of high-density lipoprotein cholesterol in a healthy elderly population. *Metabolism* 34:519–523, 1985.
19. Hackman, R.M., and C.L. Keen. Trace element assessment of runners. (Abstract) *Fed. Proc.* 42:830, 1983.
20. Haralambie, G. Changes in electrolytes and trace elements during exercise. In H. Howard and J. R. Poortmans (eds.). *Metabolic Adaptation to Prolonged Exercise.* Basal: Birkhausen Verlag, 1975, pp. 340–351.
21. Haralambie, G. Serum zinc in athletes in training. *Int. J. Sports Med.* 2:135–138, 1981.
22. Haralambie, G., and J. Keul. Das Verhalten von Serum-Ceruloplasmin und Kupfer bei langdauernder Körperbelastony. Arzneimittel Forsch. 24:112–115, 1970.
23. Hetland, O., E.A. Brubak, H.E. Refsum, and S.B. Stromme. Serum and erythrocyte zinc concentrations after prolonged exercise. In Howard, H., and J. Poortmans (eds.). *Metabolic Adaptation to Prolonged Physical Exercise.* Basel: Birkhausen, 1975, pp. 367–370.

24. Hohnadel, D.C., F.W. Sunderman, Jr., M.W. Nechay, and M.D. McNeely. Atomic absorption spectrometry of nickel, copper, zinc and lead in sweat collected from healthy subjects during sauna bathing. *Clin. Chem.* 19:1288–1292, 1973.

25. Holloszy, J., P. Mole, K. Baldwin, and R. Terjung. Exercise-induced enzymatic adaptations in muscle. In Keul, J. (ed.). *Limiting Factors of Physical Performance.* Stuttgart: G. Thieme, 1973, pp. 66–80.

26. Hooper, P.L., L. Visconti, P.J. Garry, and G.E. Johnson. Zinc lowers high-density lipoprotein-cholesterol levels. *J. Am. Med. Assoc.* 244:1960–1961, 1980.

27. Human Nutrition Information Service. *Primary Nutrient Data Set for USDA Food Consumption Surveys.* Release No. 1, 1986.

28. Jacob, R.A., H.H. Sandstead, J.M. Munoz, L.M. Klevay, and D.B. Milne. Whole body surface loss of trace metals in normal males. *Am. J. Clin. Nutr.* 34:1379–1383, 1981.

29. Keen, C.L., and R.M. Hackman. Trace elements in athletic performance. In Hatch, F.I. (ed.). *Sport, Health and Nutrition: Olympic Scientific Congress Proceedings.* Vol. 2. Champaign Ill. Human Kinetics, 1984, pp. 51–65.

30. Keshan Disease Research Group. Epidemologic studies on the etiologic relationship of selenium and Keshan disease. *Chin. Med. J.* (Engl. ed.) 92:416, 1979.

31. Klevay, L.M. The role of copper, zinc and other elements in ischemic heart disease. In O. Rennert and W.Y. Chan (eds.). *Metabolism of Trace Metabolism in Man.* Vol. 1. Boca Ratan, Fa.: CRC Press, 1984, pp. 129–157.

32. Klevay, L.M., L. Inman, L.K. Johnson, et al. Increased cholesterol in plasma in a young man during experimental copper depletion. *Metabolism* 33:1112–1118, 1984.

33. Klevay, L.M., S.J. Reck, and D.F. Barcome. Evidence of dietary copper and zinc deficiencies. *J. Am. Med. Assoc.* 241:1916–1918, 1979.

34. Koivistoinen, P. Mineral element composition of Finnish foods: N, K, Ca, Mg, P, S, Fe, Cu, Mn, Zn, Mo, Co, Ni, Cr, F, Se, Si, Rb, Al, B, Br, Hg, As, Cd, Pb, and Ash. *Acta Agri. Scand.* (Suppl.) 22, 1980.

35. Kozlovsky, A.S., P.B. Moser, S. Reiser, and R.A. Anderson. Effect of diets high in simple sugars on urinary chromium losses. *Metab.* 35:515–518, 1986.

36. Krotkiewski, M., M. Gudmundsson, P. Backstrom, and K. Mandroukas. Zinc and muscle strength. *Acta Physiol. Scand.* 116:309–311, 1982.

37. Levander, O.L. Considerations on the assessment of selenium status. *Fed. Proc.* 44:2579–2583, 1985.

38. Liesen, H., B. Dufaux, and W. Hollman. Modification of serum glycoproteins in the days following a prolonged physical exercise and the influence of physical training. *Eur. J. Appl. Physiol.* 37:243–254, 1977.

39. Lukaski, H.C., W.W. Bolonchuk, L.M. Klevay, D.B. Milne, and H.H. Sandstead. Maximal oxygen consumption as related to magnesium, copper and zinc nutriture. *Am. J. Clin. Nutr.* 37:407–415, 1983.

40. Lukaski, H.C., W.W. Bolonchuk, L.M. Klevay, D.B. Milne, and H.H. Sandstead. Changes in plasma zinc content after exercise in men fed a low-zinc diet. *Am. J. Physiol.* 247 (*Endocrinol. Metab.* 10):E88–E93, 1984.

41. Mitchell, H.H., and T.S. Hamilton. The dermal excretion under controlled environmental conditions of nitrogen and minerals of human subjects with particular reference to calcium and iron. *J. Biol. Chem.* 178:345–361, 1949.

42. National Academy of Sciences. *Recommended Dietary Allowances.* 9th ed., Washington, D.C.: National Academy Press, 1980, pp. 1–185.

43. National Research Council Subcommittee on Zinc. *Zinc.* Baltimore: University Park Press, 1979.

44. Oh, S.H., J.T. Deagen, P.D. Whanger, and P.H. Weswig. Biological function of metallothionein. V. Its induction in rats by various stresses. *Am. J. Physiol.* 234: (*Endocrinol. Metab. Gastrointes. Physiol.* 3): E282–E285, 1978.

45. Ohla, A.E., V. Klissouras, J.D. Sullivan, and S.C. Shoryna. Effect of exercise on concentration of elements in serum. *J. Sports Med.* 22:414–425, 1982.

46. O'Leary, M.J., C.J. McClain, and P.V.J. Hegarty. Effect of zinc deficiency on the weight, cellularity and zinc concentration of different skeletal muscles in the postweanling rat. *Br. J. Nutr.* 42:487–495, 1979.

47. Pekarek, R.S., R.W. Wannemacker, and W.R. Beisel. The effect of leucocytic endogenous mediator (LEM) in the tissue distribution of zinc and iron. *Proc. Soc. Exp. Biol. Med.* 140:685–688, 1972.

48. Prasad, A.S., G.J. Brewer, E.B. Shoomaker, and P. Rabbani. Hypocupremia induced by zinc therapy in adults. *J. Am. Med. Assoc.* 240:2166–2168, 1978.

49. Reiser, S., J.C. Smith Jr., W. Mertz, J.T. Holbrook, D.J. Scholfield, A.S. Powell, W.K. Canfield, and J.J. Canary. Indices of copper status in humans consuming a typical American diet containing either fructose of starch. *Am. J. Clin. Nutr.* 42:242–251, 1985.

50. Richardson, J.H., and P.D. Drake. The effects of zinc on fatigue of striated muscle. *J. Sports Med.* 19:133–134, 1979.

51. Rusin, V.Y., V.V. Nasolodin, and I.P. Gladkikk. Changes in some morphological and biochemical blood indices of adolescents involved in or not involved in sports. *Gigienai Sanitanya* 7:31–23, 1980.

52. Rusin, V.Y., V.V. Nasolodin, and V.A. Varobev. Iron, copper, manganese and zinc metabolism in athletes under high physical pressure. *Vapr. Pitan* 4:15–19, 1980.

53. Schroeder, H.A., D.V. Frost, and J.J. Balassa. Essential trace metals in man: Selenium. *J. Chron. Dis.* 23:227–243, 1970.

54. Schubert, A., J.M. Holden, and W.R. Wolf. Selenium content of a core group of foods based on a critical evaluation of published analytical data. *J. Am. Diet. Assoc.* 87:285–299, 1987.

55. Shamberger, R.J. Antioxidation and trace elements

in cancer-epidemiologic review. In Boostrom, H., and N. Ljungstedt (eds.). *Trace Elements in Health Disease.* Stockholm: Skandia Group, 1985, pp. 155–171.

56. Smith, J.C. Jr., E.R. Morris, and R. Ellis, Zinc. Requirements, bioavailabilities and recommended dietary allowances. In Prasad, A.A. (ed.). *Zinc Deficiency in Human Subjects.* New York: Alan R. Liss, 1983, pp. 147–169.

57. Solomons, N.W., and L.H. Allen. The functional assessment of nutritional status: Principles, practice, and potential. *Nutr. Rev.* 41:33–50, 1983.

58. Spencer, H., L. Kramer, E. Perakis, C. Norris, and D. Osis. Plasma levels of zinc during starvation. (Abstract) *Fed. Proc.* 41:347, 1982.

59. Underwood, E.J. *Trace Elements in Human and Animal Nutrition.* 4th ed., New York: Academic Press, 1977.

60. Vallerand, A.L., J-P. Cuerrier, D. Shapcott, R.J. Vallerand, and P.F. Gardiner. Influence of exercise training on tissue chromium concentrations in the rat. *Am. J. Clin. Nutr.* 39:402–409, 1984.

61. Van Rij, A.M., C.D. Thomson, J.M. McKenzie, and M.F. Robinson. Selenium deficiency in total parenteral nutrition. *Am. J. Clin. Nutr.* 32:2076–2079, 1979.

62. Wolf, W. Assessment of inorganic nutrient intake from self-selected diets. In Beccher, G. R., (ed.). *Human Nutrition Research.* Totawa, N.J.: Allanhold Osum and Co., 1981, pp. 175–196.

63. Young, S., and R.F. Keeler. Nutritional muscular dystrophy in lambs: Effect of muscular activity on the symmetrical distribution of lesions. *Am. J. Vet. Res.* 23:966–971, 1962.

Chapter 14

DRUG-NUTRIENT INTERACTIONS

Zebulon V. Kendrick, Ph.D., and David T. Lowenthal, M.D., Ph.D.

The interaction of pharmacological agents (drugs) with nutrients is undesirable if it adversely influences the nutritional status of an individual or results in poor bioavailability of the drug. The physiological stress of exercise training, particularly in hot, humid environmental conditions with consequent water loss, may further complicate drug–nutrient interactions in active adults. Foods or beverages may also interact with drugs to produce variable effects [20, 27, 31]. An example of this is licorice extract, which may aggravate high blood pressure and produce hypokalemia. Food enhances the absorption of propranolol and metoprolol. Alcohol produces a variety of adverse nutrient reactions influencing vitamin and mineral absorption and substrate utilization [23, 51]. Mineral oil, a laxative, may interfere with fat-soluble vitamin absorption. In many cases however, nutrient or food intake may enhance drug bioavailability. Because of the frequency and clinical importance of adverse drug–nutrient and drug–drug interactions, little attention has been given to the clinically desirable aspects of these interactions.

It is not possible to examine all the references dealing with the desirable and undesirable drug–nutrient interactions in this review. Instead the focus has been narrowed to the nutrient interactions affecting three populations: the general public, athletes, and cardiovascular patients. In these three populations the nutrients affected by drugs and the dietary modifications required to lessen undesirable interactions are described.

SITES OF DRUG–NUTRIENT INTERACTIONS

Drugs may interact with nutrients in one or more of the following ways: (a) impairing gastrointestinal nutrient absorption, (b) increasing nutrient clearance and excretion by the kidney, (c) acting as agonists or antagonists to nutrients, (d) inducing liver microsomal enzymes responsible for drug biotransformation, (e) displacing nutrients from carrier proteins, and/or (f) interacting with hormone systems, thereby influencing substrate and nutrient requirements. Drugs may also influence the overall nutritional status by exerting an inhibitory control over appetite.

Nutrients may also influence the absorption, biotransformation, and/or excretion of drugs [31, 82]. Most gastrointestinal absorption occurs directly from the lumen into the adjacent capillary network. High-protein liquid meals and high-glucose liquid meals enhance and diminish splanchnic blood flow, respectively, altering the rate of nutrient absorption [8].

Hot meals, meals high in fat, and carbohydrate, and high protein meals have all been demonstrated to have variable effects in slowing gastric emptying [17, 47]. A delay in gastric emptying time can delay drug absorption and can also adversely influence the bioavailability of drugs that are acid labile or unstable in the presence of gastric enzymes [82]. Absorption of many antibiotics and of aspirin will be delayed if the drug is administered at mealtime. Milk and dairy products, as well as diets rich in divalent and trivalent cations, have been demonstrated to markedly diminish the absorption of penicillin and tetracyclines [54,56].

Food may increase the absorption of some drugs. Two important antihypertensive agents, propranolol and metoprolol, show increased absorption when a meal is consumed concurrently with therapy [55]. The greater dissolution of these drugs by food-stimulated gastric processes probably accounts for the increase in absorption.

The excretion of some drugs by the kidneys may be altered by dietary modifications. The mode of action is by changes in urinary pH. The ionized form of drugs is more readily excreted, whereas un-ionized forms of drugs are more readily absorbed through the renal tubule and reenter the circulation. The consumption of food usually does not alter urinary pH. However, excessive consumption of acid residue-producing foods, such as most meats, breads, cheeses, nuts (except almonds), and wheat breakfast products, may result in urinary acidification. Foods that may result in alkalinization of urine are almonds and chestnuts, dairy products, and some fruits and vegetables. A more complete list of the foods that may influence urinary pH may be found in a review by Krause and Mehan [42].

Weight loss by athletes may be severe [2, 70], and psychological profiles of these athletes may resemble those of anorexics [43, 90]. Dramatic weight loss in exercising individuals may lead to marked deficiencies in nutrient intake and endogenous stores of vitamins and minerals, thereby adversely altering nutritional status. The implementation of pharmacological interventions may further aggravate the nutritional status of these individuals. Fasting and the use of very-low-calorie diets may result in hypoglycemia in athletes. Carbohydrate restriction and severe caloric deficit may lead to ketosis which, in turn, may result in nausea, loss of appetite, and a ketone-induced acidosis. Unquestionably, these conditions influence normal gastrointestinal, renal, hepatic, and cardiovascular physiological responses to exercise and stress. The influences of very-low-calorie diets on humans and exercise interactions are reviewed in Wadden, Stunkard, and Brownell [87] and in Thompson et al. [79].

ANTACIDS AND LAXATIVES

Most gastrointestinal problems for which antacids and laxatives are taken have a psychological origin. Self-medication of these frequently occurring problems occasionally leads to chronic use of antacids or laxatives and to untoward drug–nutrient interactions.

Antacids

Athletes and lay competitors may often experience gastric disturbances such as "sour stomach," "heartburn," "butterflies," and indigestion prior to athletic competitions. Antacids are usually self-prescribed for nonspecific gastrointestinal symptoms, peptic ulcers, or reflux esophagitis.

Antacids vary in their ingredients, their acid-neutralizing ability, and probably their clinical effects [19]. Antacids either neutralize or remove acid from the gastric contents. Antacids are often referred to as systemic or nonsystemic. Systemic antacids produce a metabolic alkalosis through appreciable cation absorption. Nonsystemic antacids have insoluble basic compounds that are not absorbed. Antacids may indirectly suppress gastric activity when taken in sufficient quantity to elevate the pH of the gastric contents above 5 and inactivate the pepsin secretion at pH of 7 to 8 [62]. The alkalosis induced by chronic use of systemic antacids may have pronounced influences on normal gastrointestinal function and dissolution of drugs. These agents may influence normal digestive processes of foods and availability of other drugs (see Table 1).

Aluminum hydroxide and magnesium hydroxide are regarded as nonsystemic antacids. Aluminum hydroxide is constipating, and magnesium hydroxide can induce diarrhea. Often these compounds are combined to cancel the undesirable effects (e.g., in Maalox®, DiGel®, and Gelusil®). Aluminum antacids bind to phosphate in the intestines and thereby reduce phosphate absorption, which may lead to hypophosphatemia, osteomalacia, and impaired erythrocyte function [72]. Aluminum antacids also decrease magnesium absorption and may result in hypomagnesemia and hypercalciurea. These antacids may reduce glucose, amino acid, and vitamin A and C absorption; how-

ever, these effects are probably minimal as long as the antacid is not taken in conjunction with other pharmacological agents that may influence one or more of these nutrients. Some magnesium is absorbed when magnesium hydroxide (Milk of Magnesia) or magnesium oxide antacids are consumed.

Calcium carbonate and sodium bicarbonate are excellent antacids but, because of their systemic absorption, they can cause metabolic alkalosis. Calcium carbonate intake will result in increased calcium absorption and may produce hypercalcemia. Sodium bicarbonate can cause sodium retention and overload resulting in edema and/or increased blood pressure. Bicarbonate ingestion may diminish vitamin B_{12} absorption. These types of antacids may not be as efficacious as other antacids because of their gastric hypersecretory action (acid rebound).

Table 1. ANTACID AND ANTIULCER MEDICATION

DRUG (PREPARATION)	NUTRIENT EFFECT(S)	MECHANISM OF INTERACTION	COMMENTS
Cimetidine (Tagamet®)	Decreased vitamin B12 absorption	May inhibit intrinsic factor	Decreases parietal cell acid secretion
Sucralfate (Carafate®)	Decreased phosphorus absorption	Chelation of phosphorus	Low phosphate level may influence calcium absorption
Aluminum hydroxide (Maalox®, Gelusil® Aludrox®, Amphojel®, Mylanta®)	Decreased phosphate and magnesium absorption; slight decrease in glucose, amino acid, and vitamins A and C absorption	Formation of aluminum phosphates	Hypophosphatemia, hypophosphaturia, hypercalciuria, and hypomagnesemia may occur. May interfere with tetracycline and aspirin absorption Acid rebound may follow.
Calcium carbonate (Pepto-Bismal®, Tums®, Zylase®, Kren®, Alkets®, Dicarbosil®)	Increased calcium absorption	Absorption of calcium salts	Constipation, calcinosis, and azotemia may occur after chronic use
Sodium bicarbonate (Alka-Seltzer®, Bell-Ans®, Soda Mint®)	Increased sodium absorption	Increase in circulating sodium	Sodium retention, edema, aldolosis, and milk-alkali syndrome if taken with milk
Magnesium hydroxide and oxide (Milk of Magnesia®)	Increased magnesium absorption	Formation of magnesium chloride, which is absorbed	Has saline cathartic effect. If mixed with aluminum hydroxide or calcium carbonate, the cathartic effect is lessened

Sucralfate and cimetidine are two popular prescription drugs that are successful in treating chronic gastric discomfort, reflux esophagitis, and peptic ulcers. Sucralfate, used for treatment of duodenal ulcers, may cause constipation and minor gastrointestinal disturbances and may interfere with tetracycline, cimetidine, phenytoin, and warfarin absorption [33]. Sucralfate can bind phosphorus in the gastrointestinal tract and may result in hypophosphatemia [72]. Cimetidine acts on the H_2 receptors of the gastric parietal cells to inhibit basal gastric acid secretions. It also inhibits gastric acid stimulated by food, caffeine, and insulin. Cimetidine may influence vitamin B_{12} absorption because of a potential lessening of intrinsic factor secretion. Intrinsic factor secretion is not completely blocked by cimetidine therapy. For that reason, diminished secretion of the intrinsic factor peptide needs further evaluation before any definite conclusion can be drawn concerning cimetidine's interaction with vitamin B_{12} absorption. Iron absorption could possibly be adversely influenced by the decrease in intrinsic factor even though normal acid contents exist. Intrinsic factor secretion and normal acid contents are required for adequate iron absorption. Additionally, iron and calcium compete for the same absorptive site. The use of calcium carbonate antacids may further diminish iron absorption.

Athletes and members of the public who constantly suffer from gastric discomfort may choose to alter their daily food intake patterns. It is well known that consuming five or six small meals rather than the traditional two or three meals reduces the symptoms of gastric discomfort and hastens the healing of peptic ulcers. The diet should consist of adequate protein, vitamin C, and zinc to maximize healing if ulcerations have occurred [66]. A well-planned diet does not necessitate supplementation of these nutrients. Aspirin and drugs that may cause gastric distress should be avoided by anyone who has persistent gastric discomfort, as should caffeine-containing beverages and alcohol. Some reports have suggested that upper gastrointestinal tract bleeding may occur during long-distance running [59, 70]. Aspirin or other gastric mucosa-irritating compounds may initiate or further aggravate this problem. The use of antacids, sucralfate, or cimetidine may serve prophylactically to reduce the risk of upper gastrointestinal bleeding during long-distance running.

The preferred antacid is the one having the greatest acid-neutralizing effect combined with the least effect on intestinal function. Attention should also be given to the danger of hypercalcemia and sodium retention in combining exercise with consumption of the systemic antacids.

Laxatives

Laxatives and cathartics are drugs that induce bowel movement, and are often used by athletes who have to "make weight." Most of these drugs are self-prescribed, and the frequency of consumption far exceeds the valid indications for their use. The term "laxative" implies the elimination of a soft, formed stool, whereas the term "cathartic" refers to fluid evacuation. There are five classifications of laxatives and cathartics (Table 2).

The emollients and bulk-forming laxatives respectively soften and hydrate the feces. Their effects are usually less severe than the pronounced fluid evacuation associated with the cathartics. However, interference with bile resorption, acute diarrhea, and electrolyte depletion may occur with the emollients and bulk-forming laxatives [24]. The mineral oil emollients will interfere with the absorption of water and of any fat-soluble substance. The clinical importance of a mineral oil-induced decrease in fat-soluble vitamin absorption has not been established [13]. However, the chronic use of laxatives and other nutritional practices that limit metabolism and intake of fat-soluble vitamins may result in vitamin deficiency.

Table 2. COMMONLY USED LAXATIVE PREPARATIONS

PREPARATION	DRUG	USE	NUTRIENT EFFECT(S)	MECHANISM OF INTERACTION	COMMENTS
Emollients (mineral oil, dioctyl sulfosuccinate)	MILKINOL®, Colace®, Disonate®, Fleet Enema Oil®	Fecal softeners	Mineral oil interferes with absorption of fat-soluble substances. May produce hypoprothrombinemia in pregnant women	Dioctyl sulfosuccinate is emulsifying wetting and dispersing agent. It lowers surface tension of fecal mass. Mineral oil is lipid solvent	Dioctyl sulfosuccinate may enhance mineral oil absorption if taken with it
Bulk forming (methylcellulose, bran, natural gums, psyllium)	Dialose®, Disolan Forte®, Disoplex®, Purlose®, Bassoran®, Gentlex®, Metamucil®	Fecal swelling	Acute diarrhea may occur with water, potassium, and sodium loss. Psyllium may interfere with cholesterol absorption	Increase in fecal swelling by formation of emollient gels or viscous solution. Bulk promotes peristoles and reduces transient time. Psyllium interferes with bile acid resorption	Should be taken with increased water consumption
Saline cathartics (magnesium salts and sulfates, sodium phosphates and tartrate such as Epsom salt and Milk of Magnesia)	Fleet Enema®, Haley's M-O®, Phospho-Soda®, Sal Hepatica, Vacuetts®	Increase in intestinal osmolarity; fluid evacuation	Additional magnesium absorption when renal function is depressed. Phosphates may decrease calcium in blood.	Salts slowly and incompletely absorbed; they retain water in intestines because of osmotic forces	Hypermagnesemia may result in muscle weakness and hypotension. Increased diruesis with saline cathartics may result in pronounced water loss
Contact cathartics (castor oil, phenolphthalein, and bisacodyl)	Dulcolax®, Espotabs®, Phenolax®, Ex-Lax®, Feen-A-Mint®, Correctol®	Excessive fluid evacuation; fecal hydration	Pronounced water loss. Water and electrolyte absorption inhibition resulting in hypokalemia, sodium depletion, and dehydration	May increase peristalsis by mucus irritation or by stimulation of nerve activity of intestines. Castor oil acts mainly in small intestine; others exert primary effect in large intestine	May cause intestinal cramps and increased intestinal mucus secretion. Marked individual differences in effective doses. Effect usually occurs several hours after intake. Severe gripping may occur with evacuation
Anthraquinone cathartics (senna, cascara sagrada, danthron)	Dorbane®, Gentlax® Laxaid®, Modane® Doxan®, Bassoran®, Black Draught®	Fluid evacuation	Same as for contact catharics	Acts only in large intestine. Forms glycoside compounds	

The most dramatic laxative effect is usually associated with the cathartics. The pharmacological mechanism is fluid evacuation. The resulting fluid loss and interference with electrolyte absorption may result in severe dehydration, hypokalemia, and sodium depletion, thereby affecting fluid volume and electrical excitability of the nervous system, heart, and muscle. Athletes who use cathartics to assist in "making weight" may experience more severe hypokalemia and muscle weakness if they are also consuming diuretics. If volume depletion is significant, an individual using contact cathartics chronically may experience secondary aldosteronism [22], protein loss, hypoalbuminemia, and osteomalacia of the vertebral column [30]. Certainly these consequences must be avoided by athletes.

It is not uncommon for an individual to develop a cathartic habit [27]. The use of a cathartic to make weight results in both water and fecal mass loss from the large intestine. Normal defecation may not resume for several days. Many people have inadequate information concerning normal bowel function: If a bowel movement has not occurred in 36 to 48 hours, they may use contact cathartics to stimulate evacuation. In particular in individuals restricting food intake to make weight, sufficient food digestion may not have occurred to form adequate fecal mass for a bowel movement. The use of a cathartic in this case may result in chronic cathartic use. Normal stools should be large and soft. Concern should be more for the formation of large, soft stools than for the time between bowel movements.

Constipation is a problem for many people. Some causes are resistance of the urge to defecate, dehydration, fever, and chronic use of antacids. Dietary consumption of fiber, intake of additional fluids, and moderate exercise have been suggested to enhance normal defecation. Development of successful toilet habits requires periodic attempts for relaxed periods of at least 10 minutes. Several weeks of conscientious effort may be needed.

NONSTEROIDAL ANALGESICS AND ANTIINFLAMMATORY DRUGS

Salicylates and similar nonnarcotic analgesic and antiinflammatory drugs are often used by athletes, althetic trainers, and team physicians for a variety of musculoskeletal disorders. The ease of availability and numerous therapeutic applications of nonnarcotic analgesic compounds make them one of the most commonly used groups of pharmacological agents worldwide. Aspirin, the best known nonnarcotic analgesic, is commonly used therapeutically by athletes for its potent analgesic and antiinflammatory properties.

Intolerance to aspirin has been well documented (see Table 3). Commonly cited toxic manifestations include angioedema, bronchial asthma, gastrointestinal distress (with ulceration and/or hemorrhage), hemolysis, acid–base disturbances resulting from altered respiratory stimulation, and a pronounced pyrogenic effect due to an uncoupling of oxidative phosphorylation [1, 27, 40].

The direct action of salicylates in inducing sweating enhances heat loss and thus lowers body temperature during fever states. Exercise increases the metabolic rate and thereby heat production. During long-duration exercise, the efficiency of sweating is important in thermoregulation and in maintaining adequate hydration. Inefficient sweating in hot environments may lead to dehydration and to electrolyte and acid–base disturbances when aspirin therapy is combined with endurance athletic events.

Increases of 62% and 69% in salicylate-induced sensitivity to sweating during exercise bouts for 2 hours at 25 and 35°C, respectively, have been demonstrated [81]. These findings suggest that sweating occurs at a lower rectal temperature. In a case study [25], a therapeutic dose of aspirin may have resulted in severe heat disturbances during a 100-mile race. Profuse sweating occurred and symptoms of heat illness, such as

Table 3. NONNARCOTIC, NONSTEROIDAL ANALGESICS AND ANTIINFLAMMATORY AGENTS

DRUG	NUTRIENT EFFECT(S)	MECHANISM OF INTERACTION	TOXIC EFFECTS
Salicylates, Aspirin (Ascriptin®, Bufferin®, Anacin®, Excedrin®, Vanquish®, Bayer Aspirin®)	May adversely influence water balance during period of prolonged sweating and/or exercise in hot, humid environment. Prolonged use may decrease iron and vitamin C absorption	Promotes sweating and possibly diuresis	May include tinnitus, nausea, vomiting, reduced erythrocytes and leukocytes, hemolysis, gastric and renal bleeding, asthma, acid–base disturbances, dehydration. Has pyrogenic effect
Phenylbutazone (Butazolidin®, Azolid®)	Causes sodium and chloride retention by kidneys, reduced iodine uptake by thyroid	Causes significant sodium and chloride retention by kidneys. Has uricosuric effect	May include vomiting, diarrhea, vertigo, peptic ulcers, aplastic anemia, agranulocytosis. Only short-term therapy (< 1 week) should be utilized
Acetaminophen (Tylenol®, Anacin-3®, Dristan®)	Causes nutrients to be hepatically stored or biotransformed	Hepatotoxicity influences substrate availability	Include hepatic necrosis, methemoglobinemia, and hemolytic anemia
Indomethacin (Indocin®)	Nutrient intake may decrease during therapy		May include anorexia, peptic ulcers, and asthma. May uncouple oxidative phosphorylation
Ibuprofen (Motrin®, Advil®, Nuprin®)	May cause sodium retention, decreased nutrient intake	Gastrointestinal inflammation and inhibition of renal prostaglandins may occur. May suppress appetite	May cause gastrointestinal inflammation and bleeding

chills and loss of thirst, were observed. In exercise studies in which salicylates were administered, varying results have been observed [81, 91]. It appears that aspirin administration during exercise bouts of 30 minutes in a cool environment is not sufficient to significantly increase oxygen consumption and rectal temperature above placebo controls. Aspirin administration during longer duration exercise tasks may increase oxygen consumption and rectal temperature. Because salicylate induces diuresis and enhances sweating, aspirin should be avoided in athletes who are physically or pharmacologically dehydrating to make weight and in those who experience profuse sweating.

Acid foods such as caffeine, cola drinks, citrus fruits, and juices should be avoided during aspirin therapy because of the increase in gastric discomfort. Interaction between caffeine and aspirin may result in a more marked diuresis, thus promoting water loss. Diuresis and sweating may be further stimulated when aspirin and alcohol are combined. Alcohol induces a pronounced diuresis and is a promoter of sweating [27, 51]. Alcohol may further aggravate the gastric problems associated with aspirin and increase blood loss from the gastrointestinal system. Distance competitors should avoid the use of a combination of beer (for electrolyte repletion) or caffeine (as a performance enhancer) with aspirin because of the potential of enhanced gastric discomfort, dehydration, and severe heat stress.

Phenylbutazone has a prominent antiinflammatory effect. It is poorly tolerated by many patients, and close medical supervision is required with its use. The drug causes significant retention of sodium and chloride with a marked reduction in urine formation. Because this uricosuric effect is common, the drug should be avoided during exercise. Acute renal failure due to urate deposition in the tubules may occur if exercise is continued, especially in hot, humid environments [41]. Acute renal failure may be a result of increased levels of hematin and uric acid, which compete with lactic acid for excretion. Exercise increases blood lactate levels, which can lead to dangerously high levels of uric acid in renal interstitial fluid. Urinary uric acid levels increase with phenylbutazone and during exercise. Muscle production of uric acid is further enhanced in hot, humid environments. The interaction between phenylbutazone and exercise may result in uric acid precipitation by the nephron and thus in acute renal failure.

Acetaminophen may be the drug of choice for individuals sensitive to aspirin. Hepatotoxicity is the most severe adverse effect associated with acetaminophen therapy. Acetaminophen may be associated with methemoglobinemia and hemolytic anemia.

Indomethacin, like aspirin, is an effective antiinflammatory agent. However, up to 50% of those undergoing therapy may experience untoward effects [27]. Anorexia, nausea, and peptic ulcers, often with bleeding and perforation, are common gastrointestinal complaints and complications. Diarrhea may also occur, which may compromise water balance. Overall, indomethacin is probably no better than aspirin for its antiinflammatory value. However, significant numbers of patients have experienced relief with indomethacin therapy when aspirin was not effective.

Ibuprofen, like other antiinflammatory agents, may cause gastrointestinal discomfort with vomiting. Heartburn is not unusual with ibuprofen therapy. Ibuprofen may decrease appetite, influencing nutrient intake, and may cause fluid retention. Ibuprofen is usually better tolerated than aspirin but can cause inflammation of the gastrointestinal mucosa and bleeding [44]. Ibuprofen may decrease renal function and cause sodium retention [12] and, in combination with diuretics or when given to diabetics, increase in risk of renal toxicity [6].

Most of the nonsteroidal antiinflammatory and analgesic compounds just mentioned may cause gastrointestinal discomfort and depress appetite. Acidic foods and caffeinated beverages should be avoided during nonsteroidal analgesic and antiinflammatory therapy. Water balance may be adversely influenced with aspirin because of diuresis and induced sweating. Indomethacin and salicylates have been demonstrated to uncouple oxidative phosphorylation, thereby increasing heat production. Exercise training should be avoided during phenylbutazone therapy.

CAFFEINE

Caffeine, a theophylline congener, has long been considered an ergogenic aid and/or a doping agent that can elicit physiological changes to enhance work capacity or athletic performance. Caffeine may exert a pronounced influence on substrate mobilization and utilization during prolonged work by stimulating adipocyte lipolysis [3, 14, 18] via the activation of lipase [18]; by altering glucose homeostasis; by inducing a hyperglycemic action [78]; by activating liver phosphorylase [5]; or by affecting muscle triglyceride utilization [16] and fatty acid availability. Caffeine is supposed to alter these substrates via inhibition of phosphodiesterase, which alters the concentration of cyclic adenosine monophosphate [10] and increases plasma catecholamine levels [84].

Caffeine mobilizes adipocyte fatty acids, increasing lipid availability and, in turn, a greater potential for exogenous lipid oxidation by working muscle [34, 60, 84]. An increase in oxidation of free fatty acids at the same work intensity may suppress glycogen degradation, thereby "sparing" glycogen

[14, 34]. The sparing of muscle glycogen would be due in part to the high rates of fatty acid oxidation, which may inhibit the activities of phosphofructokinase and pyruvate dehydrogenase reactions [64].

Caffeine has been demonstrated to decrease the perception of drowsiness and increase the perception of alertness, and possibly to reduce the perception of fatigue during prolonged work [26, 34]. The exact mechanisms responsible for the decreased perception of fatigue are unclear, but possibly involve reduction in neuronal thresholds [88], influence on central catecholamine receptors, and/or a direct effect on the adrenal medulla [4].

Caffeine and theophylline have a pronounced diuretic action [27]. This action may be due to direct action on the renal tubule or increased renal flow and glomerular filtration. The diuretic action of caffeine does not significantly augment potassium excretion.

Caffeine consumption may result in a prolonged augmentation of gastric secretion [68]. An athlete with known gastrointestinal problems or peptic ulcers should avoid caffeine products such as coffee, teas that contain caffeine, cola drinks, and over-the-counter pharmacological agents that contain caffeine such as Anacin®, Dexatrim®, Excedrin Extra Strength®, No Doz®, and Vanquish®. These compounds may cause further gastrointestinal irritation.

ALCOHOL

Alcohol is classified as a drug, although it is widely used as a beverage by people of all ages [23]. Clinically, alcohol or ethanol may be used in parenteral nutrition because of its well-known nitrogen-sparing effect. However, the ethanol intake is low and with amino acid therapy is not sufficient to maintain nitrogen balance. This is probably due to the carbohydrate requirement for an anabolic response [45].

Malabsorption of vitamins is well documented among alcoholics and is associated with active or binge consumption of alcohol. Thiamine absorption is significantly impaired during alcohol binging [80]. The uptake of folic acid by the jejunum is diminished during binging [28], therefore vitamin B_{12} nutriture is also affected. It is well known that alcohol also depletes riboflavin, niacin, ascorbic acid, and pyridoxine, as well as magnesium and zinc [66]. Alcohol in low doses may result in greater gastric acid secretion; at higher doses, gastric secretions and peptic activity diminish. Strong alcoholic drinks are often very irritating to the mucosa and may cause erosive gastritis [46]. These gastrointestinal problems may lead to nutritional deficiencies. Alcohol may inhibit gluconeogenesis by the liver and decrease hepatic release of glucose [69].

In long-distance races, runners depend on free fatty acids and triglycerides for energy. Alcohol will raise the levels of circulating free fatty acids, but will also inhibit the oxidation of this substrate [48]. Metabolism of the ethanol-oxidation system accounts for 20 to 30% of alcohol metabolism and does not generate any energy. Alcohol plus an accumulation of reduced nicotinamide adenine dinucleotide (NADH) may prevent gluconeogenesis, thereby resulting in hypoglycemia in an exercising individual.

Lactate accumulation secondary to alcohol ingestion will block uric acid secretion. In the state of volume contraction and renal hypoperfusion experienced by distance runners, uric acid retention with or without alcohol may be a consequence of muscle catabolism and may play a pathogenic role in rhabdomyolysis.

Alcohol is also a myocardial depressant. Impaired myocardial performance parameters, such as a decrease in stroke work with concomitant increase in left ventricular end diastolic pressure and in the left ventricular work and tension time index, have been reported after alcohol ingestion [7, 15, 65]. Heart rate and cardiac output at rest and during submaximal exercise are reported to be higher after ingestion of alcohol, whereas the total arteriovenous oxygen difference and total peripheral resistance decrease.

ORAL CONTRACEPTIVES

Oral contraceptives, or birth control pills, contain both estrogen and progesterone derivatives. Oral contraceptives may be classified as combination types and sequential types. The combination types contain both estrogen and progestin and are administered daily for 20 to 22 days of each menstrual cycle. The sequential types contain only estrogen for the initial phase of the cycle and both estrogens and progestin during the luteal phase of the cycle.

It is not uncommon for athletic women, in particular those participating in endurance events, to experience menstrual irregularity or amenorrhea. Such women should be evaluated by their gynecologist. Often, hormonal replacement of estrogen and/or progesterone may be advised. If the hormonal defect is due to a progesterone deficiency, the athlete may be placed on progesterone treatment. If the deficiency is due to deficiency of both estrogen and progesterone, the athlete may be placed on combined estrogen and progesterone therapy. It is important to note that estrogen therapy in the absence of endogenous or exogenous progesterone increases the incidence of endometrial cancer and possible breast cancer.

Numerous articles suggest that oral contraceptives may exert both metabolic and nutritional effects in women. These agents may also alter vitamin and mineral needs [77]. Vitamin B_{12} levels are lowered by chronic intake of oral contraceptives [73]. However, absorption of vitamin B_{12}, as determined by the Schilling test, appears to be unaltered with oral contraceptive medication. The differences in vitamin B_{12} levels may be due to differences in folate metabolism.

Folate deficiency and megaloblastic anemia are potential untoward effects of oral contraceptive use [66]. In some cases the folate-induced anemias were reversed when oral contraceptives were discontinued or supplemental folic acid was provided.

The ascorbic acid content of leukocytes and platelets is significantly lowered in women on oral contraceptives [9]. The plasma ascorbic acid level is decreased, and oral contraceptives may increase ascorbic acid catabolism or tissue uptake.

The nutritional requirement for riboflavin and pyridoxine (vitamin B_6) is also increased in women taking oral contraceptives. When pyridoxine is required for normal tryptophan metabolism, a decrease in level of pyridoxine would make the need for riboflavin greater. Riboflavin is involved in the oxidation of pyridoxine to its active form [86].

A pathological concern for women on oral contraceptives is the increased incidence or risk of thromboses. The risk appears to be related to the estrogen content of the oral contraceptive [32]. Oral contraceptives may increase serum vitamin K-dependent clotting factors as well as other clotting factors. As a result, the need for vitamin K may be lessened in women taking oral contraceptives.

A major nutritional problem in postmenopausal women is osteoporosis, in whom estrogen has been reported to increase calcium absorption [11]. The wide scope of the etiology and therapies of osteoporosis precludes further discussion in this review.

DRUGS USED IN THE MANAGEMENT OF CARDIOVASCULAR DISEASE

Diuretics

Thiazides bring about a decrease in peripheral resistance and plasma volume. Thiazide-like diuretics increase urinary excretion of sodium, chloride, and water by inhibiting sodium resorption in the early distal tubule. Appreciable augmentation of potassium excretion, which can lead to hypokalemia, accompanies the inhibition of sodium resorption (see Table 4). Significant hypokalemia results in moderate S-T-segment depression, cardiac irritability, and skeletal muscle fa-

Table 4. DRUGS USED IN THE MANAGEMENT OF CARDIOVASCULAR DISEASE

DRUG (PREPARATION)	NUTRIENT(S) AFFECTED	MECHANISM OF INTERACTION	COMMENTS
Thiazides (metolazone, quinethazone, Chlorthalidone®)	Sodium, potassium, chloride, water, glucose	Inhibition of sodium resorption in early distal tubule	Serum potassium level may decrease during long-term therapy. Mild hypochloremic alkalosis may occur. Increased level of uric acid and glucose. Potassium supplements often required.
Loop diuretics (furosemide, ethacrynic acid, bumetanide)	Sodium, potassium, chloride, magnesium, calcium, water. Secondarily, glucose, amino acids	Inhibition of sodium and chloride resorption in ascending loop of Henle	Rapid onset, short acting. Hyperuricemia may occur. All cause decrease in glucose tolerance and amino acid transport and may cause hyperglycemia
Potassium-sparing diuretic (triamterene, amiloride, spironolactone)	Potassium, sodium, chloride, water	Sprionolactone is competitive inhibitor of aldosterone. Triamterene acts directly on distal segment to reduce sodium resorption.	Potassium supplement may result in severe hyperkalemia
Beta-adrenergic blockers (propranolol [Inderal®] Atenolol®, Metoprolol®, Pindolol®)	Primary influence may be on substrate availability mediated by sympathomimetic amines	Block action of sympathomimetic amines on beta-adrenergic receptors	Fatigue a common complaint
Central agonists: clonidine, methyldopa (Catapres®, Aldomet®)	Increased water intake	Dry mouth may inhibit desire for food. Decrease in sympathetic output may influence substrate utilization during exercise.	Central but not peripheral salivation inhibited, resulting in dry mouth. Methyldopa may cause hemolytic anemia
Angiotensin-converting enzyme inhibitors (Captopril®, Saralasin®)	May affect water balance. May cause hyperkalemia	Inhibition of angiotensin II and plasma aldosterone. Taste perception may be diminished or lost.	Because of potential hyperkalemia, hypokalemia due to other causes must be documented before potassium supplements or potassium-sparing diuretics are prescribed.
Calcium channel blockers (verapamil nifedipine)	Decreased nutrient intake	Nausea and constipation	
Digitalis: digoxin (Lanoxin®)	Electrolytes, especially potassium. Decreased nutrient intake.	Digitalis-induced arrhythmias are more frequent with potassium-depleting diuretics	Nausea and vomiting are early signs of digitalis toxicity. Systemic antacids should be avoided when patient is undergoing digitalis therapy

tigue. Long-term diuretic treatment may also be associated with a mild degree of hypochloremia. The effects of diuretic therapy may become more pronounced when patients or athletes self-prescribe low-carbohydrate, low-calorie diets that increase sodium excretion. Any person on diuretic therapy should use dietary modifications only as prescribed by a physician and should be monitored closely if dietary modification is severe.

The loop-acting, high-ceiling diuretics act on the ascending limb of the loop of Henle. Their diuretic effect is much greater than that of the thiazides (Table 4). The increased potassium excretion in the distal segment of the nephron is proportional to the flow rate through this segment. Furosemide increases urinary calcium more than urinary sodium, while ethacrynic acid increases urinary calcium and sodium to similar degrees.

The mechanisms of action of the potassium-sparing diuretics are different. Aldosterone acts in the distal segment of the tubule, causing resorption of sodium and chloride in exchange for potassium. Spironolactone blocks the aldosterone effect, enhances diuresis, and conserves potassium. Triamterene and amiloride act directly on the distal segment of the tubule, independent of aldosterone, reducing sodium resorption and sparing potassium. Amiloride's action is enhanced when it is used in combination with a thiazide diuretic.

Diuretic-induced potassium loss can be treated with supplemental potassium, spironolactone, triamterene, or amiloride. Potassium tablets can cause gastrointestinal tract ulcerations, bleeding, or obstruction. Oral potassium supplements can cause severe or fatal hyperkalemia [35]. Potassium-rich foods such as orange juice, bananas, wheat bran, beans, shrimp, and some fish may provide adequate potassium replacement.

Diuretics may be abused by athletes to make weight. The athlete may experience hypokalemia during acute administration and the severity may be more pronounced if the athlete is restricting water intake or is concurrently on a low-carbohydrate diet.

Central Alpha-Adrenergic Agonists

Both clonidine and alpha-methyldopa (methyldopa) decrease central and peripheral outflow of catecholamines [63]. This results in reduction of plasma norepinephrine at rest and during exercise [49, 85].

Dry mouth is a chronic complaint with use of this class of drugs (Table 4). This may result in greater fluid intake and a decreased appetite and possible anorexia. The sensation tends to decrease with time, but does not disappear during chronic therapy. Plasma renin activity is depressed with the body at rest, reflecting the influence of these drugs on the sympathetic nervous system. Sensitivity to alcohol is increased with alpha-agonist therapy, because of drowsiness or sedation induced by the alpha-agonist. Alcohol thus should be avoided. In several studies [49, 50, 67], the exercise-associated changes seen in serum potassium, renin, and aldosterone have been observed in normal volunteers following single and multiple doses of clonidine and methyldopa. Increases in potassium during dynamic exercise in subjects taking clonidine or methyldopa paralleled the responses in subjects taking a placebo. With both clonidine and methyldopa, plasma renin concentration was suppressed at rest and the expected increase was blunted during exercise at maximum dosages. The plasma aldosterone level apparently showed no significant difference with the drugs compared with placebo, increasing during exercise in all groups.

Beta-Adrenergic Blockers

The most pronounced nutritional interactions with beta-adrenergic blockers are with the metabolic effects of these drugs. Propranolol in single and multiple doses has been reported to cause an increase in serum potassium level that is significantly greater than with placebo during exercise [49].

To determine the origin of the fatigue observed during exercise in normal, active individuals receiving beta-blockade (in contrast to drug-induced longevity in exercise of cardiac patients), Lundborg et al. [52] examined specific metabolic effects of beta-blockade. After disruption of neuromuscular transmission and decreased blood flow to working muscles were ruled out as causes of subject fatigue, these investigators targeted exercise substrate limitation, that is, glucose and nonesterified fatty acid availability, as the fatiguing mechanism. In fact, blood glucose level was reduced during bicycle activity of subjects receiving propranolol or metoprolol. This was followed by rapid rises in glucagon levels with drug therapy; the reduction most likely results from decreased muscle glycogenolysis, a beta-adrenoreceptor-mediated process.

Sympathomimetic amines and sympathetic nerve activity stimulate the release of renin from the juxtaglomerular apparatus of the kidney. The beta-adrenergic blocking drugs antagonize the release of renin. Renin is responsible, in part, for maintaining blood volume, and its suppression may influence water balance in the body and potassium disposition secondary to lower levels of angiotensin II and aldosterone.

Angiotensin-Converting Enzyme Inhibitors

The use of the angiotensin-converting enzyme inhibitors will reduce plasma angiotensin II and aldosterone levels significantly at rest and during physical activity (Table 4) [53, 61]. These drugs may alter the homeostatic control mechanisms for water balance because of the depression of the angiotensin–renin mechanism. In severe congestive heart failure, Captopril in combination with furosemide therapy reverses severe hyponatremia [58], and increased serum sodium concentration may occur with this drug combination [21].

The decrease in aldosterone production may lead to an increase in serum potassium level. Potassium supplements and potassium-sparing diuretics should be administered only for documented hypokalemia because of the potential significant increase in serum potassium level. In some patients, food intake may be decreased and weight loss may occur during Captopril therapy, due to a significant diminution or loss of taste.

Calcium Antagonists

The calcium antagonists verapamil and nifedipine have different clinical uses, the former as an antiarrhythmic agent particularly in paroxysmal atrial tachycardia and as a drug for chronic stable angina, the latter in treatment of angina and in postmyocardial infarction and coronary artery bypass graft management to prevent further ischemia and augment collateral myocardial flow [75]. These drugs may be used in rehabilitation of cardiac patients. The most common complaint that may affect nutritional status is that of nausea and constipation.

Digitalis, Nitrates, and Antiarrhythmias

Digitalis compounds are often administered in conjunction with potassium-depleting diuretics, which may contribute to drug-induced arrhythmias. Antacids will interfere with digitalis absorption, and calcium (found in calcium carbonate antacids) may produce arrhythmias in digitalized patients. Common toxic manifestations of digitalis therapy are nausea and vomiting, which may influence food intake.

The nitrates, represented by nitroglycerin and isosorbide dinitrate, have a number of hemodynamic effects, mostly attributable to their venodilatory actions. The major side effect that may affect nutritional status is nausea. It is important to note that orthostatic hypotension may be accentuated by alcohol when nitrate therapy is required.

The antiarrhythmics, quinidine and procainamide, may influence nutritional status by affecting the gastrointestinal system. Diarrhea, abdominal pain, nausea, and vomiting are commonly expected adverse reactions to quinidine. Procainamide may induce a bitter taste and thereby influence nutrient intake.

PERFORMANCE ENHANCERS

Anabolic Steroids

Androgens have been given to victims of starvation and to debilitated patients with chronic disease to help induce a state of positive nitrogen balance. The anabolic steroids are less virilizing than is pure testosterone and are used today by weight lifters, shot putters, discus throwers, wrestlers, and football players. The rationale for their use is that they enhance performance by increasing muscle mass, strength, and body weight, especially if consumed with a diet high in protein [37, 38, 57, 76]. Wright [89] has published an excellent review.

Body weight, total body potassium and nitrogen content, muscle size, leg performance, and strength increased significantly in men who took methandienone but not while they took placebo [29]. The increase in total body nitrogen content implies that the weight gain is not just intracellular fluid. The increases in body potassium and nitrogen are too great in proportion to weight gain for this to be attributed to gain of normal muscle or other lean tissue. Thus, the appearance may be anabolic but the weight gain produced is not entirely an increase in muscle protein mass.

The adverse effects of anabolic steroids should suffice to keep athletes from using them. Most notable among these adverse effects are the following: hepatic dysfunction, including cirrhosis of the liver and hepatocellular carcinoma (seen in aplastic anemia); decreased libido; testicular or ovarian atrophy; clitoral hypertrophy; gynecomastia; salt and water retention; and hypertension. Anabolic steroids may also cause premature closure of the epiphyses [36, 71].

Corticosteroids

Corticosteroids may be used as antiinflammatory agents that allow an athlete to continue to compete during episodes of severe musculoskeletal injury. These agents will impair calcium transport and lower serum calcium levels. Because of the effects on calcium balance, postmenopausal women should avoid these agents. These drugs also decrease uptake of amino acids from the gastrointestinal tract and promote renal secretion of amino acids [27, 31]. A high-protein diet can be helpful in the reestablishment of a positive nitrogen balance.

Amphetamines and Related Stimulants

It is well known that amphetamines and related stimulants are consumed in large doses by athletes. Their effects are controversial and dangerous [39, 74]. Their original medical indication was to induce anorexia for weight control, but they are no longer recommended for this purpose. They have been found useful in the treatment of narcolepsy and hyperactivity in children. The customary dosage of benzadrine or dexadrine is 15 mg, but professional football players allegedly consume 150 mg of amphetamines per game (83). The short-term effects of the average dose (15 mg) include a decrease in appetite, a dramatic increase in alertness and confidence, an elevation in mood, an improvement in physical performance and concentration, and a decrease in the sense of fatigue; yet associated with this is the feeling of anxiousness or of generally being on "a high."

Cocaine has an effect similar to that of the amphetamines, but the subjective symptoms of the drug are more intensely felt. This may be due to the fact that the way in which cocaine is taken results in a more rapid onset of action and a shorter duration of effect for the average dosage. Short-term effects of large amounts of cocaine are similar to those of the amphetamines. However, an initial tachycardia may become slow and weak and the tachypnea may become shallow and slow.

SUMMARY

An example of the interactions between nutrients and drugs is demonstrated clinically for antacids and laxatives; nonsteroidal analgesics and antiinflammatory drugs, including aspirin; caffeine; alcohol; oral contraceptives; diuretics; steroids; and other drugs. Many of these can have adverse effects on skeletal muscle, the heart, and the kidneys. Interactions may result in heat distress, rhabdomyolysis, electrolyte disturbances, and renal failure during exercise. The influence of each of these pharmacological agents alone may have on nutritional status may be small, but in combination the drugs may induce untoward interactions that insult the body. The drugs highlighted in this chapter are used for a variety of musculoskeletal injuries, cardiovascular disease, and gastrointestinal dysfunction and sometimes by athletes to "make weight." Interactions between the drugs themselves and with nutrient bioavailability and substrate metabolism have been discussed.

REFERENCES

1. Ali Abrishami, M., and J. Thomas. Aspirin intolerance, a review. *Ann. Allergy* 39:28–37, 1977.
2. Bassler, T. J. Body build and mortality. [Letter] *JAMA* 26:244–1437, 1980.
3. Bellet, S., A. Kershbaum, and E. Finck. Response of free fatty acids to coffee and caffeine. *Metabolism* 17:702–707, 1968.
4. Berkowitz, B., and S. Spector. Effect of caffeine and theophylline on peripheral catecholamines. *Eur. J. Pharmacol.* 13:193–196, 1971.
5. Berthet, J., E.W. Sutherland, and T.W. Rall. The assay of glucagon and epinephrine with use of liver homogenates. *J. Biol. Chem.* 229:351–354, 1957.
6. Blackshear, J.L., M. Davidman, and M.T. Stillman. Identification of risk for renal insufficiency from nonsteroidal anti-inflammatory drugs. *Arch. Intern. Med.* 143:1130–1134, 1983.
7. Blomquist, G., B. Saltin, and J.H. Mitchell. Acute

8. effects of ethanol ingestion on the response to submaximal and maximal exercise in man. *Circulation* 42:463–470, 1970.
8. Brandt, J.L., L. Castleman, H.D. Ruskin, J. Greenwald, and J. Kelly. The effect of oral protein and glucose feeding on splanchnic blood flow and oxygen utilization in normal and cirrhotic subjects. *J. Clin. Invest.* 34:1017–1025, 1955.
9. Briggs, M., and M. Briggs. Vitamin C requirement and oral contraceptives. *Nature* 238:277, 1972.
10. Butcher, R.W., and E.W. Sutherland. Adenosine 3′,5′-phosphate in biological materials. *J. Biol. Chem.* 237:1244–1250, 1962.
11. Caniggia, A., Gennari, C., and Borello, G. Intestinal absorption of calcium 47 after treatment with oral oestrogen, gestogens in senile osteoporosis. *Br. Med. J.* 4:30–32, 1970.
12. Ciabattoni, G., G.A. Cinotti, A. Pierucci, B.B. Simonetti, et al. Effects of sulindac and ibuprofen in patients with chronic glomerular disease: Evidence for the dependence of renal function on prostacyclin. *N. Engl. J. Med.* 310(5):279–283, 1984.
13. Cohen, H. Mineral oil, vitamin A, and cartone: Genesis and correction of a common misconception. *J. Med. Soc.* N.J. 67:111–1115, 1970.
14. Costill, D.L., G.P. Dalsky, and W.J. Fink. Effects of caffeine ingestion on metabolism and exercise performance. *Med. Sci. Sports Exer.* 10:155–158, 1978.
15. Conway, N. Haemodynamic effects of ethyl alcohol in patients with coronary heart disease. *Br. Heart J.* 30:638–644, 1968.
16. Crass, M.F. Exogenous substrate effects of endogenous lipid metabolism in the working rat heart. *Biochem. Biophys. Acta* 280:71–81, 1972.
17. Davenport, H.W. *Physiology of the Digestive Tract.* 3rd ed. New York: Year Book Medical Publishers, 1972.
18. Dole, V.P. Effect of nucleic acid metabolites on lipolysis in adipose tissue. *J. Biol. Chem.* 235:3125–3130, 1961.
19. Drake, D., and D. Hollander. Neutralizing capacity and cost effectiveness of antacids. *Ann. Intern. Med.* 94:215–217, 1981.
20. Dukes, M.N.G. (ed.). *Meyler's Side Effects of Drugs.* 10th ed. New York: Elsevier, 1984.
21. Dzau, V.J., and N.K. Hollenberg. Renal response to captopril in severe heart failure: Role of furosemide in natriureses and reversal of hyponatremia. *Ann. Intern. Med.* 100:777–782, 1984.
22. Fleischer, N., H. Brown, D.Y. Graham, and S. Delena. Chronic laxative-induced hyperaldosteronism and hypokalemia simulating Bartter's syndrome. *Ann. Intern. Med.* 70:791–798, 1969.
23. Fleming, C.R., and J.A. Higgins. Alcohol: Nutrient and poison (editorial) *Ann. Intern. Med.* 87(4):492–493, 1977.
24. Forman, D.T., J.E. Garvin, J.E. Forestner, and C.B. Taylor. Increased excretion of fecal bile acids by oral hydrophilic colloid. *Proc. Soc. Exp. Biol. Med.* 127:1060–1063, 1968.
25. Fred, H.L. Reflections on a 100-mile run: Effects of aspirin therapy. *Med. Sci. Sports Exer.* 12(3):212–215, 1980.

26. Goldstein, A., R. Warren, and S. Kaizer. Psychotropic effects of caffeine in man. I. International differences in sensitivity to caffeine-induced wakefulness. *J. Pharmacol. Exp. Ther.* 149:156–159, 1965.

27. Goodman, L.S., and A. Gillman. *The Pharmacological Bases of Therapeutics.* 5th ed. New York: Macmillan, 1975.

28. Halsted, C.H., E.A. Robles, and E. Mezey. Decreased jejunal uptake of labeled folic acid (^{3}H-PGA) in alcoholic patients: Roles of alcohol and nutrition. *N. Engl. J. Med.* 285:701–706, 1971.

29. Harvey, G.R., A.V. Knibbs, L. Burkinshaw, D.B. Morgan, et al. Effects of methandienone on the performance and body composition of men undergoing athletic training. *Clin. Sci.* 60:457–461, 1981.

30. Heizer, W.D., A.L. Warshaw, T.A. Waldman, and L. Laster. Protein-losing gastroenteropathy and malabsorption associated with factitious diarrhea. *Ann. Intern. Med.* 68:839–852, 1968.

31. Hethcox, J.M., and W.F. Stanaszek. Interactions of drugs and diet. *Hosp. Pharmacol.* 9:(10):373–377, 380–383, 1974.

32. Inman, W.H., M.P. Vessey, B. Westerholm, and A. Engelund. Thromboembolic disease and steroidal content of oral contraceptives: A report to the Committee on the Safety of Drugs. *Br. Med. J.* 2:203–209, 1970.

33. Ishimori, A. Safety experience with sucralfate in Japan. *J. Clin. Gastroenterol.* 3 (Suppl. 2):169–173 1981.

34. Ivy, J.L., D.L. Costill, W.J. Fink, and R.W. Lower. Influence of caffeine and carbohydrate feedings on endurance performance. *Med. Sci. Sports Exer.* 11:6–11, 1979.

35. Jaffey, L., and A. Martin. Malignant hyperkalemia after amiloride/hydrochlorothiazide treatment. (Letter) *Lancet* 1:1272, 1981.

36. Johnson, F.L., J.R. Feagler, and K. G. Lerner. Association of adrenergic anabolic steroid therapy with development of hepatocellular carcinoma. *Lancet* 2:1273–1278, 1972.

37. Johnson, L.C., G. Fisher, L.J. Silvester, and C.C. Hofheins. Anabolic steroids: Effect on strength, body weight, oxygen uptake and spermatogenesis upon mature males. *Med. Sci. Sports Exer.* 4:43–45, 1972.

38. Johnson, L.C., and J.P. O'Shea. Anabolic steroids —effects on strength development. *Science* 164:957–959, 1969.

39. Karpovich, P.V. Effect of amphetamine sulfate on athletic performance. *J. Am. Med. Assoc.* 170:558, 1959.

40. Kendrick, Z.V., S.I. Baskin, A.H. Goldfarb, and D.T. Lowenthal. Effect of age and salicylate on rectal temperature during heat exposure. *Age* 8:34–38, 1985.

41. Knochel, J.P. Renal injury in muscle disease. In (ed.) *The Kidney in Systemic Disease* (Vol. 3). S.I. Landau (Ed.). New York: John Wiley, 1976, pp. 129–140.

42. Krause, M.V., and L.K. Mehan. *Food, Nutrition, and Diet Therapy.* Philadelphia: W. B. Saunders, 1979, p. 901.

43. Kron, J., J.L. Katz, G. Gorzynski, and H. Weiner.

Hyperactivity in anorexia nervosa: A fundamental clinical feature. *Comp. Psych.* 19:433–440, 1978.

44. Lanza, F.L., G.L. Royer, R.S. Nelson, T.T. Chen, C.E. Seckman, and M.F. Rack. A comparative endoscopic evaluation of the damaging effects of nonsteroidal anti-inflammatory agents on the gastric and duodenal mucosa. *Am. J. Gastroenterol.* 75:17–21, 1982.

45. Lee, H.A. The alcohol-ethanol, sorbital, xylital. In Lee, H.A. (ed.). *Parenteral Nutrition in Acute Metablic Disease.* London: Academic Press, 1974.

46. Levy, C.M., A.K. Tanribilir, and F. Smith. Biochemistry of the gastrointestinal tract and liver disease in alcoholism. In Kissin, B., and H. Beglister (eds.) *The Biology of Alcoholism* (Vol. 1). New York: Plenum Press, pp. 307–325, 1971.

47. Levy, G., and W. Jusko. Effect of viscosity on drug absorption. *J. Pharm. Sci.* 54:219–242, 1965.

48. Lieber, C.S., S.H. Robinson, and R. Glickman. Pathogenesis and early diagnosis of alcoholic liver injury. *N. Engl. J. Med.* 298:888–893, 1978.

49. Lowenthal, D.T., M.B. Affrime, B. Falkner, S. Saris, H. Hakki, et al. Potassium disposition and neuroendocrine effects of propranolol, methyldopa and clonidine during dynamic exercise. *Clin. Exp. Hypertens.-Theory Pract.* A4(9–10):1895–1911, 1982.

50. Lowenthal, D.T., M.B. Affrime, L. Rosenthal, A.B. Gould, J. Borusso, et al. Dynamic and biochemical responses to single and repeated doses of clonidine during dynamic physical activity. *Clin. Pharmacol. Ther.* 32:18–24, 1982.

51. Lowenthal, D. T., and Z.V. Kendrick. Drug-exercise interactions. *Ann. Rev. Pharmacol. Toxicol.* 25:275–305, 1985.

52. Lundborg, P., H. Astrom, C. Bengtsson, E. Fellenius, H. Von Schenck, et al. Effect of beta-adrenoceptor blockade on exercise performance and metabolism. *Clin. Sci.* 61:229–305, 1981.

53. Manhem, P., M. Bramnert, U.L. Hulthen, and B. Hokfelt. The effect of captopril on catecholamines, renin activity, angiotensin II and aldosterone in plasma during physical exercise in hypertensive patients. *Eur. J. Clin. Invest.* 11:389–395, 1981.

54. McCracken, G.H., C.M. Ginsburg, J.C. Clahsen, and M.L. Thomas. Pharmacologic evaluation of orally administered antibodies in infants and children: Effect of feeding on bioavailability. *Pediatrics* 62(5):738–743, 1978.

55. Melander, A., K. Danielson, B. Schersten, and E. Wahlin. Enhancement of the bioavailability of propranolol and metoprolol by food. *Clin. Pharmacol. Ther.* 22:108–112, 1977.

56. Neuvonen, P.J. Interactions with the absorption of tetracyclines. *Drugs* 11(1):45–54, 1976.

57. O'Shea, J.P., and W. Winkler. Biochemical and physical effects of an anabolic steroid in competitive swimmers and weight lifters. *Nutr. Rep. Intl.* 6:351–354, 1970.

58. Packer, M., N. Medina, and M. Yushak. Correction of dilutional hyponatremia in severe chronic heart failure by converting-enzyme inhibitor. *Ann. Intern. Med.* 100:782–789, 1984.

59. Papaioannides, D., C. Giotis, N. Karaqiannis, and

C. Voudouris. Acute upper gastrointestinal hemorrhage in long distance running. *Ann. Intern. Med.* 101:719, 1984.

60. Paul, P., and B. Issekutz. Role of extra muscular energy sources in the metabolism of exercising dogs. *J. Appl. Physiol.* 22:615–622, 1967.

61. Pickering, T.G., D.B. Base, P.A. Sullivan, and J.H. Laragh. Comparison of anti-hypertensive and hormonal effects of captopril and propranolol at rest and during exercise. *Am. J. Cardiol.* 49:1566–1568, 1982.

62. Piper, D.W., and B. Fenton. pH stability and activity curves of pepsin with special reference to their clinical importance. *Gut* 6:506–508, 1965.

63. Putzeys, M.R., and S.W. Hoobler. Comparison of clonidine and methyldopa on blood pressure and side effects in hypertensive patients. *Am. Heart J.* 83:464–468, 1972.

64. Randle, P.J. Endocrine control of metabolism. *Annu. Rev. Physiol.* 25:291–324, 1963.

65. Regan, T.J., A.B. Weisse, C.B. Moschos, et al. The myocardial effects of acute and chronic usage of ethanol in man. *Trans. Assoc. Am. Phys.* 78:282–291, 1965.

66. Roe, D.A. *Drug-Induced Nutritional Deficiencies.* Westport, Conn.: Avi Publishing, 1976.

67. Rosenthal, L., M.B. Affrime, D.T. Lowenthal, B. Falkner, S. Saris, et al. Biochemical and dynamic responses to single and repeated doses of methyldopa and propranolol during dynamic physical activity. *Clin. Pharmacol. Ther.* 32:701–710, 1982.

68. Roth, J.A., and A.C. Ivy. The effect of caffeine upon gastric secretion in the dog, cat and man. *Am. J. Physiol.* 141:454–461, 1944.

69. Ryan, A. Alcohol and athletes. *Physician Sports Med.* 7:38–51, 1979.

70. Sharman, I.M. Excessive weight loss in athletes. *Br. J. Sports Med.* 16(3):180, 1982.

71. Shepard, R.J., D. Killinger, and T. Fried. Responses to sustained use of anabolic steroids. *Br. J. Sports Med.* 11:170–173, 1977.

72. Sherman, R.A., E.R. Hwang, J.A. Walker, and R.P. Eisinger. Reduction in serum phosphorus due to sucralfate. *Am. J. Gastroenterol.* 78:210–211, 1983.

73. Shojania, A.M. Effect of oral contraceptives on vitamin B-12 metabolism. *Lancet* 2:932, 1971.

74. Smith, G.M., and H.K. Beecher. Amphetamine sulfate and athletic performance. *J. Am. Med. Assoc.* 170:542, 1959.

75. Stone, P.H., E.M. Antman, J.E. Muller, and E. Braunwald.Calcium channel blocking agents in the treatment of cardiovascular disorders. II. Hemodynamic effects of clinical applications. *Ann. Intern. Med.* 93:886–904, 1980.

76. Tahmindjis, A.J. The use of anabolic steroids by athletes to increase body weight and strength. *Med. J. Austr.* 1:991–993, 1976.

77. Theuer, R.C. Effect of oral contraceptive agents on vitamin and mineral needs: A review. *J. Reprod. Med.* 8:13–19, 1972.

78. Thithapandha, A., H.M. Maling, and J.R. Gillette. Effects of caffeine and theophylline on activity of rats in relation to brain xanthine concentrations. *Proc. Exp. Biol. Med.* 139:582–586, 1972.

79. Thompson, J.K., G.J. Jarvie, B.B. Lahy, and K.J. Cureton. Exercise and obesity: Etiology, physiology and intervention. *Psychol. Bull.* 91:55–79, 1982.

80. Tomasulo, P.A., R.M. Kater, and F.L. Iber. Impairment of thiamine absorption in alcoholism. *Am. J. Clin. Nutr.* 21:1340–1344, 1968.

81. Troup, J.T. The effect of acetyl-salicylic acid administration on metabolic, cardiovascular and thermoregulatory function in young males during acute exercise in hot and neutral environments. Ph.D. dissertation, Temple University, Philadelphia, 1983.

82. Tuckerman, M.M., and S.J. Turco. *Human Nutrition.* Philadelphia: Lea & Febiger, 1983.

83. Underwood, J. Brutality. 3. Speed is all the rage. *Sports Illus.* (Aug. 28) 49:30–41, 1978.

84. Van Handel, P.J., E. Burke, D.L. Costill, and R. Cote. Physiological responses to cola ingestion. *Res. Q.* 48:436–444, 1977.

85. Virtanen, K., J. Janne, and M.H. Frick. Response of blood pressure and plasma norepinephrine to propranolol, metoprolol and clonidine during isometric and dynamic exercise. *Eur. J. Clin. Pharmacol.* 21:275–279, 1982.

86. Wada, H., and E.E. Snell. The enzymatic oxidation of pyridoxine and pyridoxamine phosphates. *J. Biol. Chem.* 236:2089–2095, 1961.

87. Wadden, T.A., A.J. Stunkard, and K.D. Brownell. Very low calorie diets: Their efficacy, safety, and future. *Ann. Intern. Med.* 99:675–684, 1983.

88. Waldeck, B. Sensitization by caffeine of central catecholamine receptors. *J. Neural Transm.* 34:61–72, 1973.

89. Wright, J. Anabolic steroids and athletes. In Hutton, R.S., and D.I. Miller (eds.). *Exercise and Sport Sciences Reviews. Vol. 8.* Philadelphia: Franklin Institute, 1980, pp. 149–202.

90. Yates, A., K. Leehey, and C.M. Shisslak. Running-an analogue of anorexia? *N. Engl. J. Med.* 308:251–255, 1983.

91. Zambraski, E.J., T.A. Rofrano, and C.D. Ciccone. Effects of aspirin treatment on kidney function in exercising man. *Med. Sci. Sports Exer.* 14:419–423, 1982.

Chapter 15

INFLUENCE OF EXERCISE ON PLASMA LIPIDS AND LIPOPROTEINS

William L. Haskell, Ph.D., Marcia L. Stefanick, Ph.D., and Robert Superko, M.D.

INTRODUCTION

Physically active people appear to be at a lower risk for coronary heart disease (CHD) than their sedentary counterparts [42]. The activity associated with this reduced risk can take place either on the job or during leisure time, with a dose-response relationship apparent: Moderately active persons have a lower risk than sedentary persons, and the most active have the lowest risk. A variety of biological changes ascribed to exercise have been proposed as possible mechanisms by which exercise contributes to this lower heart disease risk. One of the more popular considerations is exercise-induced changes in lipoprotein metabolism.

During the 1950s and 1960s, numerous investigators evaluated the relationship between physical activity status and plasma total cholesteral (T-C) or triglyceride (TG) concentrations. Most of these studies failed to provide convincing evidence that changes in habitual exercise, independent of changes in diet or body weight, produced significant changes in T-C, but did demonstrate that elevated TG concentrations frequently were normalized by endurance-type exercise [16]. In several studies during this period, a significant positive relationship was noted between exercise status and the amount of cholesterol transported as part of alpha- or high-density lipoproteins [1]. These data were essentially ignored until 1975, when a potential role for high density lipoprotein (HDL) in reverse cholesterol transport and reduced atherosclerotic risk was presented by Miller and Miller [35]. During the past decade, the relationships between activity status and plasma concentrations of the various lipoproteins and their subfractions have been extensively investigated, with emphasis placed on the role of exercise in the regulation of HDL.

This chapter is designed to provide a general overview of the relationships between exercise and the plasma concentration and composition of plasma lipoproteins. Special consideration has been given to the role of lipase enzymes in mediating the exercise responses and to selected other factors such as adiposity, nutrient intake, alcohol consumption, and cigarette smoking that may modulate the effects of exercise. Much of the data cited were collected on clinically healthy young or middle-aged men, but results from selected studies on younger and older men, women, and patients are also considered.

LIPOPROTEIN COMPOSITION AND FUNCTION

To more clearly address the influence of exercise on plasma lipoproteins, a brief review of their composition and function is provided. Comprehensive reviews of lipoprotein metabolism have been published recently [46].

Lipoproteins are the transport vehicles for both endogenously synthesized and exogenous (dietary) lipids; they contain cholesterol, triglyceride, phospholipid, and protein. They are discrete, water-soluble macromolecular complexes that are in dynamic equilibrium among themselves, with a continuous exchange of lipid, phospholipid, and protein. Lipoproteins can be classified on the basis of their gravitational density into four basic classes: chylomicrons, very-low-density lipoproteins (VLDL), low-density lipoproteins (LDL), and high-density lipoproteins (HDL). The HDL class frequently is analyzed as two separate subfractions, HDL_2

($F_{1.20}$, 3.5–9.0) and the more dense HDL_3 ($F_{1.20}$, 0–3.5), while the LDL category is separated into small LDL (sf 0–7), large LDL (sf 7–12), and intermediate-density lipoproteins (IDL; sf 12–20). In this classification, VLDL is considered sf 20–400 (see Table 1).

Thus far, approximately 16 protein constituents (apolipoproteins) have been characterized. They include apolipoprotein A (A-I, A-II, A-IV), several forms of apolipoprotein B (B_{48}, B_{100}), apolipoprotein C (C-I, C-II, C-III), apolipoprotein D, and several forms of apolipoprotein E. The biological functions of these proteins are still under investigation, but they are known to contribute to the stability of the lipoprotein particles, to provide recognition sites for cell membrane receptors, and to act as cofactors for the enzymes lipoprotein lipase and lecithin-cholesterol acyltransferase, both of which are involved in specific lipoprotein synthesis or catabolism and may be influenced by exercise. Apolipoproteins tend to be associated with

Table 1.   CHARACTERISTICS OF THE MAJOR LIPOPROTEINS IN HUMAN PLASMA.

CHARACTERISTIC	LIPOPROTEIN CLASS*			
	HDL	LDL	VLDL	Chylomicrons
Ultracentrifugal density (g/ml)	1.21–1.063	1.063–1.006	1.006–0.95	<0.95
Flotation rate (sf, Svedborg units)	—	0–20	20–400	>200
Size (Å)	50–150	215–220	300–800	400–10,000
Composition (% weight)				
Protein	45–55	18–22	6–10	1–2
Triglyceride	2–7	4–8	50–65	85–95
Cholesterol				
Free	3–5	6–8	4–8	1–3
Ester	12–20	45–50	16–22	2–4
Phospholipid	26–32	18–24	15–20	3–6
Apoprotein classification				
Major	A–I, A–II	B	B, C–III, E	B, C–I, C–II, C–III
Minor	C–III, B, C–I, C–II, E, D, E, F, apolp (a)	C–I, C–II, apolp (a)	A–I, A–II, D–I, C–II	A–1, A–II, A–IV, E, H
Source of lipoproteins				
Major	Intestine	Plasma	Liver	Intestine
Minor	Liver	—	Intestine	—

*HDL, high-density lipoproteins; LDL, low-density lipoproteins; VLDL, very-low-density lipoproteins.

specific lipoproteins and are identified on the basis of their individual antibody-binding characteristics (Table 1). They are produced primarily by the intestinal mucosa and liver. Apolipoprotein A-II and some amount of B and C are produced in the intestine, whereas the liver is the major source of apolipoproteins A-I, B, C, and E.

It now appears that cholesterol accumulation in peripheral tissues is the result of the net effect of cholesterol transport to and away from these tissues (Figure 1). Very-low-density lipoproteins synthesized in the liver and chylomicrons of intestinal origin are transported to extrahepatic tissue, where they are delipidated by LPL (located in the endothlelial surface of capillaries located in adipose tissue and skeletal muscle) with glycerol and free fatty acids taken up by peripheral tissue for storage or use as an energy substrate. Catabolism of some chylomicrons is also activated by hepatic lipase. The delipidated VLDL is taken up by specific receptors located on peripheral and hepatic cells and catabolized. The primary end product of this VLDL catabolism is LDL, the major cholesterol-carrying lipoprotein in normal human plasma. Most LDL appears to be derived from VLDL catabolism, but some is directly synthesized. Low-density

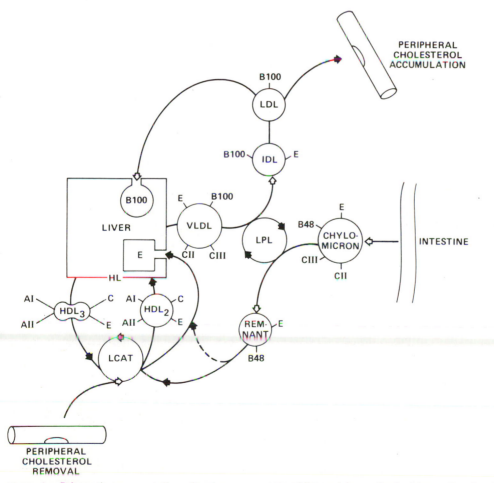

Figure 1. Schematic representation of major components of lipoprotein synthesis, transport, and catabolism. See text for discussion.

lipoproteins can be catabolized in various cells by both receptor-dependent and receptor-independent mechanisms. Once LDL binds to a receptor, it is internalized and degraded. The free cholesterol resulting from this degrading inhibits the activity of 3-hydroxy-3-methylglutoryl coenzyme A reductase, the rate-limiting enzyme in intracellular cholesterol synthesis.

High-density lipoproteins appear to be synthesized from VLDL remnants (Apo E, Apo C, and phospholipids), lipid being transferred to the remnants by the action of lecithin-cholesterol acyltransferase. Direct production of HDL occurs in both the liver and the intestine. In addition, HDL serves as an acceptor of lipid, especially free cholesterol, from various tissues. High-density lipoprotein is the substrate for lecithin-cholesterol acyltransferase, which catalyzes the conversion of both free cholesterol ester and lecithin to lysolecithin. Cholesterol esters are transferred from HDL to other lipoproteins nonspecifically, as well as by a cholesterol-ester transfer protein. The hepatic lipase enzyme probably is involved in converting HDL_2 to HDL_3, hepatic uptake of cholesterol occurring during this process.

RELATIONSHIP OF HABITUAL ACTIVITY AND PLASMA LIPOPROTEIN CONCENTRATIONS

Plasma Total Cholesterol

The concentration of cholesterol in the plasma or sera of physically active persons frequently is not different from that observed in age-, sex-, and body composition-matched sedentary controls. This is not to say that the metabolism or composition of cholesterol might not be different in these two groups, but no clinically important differences have been systematically revealed in either cross-sectional or longitudinal studies in which T-C has been the primary measure of interest.

When endurance-trained athletes have been compared with sedentary controls or the general population, their mean T-C concentrations usually are within 5% of one another, the difference being significantly different ($P<.05$) less than one-third of the time. Athletes for whom such comparisons have been made include men and women runners, cross-country skiers, ice skaters, soccer players, and tennis players [47]. In those studies reporting lower T-C values for endurance athletes, the athletes tend to be very active (usually running more than 30 km/week or the equivalent amount of training in terms of energy expenditure) and are very lean. Speed- or power-trained athletes not using anabolic steroids generally do not have T-C concentrations significantly different from those of nonathletes [9].

Within the general population, men or women reporting themselves physically active either on the job or during leisure time have T-C concentrations similar to their inactive peers. This lack of difference exists even when the activity is as vigorous and sustained as that performed by lumberjacks, whose daily caloric expenditure frequently exceeds 5000 calories [8]. Also, when the data are adjusted for factors such as body weight, body mass index, or nutrient intake, significant relationships between exercise status and T-C are not uncovered [13]. In fact, such statistical adjustments, especially for weight and nutrient intake, usually reduce the strength of any exercise and T-C relationship. Indeed, when persons are classified according to their functional capacity and the more fit have lower T-C concentrations, much of this difference can be accounted for by greater adiposity in the less fit [5].

In very few studies that have included a sedentary control group for comparison has exercise training resulted in a significant reduction in plasma T-C concentrations. In some studies changes have been reported, but they usually are quite small or major questions regarding changes in nutrient intake, weight changes, or laboratory standardization go unanswered. It is worth noting, however, that in 14 sedentary middle-aged men who increased their activity over 2 years by running approximately 12 miles/week, they decreased their body fat content from 21.6 to 18% and at the same time increased their caloric intake by an average of 400 cal/day [64]. During this time their mean T-C concentration decreased from 216 to 203 mg/dl ($P<.01$) while their HDL-C concentration significantly increased (49.8 to 53.9 mg/dl; $P<.01$). Changes in T-C concentrations were highly correlated with both running mileage and weight loss, indicating exercise-induced weight loss may produce some lowering in plasma T-C concentration.

Low-Density Lipoprotein Cholesterol

It now appears quite unlikely that exercise, without a change in body composition or diet, has clinically significant impact on plasma LDL-C concentration. The difference in LDL-C between endurance-trained athletes and sedentary controls usually is within 10%, the significantly lower values being reported for athletes in some but not all studies [47]. When lower values have been reported, they most frequently occur in very lean runners; tennis and soccer players have values similar to sedentary peers. Weight or speed-type training appears not to alter LDL-C concentrations [9]. Among the general population, reported activity status for men or women is not related to plasma LDL-C concentration [13].

The results of well-designed training studies on LDL-C are consistent with the more prevalent findings of the cross-sectional observations; the changes in LDL-C concentration with endurance training usually are relatively small (<8%) and only occasionally are they statistically significant. There is some evidence that greater amounts of exercise are more likely to produce significant decreases in LDL-C, but no systematic dose-response relationship has been established, nor does the role of body composition change as a result of exercise. Similar

results have been reported for women [4] and adolescents [30].

Data are limited on the effects of exercise training in patients with elevated LDL-C concentrations. No systematic relationship was observed between reported activity or treadmill test duration and LDL-C concentrations among the type II hyperlipidemia patients participating in the Lipid Research Clinic's coronary primary prevention trial [11]. Endurance exercise training by hypertriglyceridemic patients [27] or those with either ischemic heart disease [2] or renal failure [10] did not significantly alter LDL-C. In overweight persons, weight loss by exercise has not been markedly effective in decreasing LDL-C concentrations [49].

The traditional measurement of LDL-C is a composite of both LDL (Sf 0–12) and IDL (Sf 12–20) lipoprotein particles. Further, heterogeneity within the LDL particles is apparent when they are subjected to density gradient ultracentrifugation. Various separations have been proposed, the simplest one being the separation of LDL into "small" (Sf 0–7) and "large" (Sf 7–12) particles. Preliminary data comparing endurance-trained men with nonrunners of a similar age (but slightly greater body mass) have demonstrated a significantly lower concentration of small LDL in the runners (138 vs. 228 mg/dl; $P<.001$) but no difference in the concentration of large LDL (137 vs. 134 mg/dl; $P = .85$) [60] That endurance exercise might alter the composition of LDL was then investigated in a 1-year training study, but none of the changes in LDL-C, IDL-C, or LDL subspecies were significant [63]. The lack of consistency in the results of these two studies may be due to differences in the amount and intensity of exercise performed, the length of time over which training occurred, or differences in other characteristics that influence LDL metabolism (adiposity, diet, or heredity). Since the atherogenicity of LDL appears to vary among the various subspecies, further investigation as to any effects of exercise on subspecie metabolism should receive high priority.

High-Density Lipoprotein Cholesterol

Compared with sedentary persons or the general population, endurance-trained men and women consistently demonstrate significantly higher HDL-C concentrations. The typical mean difference for HDL-C between endurance athletes and control subjects ranges from 10 to 20 mg/dl, or 20 to 36% [Figure 2]. While such differences have been reported most frequently for long-distance runners, they also have been observed for nordic skiers, speed skaters, soccer players, and tennis players [65]. Sprinters and weight-trained athletes who perform little endurance-type exercise have HDL-C concentrations similar to those of sedentary controls [9], whereas use of androgenic hormones by weight-training athletes significantly lowers HDL-C concentrations [17]. The higher HDL-C in endurance athletes is not due to an acute increase in response to vigorous exercise, since even several hours of running usually does not significantly alter plasma HDL-C concentrations [58]. In the few studies in which HDL-C values were not different for endurance athletes and less active persons, either the total cholesterol concentration in the runners was exceptionally low (with a very high HDL-C/total cholesterol ratio; >.30 or the HDL-C concentration of the control subjects was unusually high.

Within the general population, HDL-C varies with level of habitual activity, ranging from "subnormal" values for patients enduring bed rest because of spinal cord injury [38] values that approach those of endurance athletes in persons with very physically demanding jobs, such as Finnish lumberjacks [29]. The differences in most of the general population that can be accounted for by exercise, when the effect of other factors such as body mass, alcohol use, and cigarette smoking are taken into account, are quite small and usually do not exceed 5 to 10% [13]. As in the cross-sectional comparison of athletes, the higher HDL-C concentrations in more active persons are associated with lower plasma TG concentrations and tend to be highest in the most active persons, who are also quite lean.

So far, longitudinal studies have provided equivocal evidence that endurance or aerobic-type exercise training results in increased HDL-C concentration [59]. Of the more than 30 training studies now published, approximately half have demonstrated a significant increase in those subjects assigned to an exercise training group. These results include healthy men and women, obese subjects, hyperlipidemic patients, and patients with coronary heart disease. Analysis of these studies has not provided clear-cut evidence why such inconsistencies exist. Differences cannot be totally accounted for by variations in baseline values, training regimen, dietary intake including alcohol, body composition, or cigarette smoking. However, evidence exists that the amount of train-

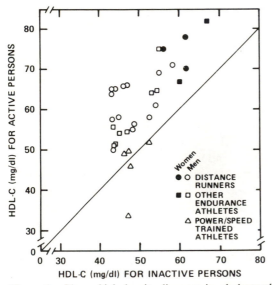

Figure 2. Plama high-density lipoprotein cholesterol (HDL-C) concentration for well-trained men and women athletes versus inactive control subjects. The values above the line of identity indicate higher values for the athletes. (Data from 32 cross-sectional studies reviewed by Wood, P.D., P.T. Williams, and W.L. Haskell. Physical activity and high density lipoproteins. In Miller, N.E., and G.J. Miller (eds.). *Clinical and Metabolic Aspects of High Density Lipoproteins.* Amsterdam: Elsevier, 1984.

ing per week and the length of the training program may be related to the magnitude of HDL-C increase [59, 61]. Several studies have demonstrated a highly significant correlation between the magnitude of the increase in exercise and the increase in HDL-C concentration. However, when the change in HDL-C concentration with exercise training for 28 studies reviewed by Wood, Williams, and Haskell [65] is plotted against the number of weeks of training in each study, no strong association is apparent (Figure 3). This relationship is not altered when the changes in HDL-C are expressed as a percentage from baseline. At 10 weeks of training or less, as many studies have reported a decrease in HDL-C as have reported an increase. All studies of greater than 12 weeks duration observed an increase in HDL-C (not all of these increases were significant at $P<.05$), with no relationship apparent between HDL-C increase and training program duration between 12 and 52 weeks.

The subfractions of HDL, especially HDL_2 and HDL_3, have been of substantial clinical interest due to apparent differences in their biological functions and their differential responses to various interventions. For example, the higher plasma HDL concentrations in women are primarily due to a higher HDL_2 mass, and both HDL_2 cholesterol and the major HDL_2 protein, apolipoprotein A-I, are negatively associated with coronary atherosclerosis, whereas HDL_3 has not yet been shown to related coronary heart disease risk. Some of the differences reported from various laboratories on factors regulating HDL subfractions can be attributed to a laboratory methodology that is still evolving and to different definitions for the HDL_2 and HDL_3 particle regions.

Comparisons of endurance-trained athletes and sedentary controls generally have demonstrated a higher HDL_2 mass or HDL_2-C concentration in more active persons, without major differences being observed for HDL_3-C [60]. Most data demonstrating higher HDL_2 values for trained athletes are derived from studies of male endurance runners, but similar results have been reported for physically active military students in whom HDL_2-C was significantly correlated with exercise capacity ($r = .52$), whereas HDL_3 was negatively correlated ($r = .22$) [25]. An exception has been the report that physical activity across the full spectrum from bed rest to endurance running is related similarly to HDL_2-C and HDL_3-C [28].

Sedentary healthy men [43] and cardiac patients [2] who undertake a program of endurance training have demonstrated significant increases in HDL_2-C concentration. Also, increases in HDL_2 mass were significantly correlated with distance run ($r = 0.41$) and increased maximal oxygen uptake ($\dot{V}o_2max$) ($r = 0.39$) in men who participated in an endurance training program for 1 year [63].

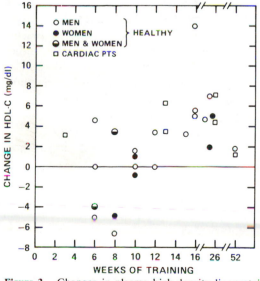

Figure 3. Changes in plasma high-density lipoprotein cholesterol (HDL-C) concentration with an endurance exercise training program ranging from 3 to 52 weeks in duration. (Data from 29 endurance training studies reviewed by Wood, P.D., P.T. Williams, and W.L. Haskell. Physical activity and high density lipoproteins. In Miller, N.E., and G.J. Miller (eds.). *Clinical and Metabolic Aspects of High-Density Lipoproteins.* Amsterdam: Elsevier, 1984.

Plasma Triglycerides

Most endurance-trained athletes have a very low fasting plasma TG concentration, values typically being below 100 mg/dl for men and 80 mg/dl for women. Low values, compared with those for sedentary controls or the general population, have been reported for long-distance runners, cross-country skiers, and tennis players. The low plasma TG concentration observed for endurance athletes is especially impressive for older athletes, in whom mean values may be only 75 to 80 mg/dl, compared with the 150 mg/dl values for sedentary men of a similar age [32]. Contributing to the lower TG concentration in these athletes is their tendency to be very lean. In studies that do not find lower plasma TG concentrations for endurance athletes, the values for the comparison group usually are low as well. Very active women have low TG concentrations even when using oral contraceptives [34]. Athletes involved in power or speed-type training have plasma TG concentrations similar to those of inactive people unless they are using anabolic steroids, which tend to elevate TG concentrations. Limited information has been published on the relationship between plasma TG concentration and habitual exercise status in the general population. Lower values have been reported for people who are more active on the job or during leisure time in selected populations [13] but not in others [33].

Endurance exercise training decreases plasma TC concentrations when pretraining values are elevated [16] but not when pretraining values are relatively low (<120 mg/dl). This plasma TG lowering effect appears to have both acute and chronic components. Following a bout of vigorous endurance exercise, including a typical 45-minute training session, plasma TG concentration is temporarily decreased in most hypertriglyceridemic subjects [40]. The magnitude of this decrease is positively related to preexercise TG concentrations and the amount of exercise performed, but occurs even if the increased caloric expenditure is compensated for by an increase in caloric intake [12]. Independent of this acute lowering effect, more physically active individuals generally have a lower plasma TG concentration even when they have not exercised recently. The time course for the return of TG concentration to pretraining values during detraining has not been established.

Since, in the fasting state, most of the plasma TG is carried as part of VLDL, the major plasma TG exercise effects are seen in the VLDL. When total plasma TG concentration is modified by exercise, the VLDL TG also is changed. In the few studies where VLDL TG concentrations have been measured, they generally are low in endurance athletes and decrease with training only when pretraining values are elevated.

The amount of TG in plasma LDL is so small that accurate measurement of changes in its concentration is technically difficult and not frequently reported. Lower plasma LDL TG concentrations have been observed in long-distance runners [60], while Finnish lumberjacks were found to have higher plasma LDL TG values than sedentary workers [29]. No change in plasma LDL TG was obtained for men training either 10 [39] or 16 [54] weeks.

The higher HDL mass observed in endurance athletes appears to be due to an increase in all of its lipid constituents including TG, especially that TG found in the HDL$_2$ subfraction. As the result of a 16-week exercise training program, patients with coronary heart disease demonstrated a mean increase in HDL$_2$ TG from 0.6 to 1.2 mg/dl ($P < .02$) whereas, values for patients who remained sedentary did not change [2]. No changes were observed for HDL$_3$ TG.

Apolipoproteins

So far the effects of exercise have been investigated for only a few of the apolipoproteins, primarily A-I and A-II. A few reports are now emerging on apolipoproteins B and

E. Cross-sectional comparisons of men and women endurance-trained athletes versus sedentary controls usually have demonstrated substantially higher A-I but not A-II levels for the athletes [62]. The typical apolipoprotein A-I concentration has been approximately 30% higher for the athletes. Herbert et al. [15] reported that the plasma concentrations of apolipoproteins A-I and A-II were not different between runners and sedentary men, but, due to the increase in plasma volume of the runners, the plasma masses of the athletes were 58 and 29% greater for A-I and A-II, respectively. These increased HDL apolipoprotein masses were associated with 27% lower fractional catabolic rate in runners. Bed rest due to spinal cord injury is associated with lower apolipoprotein A-I concentrations in both men (23% lower) and women (34% lower) when compared with levels in ambulatory controls [36]. The relationship of any of the apolipoproteins to exercise status in the general population has not been reported.

Endurance exercise training generally has resulted in a significant increase in apolipoprotein A-I concentration. Men who exercised for 12 weeks increased their A-I concentrations by 10% ($P = 0.02$) [20]. However, Wood et al. [63] found no change in mean apolipoprotein A-I, A-II, or B concentrations during 1 year of exercise training: Apolipoproteins A-I and A-II were not associated with the amount of exercise performed by individuals in the training group, but the change in apolipoprotein B was negatively correlated with miles run ($r = -0.29$; $p < 0.015$).

MECHANISMS UNDERLYING EXERCISE-INDUCED CHANGES IN LIPOPROTEINS

Endurance training enhances the capacity of skeletal muscle to utilize free fatty acids as fuel during heavy exercise, partially due to well-established changes in skeletal muscle mitochondrial size, number, and enzyme activity, which improves the muscle's ability to oxidize fats. During prolonged exercise, increased energy demands of working muscles exert a major influence on plasma lipoprotein metabolism, as the muscles rely more on fat oxidation for fuel.

Enhanced Triglyceride Removal and Lipoprotein Lipase Activity

Lipoprotein lipase, located in the capillary walls of adipose tissue and skeletal muscle, particularly in slow-twitch fibers [3], increases its activity acutely during exercise [18]. Resting lipoprotein lipase activity of skeletal muscle and adipose tissue also has been shown to be elevated in athletes, relative to sedentary controls [38]. Lipoprotein lipase activity has been correlated positively with maximum oxygen uptake [53] and/or the amount of physical activity performed and has been found to be increased by endurance training [42].

Activation of lipoprotein lipase, which requires the presence of apolipoprotein C-II from HDL particles, results in hydrolysis of the core triglycerides of VLDL. Exercise-induced elevations of lipoprotein lipase activity probably underlie the reduction in plasma TG levels seen immediately following exercise [44]. Similarly the long-lasting lipoprotein lipase activity elevations, which facilitate restoration of muscle and adipose tissue triglyceride stores during the recovery period, promote plasma clearance of VLDL following exercise, thereby further reducing TG levels. Better tissue perfusion following endurance training as a result of increased capillarization of skeletal muscle would enable larger amounts of substrate, in the form of VLDL, to come into contact with capillary-bound lipoprotein lipase.

Post-heparin plasma lipoprotein lipase activity which includes enzymes released from adipose tissue and from cardiac and skeletal muscle lipoprotein lipase, has also been shown to correlate positively with HDL concentrations [38, 53], specifically HDL_2 [22,

23]. Elevation of lipoprotein lipase activity in working muscle has been shown to be accompanied by higher HDL_2-C levels in venous plasma from the muscle, relative to arterial plasma, suggesting a direct role of skeletal muscle lipoprotein lipase in exercise-related alterations in HDL_2-C [21].

Besides being formed by hydrolysis of chylomicrons and VLDL by lipoprotein lipase, HDL is also formed through the conversion of nascent, discoidal particles secreted from the liver by plasma lecithin-cholesterol acyltransferase, which transfers plasma fatty acids carried by the phospholipid lecithin to the nascent particle. HDL_2 concentrations are also increased by the action of lecithin-cholesterol acyltransferase, following lipoprotein lipase-mediated hydrolysis of HDL_3. There is preliminary evidence that the acyltransferase activity is increased by exercise, which provides another mechanism by which exercise could lead to lipoprotein changes [31].

Another possible mechanism underlying the reduced TG levels of athletes involves changes in insulin sensitivity with training. Increased insulin sensitivity has been postulated to underlie the inhibition of carbohydrate-induced hypertriglyceridemia in trained rats [66]. A reduced postprandial insulin response to a carbohydrate diet would lead to decreased hepatic VLDL TG secretion and lower plasma TG levels. This mechanism could serve a protective role against the high carbohydrate diet required in endurance exercise, and could be significant enough to help bring about the significantly lower TG concentrations of endurance-trained athletes.

Exercise, Adiposity, and Lipoproteins

Long-term endurance training usually reduces adiposity. Several authors have argued that exercise-related lipoprotein changes are actually due to a decrease in adiposity, which is strongly associated with increased HDL and decreased VLDL concentrations, rather than to a unique exercise effect. We have recently shown that weight loss, specifically fat loss, whether achieved by exercise or by caloric restriction without exercise, results in reductions in hepatic lipase activity, which is strongly associated with increases in HDL, particularly HDL_2 [31].

Hepatic lipase activity has previously been shown to be lower in athletes relative to sedentary controls [23], perhaps due to the lower adiposity of athletes, and to be reduced by training [53]. Considerable evidence supports a role for hepatic lipase activity in the metabolism of HDL, specifically in the conversion of HDL_2 to HDL_3, such that reduced hepatic lipase activity might result in reduced conversion of HDL_2 to HDL_3, with a net increase in HDL_2 [26, 52, 55]. However, exercise has also been shown to bring about HDL elevations separately and independently of weight loss [49]. We would propose that when a negative calorie balance and loss of body fat are also consequences of the exercise, a reduction in hepatic lipase activity would accompany more direct stimulating effects of the exercise on tissue lipoprotein lipase activity, thereby promoting further HDL increases, specifically HDL_2 elevations.

There is some evidence that the exercise-related fat loss involves abdominal adipose tissue sites more selectively than other sites [7]. A "male" abdominal obesity pattern has been shown to render both men and women more susceptible to the effect on lipoprotein metabolism of excess body fat, relative to a "female" gluteal-femoral pattern [24]. The waist/hip girth ratio has been shown to correlate negatively with HDL cholesterol and HDL_2 mass and positively with TG and VLDL cholesterol and mass in our laboratory [56]. Abdominal adipocytes appear to be more responsive to catecholamine-induced lipolysis than femoral fat cells [48], and exercise training reportedly increases fat cell beta-receptor sensitivity to norepinephrine, thereby possibly enhancing the lipolytic effect of catecholamines. Verification that exercise leads to alterations in fat distribution may therefore offer insights into the mechanism by which exercise leads to specific lipoprotein changes.

Exercise, Sex Hormones, and Lipoproteins

Endurance exercise tends to shift the lipoprotein profile of men to look more like that of women, raising the possibility that sex hormones might be modified by exercise. One possible mechanism through which sex hormones could exert their influence on lipoproteins concentrations is by altering tissue lipase activity. Women have been shown to have a higher mean lipoprotein lipase activity and lower hepatic lipase activity at any given physical activity level than men [37]. Exogenous estrogen has been shown to simultaneously decrease hepatic lipase activity and increase HDL_2 [45], while androgen therapy has the opposite effect in both men and women [16].

While plasma lipoprotein levels may be directly affected by hormonal influences on lipase activities, another possible means by which sex hormones could affect lipoprotein metabolism is through their long-term or cumulative impact on adipose tissue distribution, specifically with respect to abdominal versus gluteal-femoral deposition of fat. Increasing androgenicity in women, as reflected by a decrease in level of sex hormone-binding globulin and an increase in the percent of the hormone that is unbound and therefore physiologically active, has been reported to be accompanied by an increased waist/hip girth ratio, independent of and additive to degree of obesity [8]. Likewise in men, the waist/hip girth ratio correlated negatively with testosterone and sex hormone-binding globulin levels, and was seen to have a major influence on relationships between the globulin and the HDL subfractions [56].

Exercise repeatedly has been shown to affect steroid hormone levels in both men and women; however, there does not yet seem to be agreement as to the direction of the change. This probably relates to differences in intensity and duration of exercise, prior fitness status, the amount of time that has passed between the exercise and blood sampling, and, especially in women, prior hormonal status. The fact that exercise effects on lipoproteins are less consistently demonstrated in women might indicate that changes in sex hormones are of less significance for lipoprotein regulation in women, or alternatively, that exercise-induced changes in fat distribution is of less importance in women in whom sex hormones already favor a low waist/hip girth ratio. Considerable research is needed to test these hypotheses.

FACTORS INFLUENCING LIPOPROTEIN RESPONSES TO EXERCISE

The varied responses of the lipoproteins to exercise training reported here may be due to variations in selected characteristics of the study participants as well as to characteristics of the exercise regimens. It appears that a sustained increase in energy production by skeletal muscles above production at rest is a critical stimulus for exercise-induced changes in lipoprotein metabolism. The primary evidence for this conclusion is that heavy resistance-type exercise, which requires a lower rate of energy expenditure than endurance-type exercise, has less influence on plasma lipoprotein concentrations and on related enzymes. Also, in those endurance-training studies that investigated the dose-response relationship between exercise amount and magnitude of lipoprotein change, a positive association generally has been observed. However, differences in the characteristics of the exercise regimens do not account for the disparate results from many studies. Some evidence exists that larger lipoprotein changes may occur more frequently if subjects are initially very inactive or if the lipoprotein concentrations are substantially elevated, in the case of TG and VLDL, or low, in the case of HDL [59]. Also, changes may result in some persons only after an extended period of training (Figure 3).

The Synergy of Exercise and Leanness

As repeatedly stated in various sections of this chapter, being lean appears to produce many of same alterations in lipoprotein metabolism as does endurance exercise training: low VLDL and TG, high HDL-C and apolipoprotein A-I, and relatively minor effects on LDL-C and associated apolipoproteins. Whereas lipoprotein changes can occur independent of alterations in body composition, the likelihood that significant changes will result from increased activity is enhanced if the activity is accompanied by a decrease in adiposity. The greatest differences in lipoprotein profiles with exercise occur when high-volume endurance exercise is accompanied by reductions in body fat to a point where it represents less than 12% of total body mass for men and 15% for women. The exceedingly low TG and high HDL-C concentrations reported for endurance athletes who have undergone years of training probably result from the synergy of extreme leanness, fitness, and genetic endowment.

Nutrient Intake and Exercise

Some of the variations in lipoprotein responses to exercise training could be due to differences in nutrient intake among study participants. Even quite small reductions in saturated fat or cholesterol intake could account for changes in T-C or LDL-C concentrations, leading to an erroneous conclusion in some studies that these decreases were the result of increased exercise. The increase in HDL-C could be enhanced by increased alcohol intake as a means of achieving needed fluid replacement following exercise or by a sustained increase in dietary fat content. In general, however, it appears that the dietary habits of active people, especially distance runners who consume a large percentage of their calories in the form of carbohydrate, would not account for their lower TG and higher HDL concentrations. If anything, a higher carbohydrate diet would tend to increase TG and VLDL and decrease HDL-C concentrations. Increases in alcohol intake would augment the HDL-C response to exercise. Several well-executed studies have demonstrated that short-term changes in either dietary fat intake [19] or total caloric intake [28] do not significantly alter the HDL-C concentrations of very active men. Overall, while it appears that changes in plasma lipoprotein concentrations are produced by exercise independent of any change in nutrient intake, variations in nutrient intake may contribute to significant variations in lipoprotein response to similar exercise regimens.

The Attenuation Effect of Cigarette Smoking

Individuals who smoke cigarettes demonstrate an attenuated HDL-C response to exercise. Cross-sectional studies have demonstrated that physically active men and women who smoke have significantly lower HDL-C concentrations than do their non-smoking counterparts, the mean difference ranging from 8 to 20% (50, 51). These differences exist when adjusted for body fatness and alcohol intake. Preliminary data also support the notion that when sedentary men initiate an exercise program, the magnitude of the HDL-C change that occurs will be influenced by their smoking status. The increase in HDL-C and HDL-C$_2$ following exercise training by cardiac patients was substantially less in those patients who continued to smoke compared with those who reduced their smoking or were nonsmokers [6]. This attenuation effect of smoking may be due to the lower lipoprotein lipase activity reported in cigarette smokers, but other changes in the circulation and metabolism of smokers produced by nicotine and carbon monoxide may also be responsible.

SUMMARY

Men and women who self-select participation in vigorous endurance-type exercise generally have plasma lipoprotein profiles consistent with a lower risk for coronary heart disease. Less clear is how much of this potential benefit can be achieved by exercise regimens that are acceptable and within the capacity of most sedentary adults. The major alterations resulting from exercise are a reduction in plasma triglyceride concentration and an increase in high-density lipoprotein (HDL) mass, due especially to increases in HDL_2 cholesterol and apolipoprotein A-I. The percent of plasma total cholesterol (T-C) contained in HDL-C, or the ratio of HDL-C to low-density lipoprotein (LDL)-C, considered to be good lipoprotein risk predictors for coronary heart disease, frequently are increased by endurance exercise. Plasma LDL-C concentration decreases in some situations but seems less amenable to changes with exercise than does plasma triglyceride or HDL-C. Modification of enzymes involved in triglyceride and cholesterol synthesis and catabolism (lipoprotein lipase, hepatic lipase, and lecithin-cholesterol acyltransferase) most likely mediate the exercise-induced changes in lipoproteins. The high rate of energy turnover in skeletal muscle and the increase in adrenergic drive during endurance exercise probably are responsible for the changes in the activity of these enzymes.

Future research should be directed at establishing how exercise modifies the activity of lipoprotein and hepatic lipase and of lecithin-cholesterol acyltransferase, as well as other enzymes and hormones that contribute to the regulation of lipoprotein metabolism and probably are influenced by exercise. As our understanding of the function of the more recently identified apolipoproteins and the LDL subfractions is increased, it should be determined if exercise modifies their me-

tabolism. Of a more applied nature is the need to better define the dose-response relationship between various exercise regimens and changes in specific lipoprotein components, and eventually to determine if the exercise-induced changes in lipoproteins are casually linked to a reduction in atherosclerosis and clinical manifestations of coronary heart disease.

REFERENCES

1. Altakruse, E.B., and J.H. Wilmore. Changes in blood chemistries following a controlled exercise program. *J. Occup. Med.* 15:110–113, 1973.
2. Ballantyne, F., R. Clark, H. Simpson, and D. Ballantyne. The effect of moderate physical exercise on the plasma lipoprotein subfractions of male survivors of myocardial infarction. *Circulation* 65:913–918, 1982.
3. Borensztajn, J., M.S. Rone, S.P. Babirak, J.A. McGarr, and L.B. Oscai. Effect of exercise on lipoprotein lipase activity in rat heart and skeletal muscle. *Am. J. Physiol.* 229:392–397, 1975.
4. Brownell, K.D., P.S. Bachorik, and R.S. Ayerle. Changes in plasma lipid and lipoprotein levels in men and women after a program of moderate exercise. *Circulation* 65:477–484, 1982.
5. Cooper, K.H., M.L. Pollock, R.P. Martin, S. White, A. Linnerud, and A. Jackson. Physical fitness levels vs. selected coronary risk factors. *JAMA* 236:166–169, 1976.
6. Cowan, G.O. Influence of exercise on high-density lipoprotein. *Am. J. Cardiol.* 52(4):13B–19B, 1983.
7. Despres, J.P., C. Bouchard, A. Tremblay, R. Savard, and M. Marcotle. Effects of aerobic training on fat distribution in male subjects. *Med. Sci. Sports Exer.* 17:113–118, 1985.
8. Evans, D.J., P.G. Hoffmann, R.K. Kalkhoff, and A.H. Kissebah. Relationship of androgenic activity to body fat topography, a fat cell morphology and metabolic aberrations in premenopausal women. *J. Clin. Endocrinol. Metab.* 57:304–310, 1983.
9. Farrell, P.A., M.G. Maksud, M.L. Pollock, et al. A comparison of plasma cholesterol, triglycerides, and high-density lipoprotein cholesterol in speed skaters, weightlifters and non-athletes. *Eur. J. Appl. Physiol.* 481:77–82, 1982.
10. Goldberg, A.P., J.M. Hageberg, A.A. Delmez, M.E. Hayes, and H. Harter. Metabolic effects of exercise training in hemodialysis patients. *Kidney Int.* 18:754–761, 1980.
11. Gordon, D.J., J.L. Witztum, A. Hunninghake, S. Gates, and C.J. Glueck. Habitual physical activity and high density lipoprotein cholesterol in men with primary hypercholesterolemia. *Circulation* 67:512–520, 1983.
12. Gyntelberg, F., R. Brennan, J. Holloszy, G. Schon-

feld, M., Rennie, and S. Weidman. Plasma triglyceride lowering by exercise despite increased food intake in patients with Type-IV hyperlipoproteinemia. *Am. J. Clin. Nutr.* 30:716–720, 1977.

13. Haskell, W.L., H.L. Taylor, P.D. Wood, H. Schrott, and G. Heiss. Strenuous physical activity, treadmill exercise test response and plasma high-density lipoprotein cholesterol: The Lipid Research Clinic Program Prevalence Study. *Circulation* 62(Suppl. IV):53–61, 1980.

14. Hazzard, W.R., S.M. Haffner, R.S. Kushwaha, D. Applebaum-Bowden, and D.M. Foster. Preliminary report: Kinetic studies on the modulation of high-density lipoprotein, apolipoprotein, and subfraction metabolism by sex steroids in post-menopausal woman. *Metabolism* 33:779–784, 1984.

15. Herbert, P.N., A.N. Bernier, E.M. Cullinane, et al. High-density lipoprotein metabolism in runners and sedentary men. *JAMA* 252:1034–1037, 1984.

16. Holloszy, J.O., J.S. Skinner, G. Toro, and T.K. Cureton. Effects of a six-month program for endurance exercise on serum lipids of middle-aged men. *Am. J. Cardiol.* 14:753–760, 1964.

17. Hurley, B.F., A.R. Seals, J.M. Hagberg, et al. High-density lipoprotein cholesterol in bodybuilders vs. powerlifters: Negative effects of androgen use. *JAMA* 252:507–513, 1984.

18. Kantor, M.A., E.M., Cullinane, P.N. Herbert, and P.D. Thompson. Acute increase in lipoprotein lipase following prolonged exercise. *Metabolism* 33:454–457, 1984.

19. Kiens, B., P. Gad, H. Lithell, and B. Vessby. Minor dietary effects on HDL in physically active men. *Eur. J. Clin. Invest.* 11:265–271, 1981.

20. Kiens, B., I. Jorgenson, S. Lewis, et al. Increased plasma HDL-cholesterol and Apo A-I in sedentary middle-aged men after physical conditioning. *Eur. J. Clin. Invest.* 10:203–209, 1980.

21. Kiens, B., and H. Lithell. Lipoprotein metabolism related to adaptations in human skeletal muscle. (Abstract) *Clin. Physiol.* 5(4):108, 1985.

22. Krauss, R.M., R.I. Levy, and D.S. Fredrickson. Selective measurement of two lipase activities in postheparin plasma from normal subjects and patients with hyperlipoproteinemia. *J. Clin. Invest.* 54:1107–1124, 1974.

23. Krauss, R.M., P.D. Wood, C. Giotas, D. Waterman, and F.T. Lindgren. Heparin-released plasma lipase activities and lipoprotein levels in distance runners. (Abstract) *Circulation* 60; No. 4, Part II: 73, 1979.

24. Krotkiewski, M., P. Bjorntorp, L. Sjostrom, and U. Smith. Impact of obesity on metabolism in men and women: Importance of regional adipose tissue distribution. *J. Clin. Invest.* 72:1150–1162, 1983.

25. Kuusi, T., E.A. Nikkila, P. Saarinen, P. Varjo, and L.A. Laitinen. Plasma high density lipoprotein HDL$_2$, HDL$_3$ and postheparin plasma lipase in relation to parameters of physical fitness. *Atherosclerosis* 41:209–219, 1982.

26. Kuusi, T., P. Saarinen, and E.A. Nikkila. Evidence for the role of hepatic endothelial lipase in the metabolism of plasma high density lipoprotein in man. *Atherosclerosis* 36:589–593, 1980.

27. Lampman, R.M., J.T. Santinga, P.J. Savage, et al. Effect of exercise training on glucose tolerance, in vivo insulin sensitivity, lipid and lipoprotein concentrations in middle-aged men with mild hypertriglyceridemia. *Metabolism* 34:205–211, 1985.

28. LaPorte, R.E., G. Brenes, S. Dearwater, et al. HDL-cholesterol across a spectrum of physical activity from quadriplegia to marathon running. *Lancet* 1:1212–1213, 1983.

29. Lehtonen, A., and J. Viikari. Serum triglycerides and cholesterol and serum high density lipoprotein cholesterol in highly physical active men. *Acta Med. Scand.* 204:111–114, 1978.

30. Linder, C.W., R. DuRant, and O.M. Mahoney. The effect of physical conditioning on serum lipids and lipoproteins in white male adolescents. *Med. Sci. Sports Exerc.* 15:232–236, 1983.

31. Marniemi, J., S. Dahlstrom, M. Kuist, A. Seppanen, and E. Hiefanen. Dependence of serum lipid and lecithin: Cholesterol acyltransferase levels on physical training of young men. *Eur. J. Appl. Physiol.* 49:25–35, 1982.

32. Martin, R.P., W.L. Haskell, and P.D. Wood. Blood chemistry and lipid profiles of elite distance runners. *Ann. NY Acad. Sci.* 301:346–360, 1977.

33. Masarei, J.R.L., J.E. Pyke, and F.S. Pyke. Physical fitness and plasma HDL cholesterol concentrations in male business executives. *Atherosclerosis* 42:77–83, 1982.

34. Merians D.R., W.L. Haskell, K.M. Vranizan, et al. Relationship of exercise, oral contraceptive use and body fat to concentrations of plasma lipids and lipoprotein cholesterol in young women. *Am. J. Med.* 78:913–919, 1985.

35. Miller, G., and N. Miller. Plasma high density lipoprotein concentration and development of ischemic heart disease. *Lancet* 1:16–19, 1975.

36. Nikkila, E.A., T. Kuusi, and P. Myllynen. High-density lipoprotein and apolipoprotein A-I during physical inactivity. *Atherosclerosis* 37:457–462, 1980.

37. Nikkila, E.A., T. Kuusi, and M.R. Taskinen. Role of LPL and hepatic endothelial lipase in the metabolism of HDLs: A novel concept on cholesterol transport in HDL cycle. In Carlson, L.A., and B. Pernow (eds.). *Metabolic Risk Factors in Ischemic CV Disease*. New York: Raven Press, 1982, pp. 205–215.

38. Nikkila, E.A., M.R. Taskinen, S. Rehunen, and M. Harkonen. Lipoprotein lipase activity in adipose tissue and skeletal muscle of runners: Relation to serum lipoproteins. *Metabolism* 27:1661–1671, 1978.

39. Nye, E., K. Carlson, P. Kirstein, and S. Rossner. Changes in high-density lipoprotein subfractions and other lipoproteins induced by exercise. *Clin. Chim. Acta* 113:51–57, 1981.

40. Oscai, L.B., J.A. Patterson, D.L. Bogard, R.J. Beck, and B.L. Rothermel. Normalization of serum triglycerides and lipoprotein electrophoretic patterns by exercise. *Am. J. Cardiol.* 30:775–780, 1972.

41. Paffenbarger, R.S., R.T. Hydes, A.L. Wing, and C. Hsieh. Physical activity, all cause mortality and lon-

gevity of college alumni. *N. Engl. J. Med.* 314:605–613, 1986.

42. Peltonen, P., J. Marniemi, E. Hiefman, I. Vuori, and C. Ehnholm. Changes in serum lipids, lipoproteins and heparin releasable lipolytic enzymes during moderate physical training in man: A longitudinal study. *Metabolism* 30:518–526, 1981.

43. Rauramaa, R., J. Salonen, K. Kukkonen-Harjula, et al. Effects of mild physical exercise on serum lipoproteins and metabolites of arachidonic acid: A controlled randomized trial in middle aged men. *Br. Med. J.* 288:603–606, 1984.

44. Sady, S.P., E.M. Cullinane, P.N. Herbert, M.A. Kantor, and P.D. Thompson. Training, diet and physical characteristics of distance runners with low or high concentrations of high density lipoprotein cholesterol. *Atherosclerosis* 53:273–281, 1984.

45. Schaefer, E.J., D.M. Foster, L.A. Zech, F.T. Lindgren, H.B. Brewer, and R.I. Levy. The effects of estrogen administration on plasma lipoprotein metabolism in premenopausal females. *J. Clin. Endocrinol. Metab.* 57:262–267, 1983.

46. Schaefer, D.J., and R.I. Levy. Pathogenesis and management of lipoprotein disorders. *N. Engl. J. Med.* 312:1300–1310, 1985.

47. Schnabel, A., and W. Kindermann. Effects of maximal oxygen uptake and different forms of physical training on serum lipoproteins. *Eur. J. Appl. Physiol.* 48:263–277, 1982.

48. Smith, U. Regional differences and effect of cell size on lipolysis in human adipocytes. In Angel, A., C.H. Hollenberg, and D.A.K. Roncari (eds.). *The Adipocyte and Obesity: Cellular and Molecular Mechanisms.* New York: Raven Press, 1983, pp. 245–250.

49. Sopko, G., A.S. Leon, D.R. Jacobs, et al. The effects of exercise and weight loss on plasma lipids in young obese men. *Metabolism* 34:227–236, 1985.

50. Stamford, B.A., S. Matter, R.D. Fell, et al. Cigarette smoking, physical activity and alcohol consumption: Relationship to blood lipids and lipoproteins in premenopausal females. *Metabolism* 33:585–590, 1984.

51. Stamford, B.A., S. Matter, R.D. Fell, et al. Cigarette smoking, exercise and high density lipoprotein cholesterol. *Atherosclerosis* 52:73, 1984.

52. Stefanick, M.L., R.B. Terry, W.L. Haskell, and P.D. Wood. Relationships of changes in postheparin hepatic and lipoprotein lipase activity to HDL-cholesterol changes following weight loss achieved by dieting versus exercise. Paper presented at 6th Washington Spring Symposium, *Cardiovascular Disease '86*, May, 1986.

53. Stubbe, I., P. Hanson, A. Gustafson, and P. Nilsson-Ehle. Plasma lipoproteins and lipolytic enzyme activities during endurance training in sedentary men: Changes in high density lipoprotein subfractions and composition. *Metabolism* 32:1120–1127, 1983.

54. Sutherland, W.H.F., S.P. Woodhouse, S. Williamson, and B. Smith. Decreased and continued physical activity and plasma lipoprotein lipids in previously trained men. *Atherosclerosis* 39:307–311, 1981.

55. Taskinen, M.R., and E.A. Nikkila. High density lipoprotein subfractions in relation to lipoprotein lipase activity of tissues in man: Evidence for reciprocal regulation of HDL_2 and HDL_3 levels by lipoprotein lipase. *Clin. Chim. Acta* 112:325–332, 1981.

56. Terry, R.B., M.L. Stefanick, R. M. Krauss, W.L. Haskell, and P.D. Wood. Relationships between abdomen to hip ratio, plasma lipoproteins and sex hormones. (Abstract) *Circulation* 72; No. 4, Part II:452, 1985.

57. Thompson, P.D., E.M. Cullinane, R. Eshleman, S. Sady, and P.N. Herbert. The effects of caloric restriction and exercise cessation on the serum lipid and lipoprotein concentrations of endurance athletes. *Metabolism* 33:943–950, 1984.

58. Thompson, P.D., E. Cullinane, L.O. Henderson, and P.N. Herbert. Acute effects of prolonged exercise on serum lipids. *Metabolism* 29:662–665, 1980.

59. Tran, Z.V., and A. Weltman. Differential effects on exercise on serum lipid and lipoprotein levels seen with changes in body weight: A meta analysis. *JAMA* 254:919–924, 1985.

60. Williams, P.T., R.M. Krauss, P.D. Wood, F.T. Lindgren, C. Giotas, and K.M. Vranizan. Lipoprotein subfractions of runners and sedentary men. *Metabolism* 35:45–52, 1986.

61. Williams, P.T., P.D. Wood, W.L. Haskell, and K. Vranizan. The effects of running mileage and duration on plasma lipoprotein levels. *JAMA* 247:2674–2679, 1982.

62. Wood, P., and W. Haskell. The effect of exercise on plasma high-density lipoproteins. *Lipids* 14:417–427, 1979.

63. Wood, P.D., W.L. Haskell, S.N. Blair, et al. Increased exercise level and plasma lipoprotein concentrations: A one-year randomized controlled study in sedentary middle-aged men. *Metabolism* 32:31–39, 1983.

64. Wood, P.D., R.B. Terry, and W.L. Haskell. Metabolism of substrates: Diet, lipoprotein metabolism, and exercise. *Fed. Proc.* 44:358–363, 1985.

65. Wood, P.D., P.T. Williams, and W.L. Haskell. Physical activity and high density lipoproteins. In Miller, N.E., and G.J. Miller (eds.). *Clinical and Metabolic Aspects of High Density Lipoproteins.* Amsterdam: Elsevier, 1984, pp. 133–165.

66. Zavaroni, I., Y.-D.I. Chen, C.E. Mondon, and G.M. Reaven. Ability of exercise to inhibit carbohydrate-induced hypertriglyceridemia in rats. *Metabolism* 30:476–480, 1981.

Chapter 16

EXERCISE AND DIABETES MELLITUS

Hassan Kanj, M.D., Steven H. Schneider, M.D., and Neil B. Ruderman, M.D.

The impression that physical activity is beneficial for patients with diabetes is centuries old [56]. However, in the early 1900s many physicians felt that exercise was contraindicated in their generally poorly controlled diabetic populations [44]. Following the discovery of insulin, exercise was repopularized for the treatment of diabetes by Joslin [17] and Katsh [20], who portrayed exercise as one of the three basic modalities of therapy along with diet and insulin. Despite these recommendations, the use of exercise in an attempt to improve glycemic control has been limited. In recent years there has been a resurgence of interest in the potential role of exercise in the treatment of diabetes. It has become increasingly clear that the response to exercise, as well as the risk of serious complications, varies among subgroups of patients. A better understanding of the risks of exercise and a more sober assessment of its benefits now make possible recommendations of specific exercise prescriptions tailored to individual patients.

EFFECTS OF EXERCISE ON CARBOHYDRATE METABOLISM

The physiology and biochemistry of exercise have been reviewed in detail elsewhere in this book. Exercise places a major stress on glucose homeostasis. Peripheral uptake and utilization of glucose may increase more than 10-fold, yet the body is able to regulate plasma glucose levels so efficiently that, following 2 to 3 hours of intense exercise, plasma glucose remains at near basal levels.

In the postabsorptive state, the increased glucose utilization associated with exercise must be matched by an increase in hepatic glucose production, to prevent the development of hypoglycemia. The autonomic nervous system plays a major role in this tightly regulated process. As exercise begins, alpha-adrenergic imput into the pancreas results in an inhibition of insulin release [11]. This, in turn, stimulates hepatic glucose production both directly and by sensitizing the liver to basal levels of epinephrine and glucagon. As moderately intense exercise becomes more prolonged, increased plasma levels of glucagon and epinephrine further stimulate hepatic glucose production, and epinephrine has a restraining effect on peripheral glucose utilization (see Chapter 7).

In addition to stimulating glucose uptake acutely, the effects of exercise on glucose can persist for many hours after activity has ceased. While the sensitivity of muscle to the effects of insulin is enhanced following exercise, increased glucose uptake is partially independent of insulin-mediated glucose transport.

Physical training and high levels of aerobic exercise capacity are strongly associated with increased sensitivity to insulin, and there is a linear relationship between insulin sensitivity, measured by glucose clamp techniques, and indices of aerobic fitness. Increased insulin sensitivity during physical training is demonstrable in all age groups and can occur independently of measurable changes in body weight or composition [2, 57]. Changes in insulin receptor concentration during physical training do not account for the increased insulin sensitivity, and the physiology of these changes remains unclear. It is also unclear what the relationship is between the persistent effects of an individual exercise bout and changes related to the trained state per se.

RELATION OF PHYSICAL ACTIVITY TO GLUCOSE INTOLERANCE

Extremes of inactivity result in impaired glucose disposal; as few as 3 days of bed rest result in glucose intolerance and hyperinsulinemia in normal young men [30]. At the other extreme, cross-sectional studies have determined that endurance athletes consistently have enhanced glucose disposal and insulin sensitivity compared with normal controls [24], and there is some evidence that lifelong vigorous physical activity can partially prevent the deterioration of glucose tolerance that is normally seen with aging [47, 53]. Nevertheless, epidemiologic studies in normal populations have not consistently documented a relationship between habitual physical activity and glucose tolerance [37, 47].

EXERCISE AND PHYSICAL TRAINING IN THE TREATMENT OF DIABETES MELLITUS

The rationale for using exercise in the treatment of diabetes mellitus is based on two major considerations. The first is that the enhanced glucose disposal and insulin

sensitivity associated with regular exercise can be used to improve glycemic control. Equally important is the potential for regular exercise to diminish the propensity of the diabetic patient for accelerated artherosclerosis.

Effects of Regular Exercise in Type I Diabetes

Studies on the effects of exercise on glycemic control in patients with type I diabetes have been generally disappointing. Improved control in children during periods of increased activity such as summer camp are difficult to interpret due to the large number of confounding variables [58]. Controlled studies confirm an enhanced insulin sensitivity in patients with type I diabetes during periods of physical training [60]. Nevertheless, in most studies this has not been associated with improved glycemic control. In such patients, in whom absolute insulin deficiency is the rule, the major clinical consideration is the timing and distribution of insulin administration and the intake of food. Avoiding hypoglycemia during and following exercise is an almost universal problem in such patients. Common strategies include a decrease in insulin dosage and increased carbohydrate intake. This may partially negate the improved glycemic control that might be expected to result from the exercise-induced enhancement of insulin sensitivity.

Although most patients with type I diabetes fail to demonstrate improved glycemic control with regular exercise, some are likely to benefit more than others. These include patients less prone to hypoglycemia and those willing and able to regulate carefully the timing and amount of their exercise and to frequently self-monitor blood glucose levels to adjust their insulin dosages and feeding. Even when regular exercise fails to achieve better glycemic control, it often results in decreased insulin requirements and may still be appropriate for its psychological benefits and its potential protective effects on atherosclerosis.

Effects of Regular Exercise in Type II Diabetes

The pathophysiology of type II diabetes is heterogeneous but is often associated with peripheral insulin resistance. This resistance could be at the receptor level, which is the case in persons with mild hyperglycemia, or at the post receptor level, which occurs in those with severe hyperglycemia [39]. Thus, it is not surprising that metabolic response to regular exercise varies considerably among patients. In general, studies in patients with type II diabetes have demonstrated a modest but significant beneficial effect of regular exercise on glycemic control [46, 48, 50]. Identification of subgroups of type II patients who are particularly likely to respond to exercise is under current investigation (see section on exercise prescription).

It remains unclear to what extent the metabolic changes noted during programs of physical training are due to residual effects of individual exercise bouts or to improved aerobic "fitness" per se. We have assessed the effects of 6 weeks of physical training on a group fo 20 sedentary men with type II diabetes on a weight-maintenance diet [50]. Oral glucose tolerance was improved 12 hours, but not 72 hours, after the last exercise bout. Improved glucose tolerance correlates poorly with indices of fitness such as maximal oxygen uptake ($\dot{V}O_2$max) and muscle oxidative enzyme concentrations, and the improved insulin sensitivity associated with training as demonstrated by the glucose clamp technique often fails to correlate with measures of improved glycemic control. These findings and the tendency for glucose tolerance to deteriorate rapidly following discontinuation of an exercise program before indices of aerobic fitness decrease are most consistent with benefits being related to the summed residual effects of the individual exercise bouts (Figure 1). The trained state

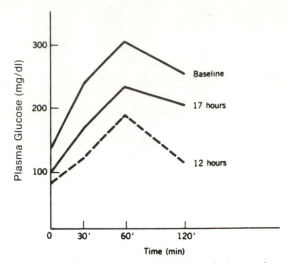

Figure 1. Glucose tolerance following a single exercise bout in a diabetic patient.

may contribute to improved metabolic control by causing an exaggerated and prolonged acute exercise response [54].

Atherosclerosis in Diabetes and the Effects of Exercise

Epidemiological studies have established that cerebrovascular, coronary, and peripheral arterial diseases are more common in diabetics than in normal persons and occur at an earlier age. The international atherosclerosis project established that the atherosclerotic process appears to be accelerated in the coronary arteries and abdominal aortas in patients with diabetes independent of sex, age, race, or the presence of hypertension [43]. A 16-year follow-up study of the prevalence of coronary heart disease among the Framingham population revealed an increased morbidity and mortality from all cardiovascular causes among the diabetic group, independent of the absolute level of glycemic control or the treatment modality [13]. In addition, diabetes eliminates the relative protection from atherosclerosis possessed by premenopausal women.

Animal studies suggest a protective effect of exercise training on the progression of atherosclerotic macrovascular disease. Kramsch and colleagues [26] have shown that exercise markedly retards the development of atherosclerosis in monkeys maintained on a high-cholesterol diet.

In humans, epidemiologic data suggest that endurance-type exercise diminishes both the mortality and morbidity from atherosclerotic vascular disease in normal subjects. Paffenberger et al.[40], in a study of Harvard graduates, noted that the incidence of first heart attacks was significantly lower in individuals with the greatest degree of physical activity. The protective effect of physical exercise was also seen among cigarette smokers, hypertensives, and a small number of patients with diabetes. Athletes were at low risk for coronary heart disease only if they had continued vigorous activity into adulthood. In the Framingham study [19], coronary heart disease incidence and mortality after 14 years were inversely related to a physical activity index in men independent of age, blood pressure, smoking, and plasma cholesterol level. While the reasons for the increased incidence of atherosclerosis in diabetics are not fully understood, a number of risk factors known to be associated with cardiovascular disease are often found in patients with diabetes mellitus and may be favorably influenced by regular exercise. These include hyperglycemia, insulin resistance, hyperlipidemia, obesity, hypercoagulable state, hypertension, and psychological stress, all of which may be potentially improved by physical training (Table 1).

Hyperglycemia and Insulin Resistance. It is not clear to what degree hyperglycemia per se contributes to macrovascular disease. The risk of coronary artery disease is increased in individuals whose fasting plasma glucose level is in the upper 2% of the normal range, but there is little further increase in relative risk with more severe degrees of hyperglycemia. A number of large epidemiologic studies, including the Framingham study, have

Table 1. ATHEROSCLEROTIC RISK FACTORS POTENTIALLY IMPROVED BY REGULAR EXERCISE IN DIABETES

Glucose intolerance
Hyperinsulinemia
Hyperlipidemia
Obesity
Coagulation abnormalities
Hypertension
Psychological stress

failed to find a relationship between atherosclerotic risk and indices of hyperglycemia. Hyperglycemia could contribute directly to atherosclerosis by altering the connective tissue and cellular components in the vessel wall and by glycosylation of proteins, and indirectly by exacerbating a number of other risk factors such as hyperlipidemia and the hypercoagulable state.

Epidemiologic studies have established that subjects with diseases of cerebral, coronary, and peripheral arteries have elevated insulin responses to an oral glucose load compared with subjects without evidence of vascular disease. In addition, three prospective studies, the Helsinki policemen study [42], the Paris study [9], and the Busselton, Australia study [61], have shown a strong correlation between insulin levels and ischemic heart disease. The relationship of insulin to atherosclerosis has been reviewed recently by Stout [55].

Regular exercise has been shown to result in decreased insulin levels in normal and obese subjects and in patients with impaired glucose tolerance [28, 31]. Many patients with type II diabetes and insulin resistance have endogenous hyperinsulinemia. Attempts at glucose control with exogenous insulin administration may result in extremely high plasma insulin levels in many such patients. In addition, many patients with type I diabetes treated with intensive insulin therapy have elevated plasma insulin levels at various times during the day. The increased insulin sensitivity that occurs during physical training in diabetes often results in a decrease in need for exogenous insulin. In patients with type II diabetes, improvements in glycemic control and glucose tolerance associated with exercise occur in the face of unchanged insulin levels, consistent with improved insulin sensitivity. Substantial reduction of endogenous plasma insulin levels in type II patients in association with exercise training may not occur in the absence of significant weight reduction, although in a small group of hyperinsulinemic patients regular exercise training may result in a significant reduction in plasma insulin levels, especially after a meal.

Hyperlipidemia. Hyperlipidemia is a common finding in patients with diabetes mellitus. The pattern depends on the severity of the metabolic derangement, the type of diabetes, and the treatment modality. Studies of patients with type II diabetes mellitus most commonly demonstrate elevations in plasma triglyceride and cholesterol levels and lower than normal levels of high-density lipoprotein (HDL)-cholesterol [23].

Cross-sectional and longitudinal studies in normal subjects have demonstrated that regular exercise can favorably alter plasma lipid levels, presumably decreasing cardiovascular risk (see Chapter 15).

Most studies of regular exercise in patients with type II diabetes have revealed a significant decrease in plasma triglyceride levels and very-low-density lipoproteins (VLDL) but much smaller and often nonsignificant changes in plasma low-density lipoproteins (LDL) and HDL-cholesterol. A major confounding factor in many studies is the role of concomitant weight reduction. While the atherogenic potential of VLDL particles is unclear, VLDL particles in patients with diabetes mellitus may be altered to become more atherogenic. Thus, lowering of VLDL levels by regular exercise may exert a beneficial effect.

In our recent clinical experience of 108 patients with type II diabetes, an average fall in plasma triglyceride level of 15% from the basal level was found over 3 months with no change in cholesterol and HDL-cholesterol

levels (unpublished data). The time course of changes in plasma triglyceride levels suggests that, as with glucose, many of the benefits of exercise training are due to the summed effects of the individual exercise bouts. Holloszy et al. [16] and Cullinane et al [7] demonstrated a decrease in plasma triglyceride levels after a bout of intensive exercise. The levels returned to basal levels after 48 to 72 hours. In the study by Schneider et al. [50], a signigicant decrease in plasma triglyceride levels was consistently noted 12 hours following a typical exercise training bout, but 72 hours later the improvement was no longer measureable (Figure 2).

In conclusion, there is little doubt that regular exercise can result in lower levels of VLDL. Attempts to elevate plasma HDL-cholesterol levels with exercise alone may require exercise of longer duration and greater intensity than is usually recommended.

Obesity. Obesity is associated with an increased frequency of atherogenic risk factors, for example, hypertension, hyperinsulinemia, and decreased HDL-cholesterol levels.

Exercise has been recommended by many investigators as an adjunct to caloric restric-

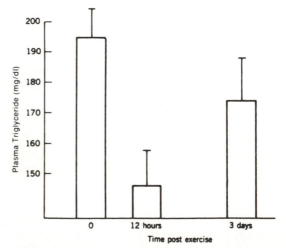

Figure 2. Effect of a single exercise bout on plasma triglyceride level.

tion in the treatment of obesity. Not only are extra calories consumed during exercise, but under certain circumstances metabolic rates may remain increased for several hours after cessation of physical activity. Neverthess, the caloric deficit induced by moderate exercise is not great and is often matched by an increase in caloric consumption. As a result, minimal if any weight reduction is achieved by exercise programs of modest intensity unless caloric intake is simultaneously controlled.

Exercise and weight reduction result in improved glucose disposal through different mechanisms [3]. With calorie restriction, enhanced glucose disposal occurs mainly via increased oxidative metabolism, whereas following exercise, glucose disposal is directed primarily at restoring depleted glycogen stores. Studies have shown that a combination of diet and physical training results in a greater increment in glucose disposal than does diet alone, although the improvement in glucose tolerance is not statistically significant [3].

Abnormalities of Coagulation and Hemostasis. Patients with diabetes mellitus suffer from a hypercoagulable state. This is associated with elevated levels of fibrinogen and factor VIII complex activity, platelet hyperaggregability, increased thromboxane and decreased prostacycline synthesis, and a depressed fibrinolytic response to a variety of stimuli [6]. It is not yet clear to what degree these changes are related to metabolic control and to what extent they are the result of vascular injury.

The potential role of the coagulation system in atherogenesis has been the focus of a number of recent studies. Studies by Wilhelmsen et al. [63] and by Kostis et al.[25] have confirmed the association between abnormalities in the coagulation system similar to those noted in diabetes and the risk of myocardial infarction. In the diabetic, however, it is unclear whether such abnormalities predate the atherogenic process or are the result of it, or both.

Whether exercise results in a coagulation profile that reduces the risk for atherosclerosis in diabetes is not known. Decreased increments in platelet aggregability, factor VIII complex activity, and other indices of activation of the coagulation cascade have been found following exercise in trained normal subjects. In our studies of type II diabetes, 6 weeks of training resulted in increased resting fibrinolytic activity [52].

Hypertension. Hypertension markedly increases the prevalence and severity of atherosclerotic vascular disease, especially in patients with diabetes. The Framingham study showed that mortality from coronary heart disease and stroke in diabetic subjects is fourfold higher if they are hypertensive [18].

There is at least circumstantial evidence that exercise training may have a beneficial effect in the treatment of hypertension. Epidemiologic studies indicate that active individuals have significantly lower systolic and diastolic blood pressure at rest than do their less active age-matched controls [38], and exercise training has been shown by some but not all investigators to result in significant lowering of blood pressure in normotensive and hypertensive subjects [15, 33]. In patients with type II diabetes mellitus, we have noted that exercise and diet treatment have been effective in reducing the blood pressure of hypertensive patients with a mean reduction of 10 to 15 mmHg in diastolic blood pressure following 4 months of training. It is interesting to note that hypertensive patients may have an increased incidence of hyperinsulinemia, and the decrease in blood pressure following exercise training correlates with a decrease in plasma insulin concentration [27].

Psychological Stress. Chronic illnesses such as diabetes mellitus may be associated with significant psychological stress, which in turn may exacerbate hyperglycemia and result in increased insulin requirements. Stress is known to increase the activity of the sympathoadrenomedullary system, elevate plasma cortisol levels, and possibly enhance secretion of glucagon and growth hormone, and may be an additional risk factor for accelerated atherosclerosis. The type and severity of stress necessary to disturb glucose metabolism are not known. Recently it was shown that sudden and short-lived psychological stimuli are unlikely to disturb metabolic control in patients with type I diabetes [22]. The impact of such events on patients with type II diabetes is still unknown.

Repeated studies have revealed improvements in some psychological parameters with regular exercise, especially reduction in perception and response to psychological stress. Measures of depression and anxiety are most likely to improve. Unfortunately, there is no evidence that potentially detrimental type A personality traits are altered by exercise training.

Aerobic Exercise Performance

In the absence of autonomic neuropathy, patients with type I diabetes generally have normal aerobic exercise capacity [14]. On the other hand, most studies of type II diabetes have demonstrated low levels of aerobic fitness as measured by Vo_2max [3, 45, 46, 50].

Whether the decreased Vo_2max in patients with type II diabetes is secondary to the metabolic abnormalities or is independent of and precedes them remains to be established. Saltin et al. [47] demonstrated a similar decrease in Vo_2max in subjects with impaired glucose tolerance without overt diabetes mellitus compared with appropriate controls with normal glucose tolerance. This suggests that the abnormality in aerobic exercise performance could precede the major metabolic disturbance of the diabetic state. Interestingly, when these subjects were followed over a 3-year period, none of the subjects who engaged in a program of long-term aerobic training developed overt diabetes. These observations raised the possibility that programs designed to increase aerobic work capacity may protect a subgroup of the population with glucose intolerance from a progression to overt diabetes mellitus.

COMPLICATIONS OF EXERCISE IN DIABETES MELLITUS

Exercise in a person with diabetes may lead to several complications, and anyone prescribing an exercise program for these patients must be aware of these (Table 2).

Hypoglycemia

Hypoglycemia is a common problem in patients treated with insulin. It is infrequently noted in patients treated with diet or oral hypoglycemic agents. The magnitude of the hypoglycemic effect of an individual exercise bout in diabetes depends on a variety of factors. It should be emphasized that clinically important episodes of hypoglycemia often occur many hours after exercise, and these late episodes may be particularly dangerous, since patients are less likely to anticipate them.

Normal individuals can exercise for many hours with little fall in plasma glucose levels. Factors that may contribute to the hypoglycemic effect of exercise in insulin-treated patients probably include:

1. Increased sensitivity to insulin.
2. Accelerated absorption of depot insulin.
3. Inability of plasma insulin concentrations to decrease during exercise.
4. Impaired counterregulatory hormone response.

An acute increase in sensitivity to insulin during exercise has been consistently reported. This phenomenon persists for many hours and may also be responsible, in part, for the late hypoglycemic episodes.

There is evidence that brisk exercise of muscles underlying depot insulin injections may accelerate the absorption of the insulin from the depot site. This is of particular importance when exercise is performed shortly

**Table 2.   COMPLICATIONS OF EXERCISE TRAIN-
ING IN DIABETIC PATIENTS**

Metabolic
  Hypoglycemia
  Hyperglycemia and ketosis
Vascular and renal
  Sequelae of occult coronary artery disease
  Worsening of retinopathy and retinal hemorrhage
  Worsening of proteinuria
Miscellaneous
  Heat and cold intolerance
  Postural hypotension
  Tendency to ignore diet
Rheumatologic and orthopedic
  Foot ulcerations, blisters, and infections
  Degenerative arthritis
  Orthopedic injury

after an injection of a short-acting insulin. In practice, this is only occasionally a clinically significant factor, and studies suggest that changing the injection site rarely results in a decreased tendency for development of hypoglycemia [21].

The presence of depot insulin prevents the decrease in plasma insulin levels that normally occurs during exercise. This might be expected to predispose patients to hypoglycemia by restraining hepatic glucose output. While this is an attractive explanation for exercise-induced hypoglycemia, recent studies suggest that moderate hyperinsulinemia is insufficient to restrain hepatic glucose output during exercise in normal subjects [4] and it has been repeatedly demonstrated [49] that maintaining the basal level of insulin by intravenous administration during exercise does not predictably result in hypoglycemia in type I diabetic patients.

Most patients with diabetes mellitus who have autonomic neuropathy suffer from an impaired counterregulatory hormone response. In addition, recent studies in patients with type I diabetes without clinical evidence of autonomic neuropathy who have suffered severe, recurrent hypoglycemia during intensive insulin therapy indicate that some of these individuals suffer from impaired glucagon and epinephrine responses to

insulin-induced hypoglycemia [62]. Whether such individuals are at increased risk for development of hypoglycemia during exercise is currently under investigation.

Patients with poorly controlled insulin-treated diabetes with variations in plasma glucose levels from day to day are particularly likely to develop exercise-associated hypoglycemia. Better glucose control may actually decrease the risk of hypoglycemia in this subgroup, but aggressive insulin therapy with "normalization" of plasma glucose levels may exacerbate the risk of hypoglycemia.

Various commonly prescribed medications could play a role in exercise-induced hypoglycemia in some diabetic patients. Beta-adrenergic blocking agents might aggravate exercise-induced hypoglycemia, especially in the subgroup of patients with an impaired glucagon response [8]. Ethanol can inhibit gluconeogenesis and, in the absence of adequate hepatic glycogen stores, predispose to hypoglycemia. Other drugs may also predispose to hypoglycemia—prostaglandin synthase inhibitors can decrease glycogenolysis [12] and angiotensin-converting enzyme inhibitors can increase the rate of glucose utilization [10]. Whether these effects are clinically significant remains to be determined.

The following guidelines may be useful for the well-controlled insulin-dependent diabetic who wishes to participate in strenuous exercise without the risk of hypoglycemia (see also Table 3).

1. During prolonged exercise the patient can take an additional 15 to 30 gm of readily absorbable carbohydrate every 30 minutes. At the end of a prolonged exercise session, a final snack of "lente" carbohydrate such as milk may help to prevent a late hypoglycemic episode.

2. In patients who use a single daily dose of intermediate-acting insulin, the dose may be decreased by 30 to 35% if strenuous exercise is performed. Some patients will need to shift to a schedule of two or more

Table 3. STEPS TO PREVENT EXERCISE-INDUCED HYPOGLYCEMIA IN INSULIN-TREATED PATIENTS WITH DIABETES

Increased consumption of carbohydrates during exercise (an extra 15 to 30 gm every 30 minutes).
After prolonged exercise, eat a snack containing protein and complex carbohydrates.
Decrease insulin dose.
Avoid late-evening exercise.
Avoid exercise shortly after an injection of regular insulin.
Inject insulin away from the most active muscles.
Self-monitor blood glucose level

doses a day with or without the addition of short-acting insulin.

3. If a combination of intermediate- and short-acting insulin is being used, the short-acting insulin may be omitted and the dose of the intermediate-acting insulin decreased by one-third prior to exercise. However, hyperglycemia may occur later in the day and a second injection of short-acting insulin may be required.

4. If only short-acting insulin is used, the dose prior to exercise can be reduced by 30 to 50%. Supplemental carbohydrate prior to, during, and following exercise may be necessary to prevent hypoglycemia.

5. Patients treated with continuous subcutaneous insulin infusion (CSII) may be at particularly high risk for hypoglycemia. When exercise follows a meal, maintaining the insulin infusion at the basal rate while eliminating the mealtime bolus usually prevents this hypoglycemic response [41].

Although these guidelines are helpful in patients whose diabetes is well controlled, the response of an individual diabetic to exercise may be unpredictable because of the heterogeneity of the diabetic population. Each patient should serve as his or her own control. Intensive home blood glucose monitoring is very useful for better glycemic control and avoidance of hypoglycemia. However, in patients in whom metabolic control is difficult to achieve, it may not be possible to institute a standardized exercise program without worsening of metabolic control.

Hyperglycemia and Ketosis

Exercise under conditions of poor metabolic control (fasting blood glucose values above 300 mg/dl) may actually worsen hyperglycemia and precipitate ketosis in type I patients [1]. Severe insulin deficiency and hyperglycemia with accompanying dehydration result in an exaggerated increase in counterregulatory hormones during exercise. In such patients, inadequate insulin levels together with elevated levels of glucagon and epinephrine cause excessive hepatic glucose production, glycogenolysis, and ketogenesis. In addition, the utilization of glucose and ketone bodies by exercising muscle may be diminished. A similar but usually less severe problem can occur in type II patients. Patients should be warned against exercise under conditions of poor metabolic control, and they should administer adequate amounts of insulin to restore good metabolic control before starting to exercise again.

Vascular and Renal Complications

Intensive exercise is a common cause of retinal hemorrhage in patients with proliferative retinopathy. This problem is usually encountered with exercise at high levels of intensity, isometric exercises, and exercise that requires Valsalva-type maneuvers. Exercise-induced increase in systolic blood pressure and increased levels of epinephrine and growth hormone during exercise may play a role. In the face of significant retinal disease, the advice of an ophthalmologist should be sought and laser treatment may be required before participation in physical activities is encouraged. Whether high-intensity exercise causes retinopathy or accelerates its clinical course is unclear. However, the perception that intensive exercise regimens are associated with acceleration of retinal changes, while unproven, is commonly held.

Proteinuria, usually transient, has been demonstrated in normal as well as diabetic individuals after exercise. Usually the degree of proteinuria is proportional to the intensity of exercise performed and the level of systolic blood pressure achieved. It is probably related to altered renal hemodynamics [35]. The possibility that exercise-induced renal hemodynamic changes that result in proteinuria might contribute to the progression of diabetic nephropathy has not been studied.

Patients with diabetes mellitus have a high incidence of atherosclerotic coronary disease, which is often asymptomatic. Strenuous exercise may be hazardous for these patients. Exercising at appropriate intensities, proper warm-up and warm-down periods, and avoidance of dehydration and exercise in extremes of temperature help to avoid such problems.

Miscellaneous Complications

Patients with significant peripheral neuropathy are at serious risk for traumatic injury to the feet because of loss of sensory function. Such patients should probably avoid exercises that result in repeated foot trauma, such as jogging. Patients engaging in activities that place their feet at increased risk must obtain proper footwear and inspect their feet after each exercise session.

Some studies have suggested a possible relationship between degenerative joint disease and diabetes mellitus [29, 59]. One could speculate that such a relationship could be related to the neuropathy and vasculopathy that accompany diabetes mellitus or to an accelerated age-related change in the collagen that has been noted in patients with diabetes mellitus [36].

Autonomic neuropathy is a common finding in patients with long-standing diabetes mellitus. This may interfere with the cardiovascular reflexes necessary to maintain the cardiac output and blood pressure during physical exertion. Such patients may be at risk for development of hypotensive episodes during or after exercise and may also be at a higher risk for dehydration, especially if they exercise on warm days. Finally, autonomic neuropathy may be associated with a deficient response of glucagon and epinephrine to hypoglycemia. Thus, patients with significant autonomic neuropathy should probably abstain from intensive exercise or competitive sports.

SELECTION OF PARTICIPANTS FOR AN EXERCISE PROGRAM

Formal exercise programs are expensive and labor intensive and have high drop-out rates. In some patients the risks of exercise may exceed the expected benefits. It is therefore important to define those individuals most likely to benefit from a formal exercise program.

In our experience, characteristics of this population include:

1. Type II diabetes mellitus.
2. Fasting plasma glucose level less than 220 mg/dl.
3. A well-maintained or elevated plasma insulin level following a glucose load.
4. Poor initial aerobic fitness.

Patients with type I diabetes mellitus who have difficulty controlling their blood sugar levels often do poorly in exercise programs and may demonstrate metabolic deterioration.

In our experience, psychological factors play an important role in patient compliance [5]. Self-referred patients and female patients have done particularly well in such programs. Male patients, who are usually more likely to be physician referred, do not do as well. Type A personality traits are a strong predictor of drop-out, especially if the patient is physician referred. Interestingly, despite the fact that exercise programs are expensive and labor intensive, the educational or economic level of the patient appears to have little impact on eventual success in such programs.

THE EXERCISE PRESCRIPTION

Young, active patients with diabetes of short duration and no evidence of vascular complications rarely require specific exercise recommendations. However, sedentary patients over the age of 40 or patients with diabetes mellitus of more than 10 years duration should have a thorough cardiovascular evaluation including resting and stress electrocardiograms before participating in an exercise program. About 10% of asymptomatic patients have significant coronary artery disease detected with a stress electrocardiogram. Following this evaluation, a prescription can be given indicating type, duration, frequency, and intensity of exercise.

Type of Exercise

Aerobic-type activities, for example, swimming, cycling, and brisk walking, are usually recommended to patients with diabetes mellitus. These exercises result in improved insulin sensitivity and enhanced glucose disposal per unit of muscle mass. Recent studies suggest that anaerobic power-type exercise, such as weight lifting, may also be associated with improved glucose disposal [34]. Here, benefits seem to be related to the increased muscle mass with little or no change in the efficiency of muscle glucose utilization. Since comparable improvements in glucose disposal have been demonstrated for anaerobic and aerobic exercise programs, at the present time it seems unnecessary to discourage the former, especially in the young patient with no evidence of vascular complications. Nevertheless, complications of exercise training occur more frequently during high-intensity an-

aerobic training, and improvements of cardiovascular risk factors other than hyperglycemia may not occur.

For older patients and for those with proliferative retinopathy, very-high-intensity exercise, strenuous calisthenics, and excessive isometric, stretching, and squatting maneuvers should be discouraged.

Intensity and Duration of Exercise

There have been few studies regarding the optimal duration of exercise necessary to maximize beneficial metabolic effects. Exercise of less than 15 to 20 minutes duration generally results in a poor training effect, whereas sessions of greater than 45 minutes are associated with an increased incidence of musculoskeletal injuries. Interestingly, rest periods of up to 90 seconds every five minutes have little effect on improved fitness for a given total amount of exercise, and frequent brief rest periods are probably a good strategy for older and more sedentary patients who cannot tolerate sustained exercise of even low intensity.

Optimization of a specific physiological or metabolic effect may require different levels of exercise intensity. In terms of glucose disposal, exercise of 30% of $\dot{V}O_2max$ or less has been associated with little benefit. At exercise intensities of greater than 50% of $\dot{V}O_2max$, improvements in glucose disposal are related to the total work performed [32]. Thus, a decrease in intensity can be compensated for to some degree by an increase in duration of exercise. Other metabolic parameters, e.g., lipid metabolism and coagulation parameters, may require work loads of different intensity and frequency. Increases in HDL-cholesterol level have generally been noted with high-intensity workloads for prolonged periods. For example, Wood and Haskell concluded that exercise equivalent to at least 8 miles per week of brisk running was required for significant elevation of HDL-cholesterol [64]. Changes in fibrinolysis appear to require work of sufficient in-

Table 4. THE EXERCISE PRESCRIPTION *

Type of exercise
  Aerobic (better cardiovascular fitness, improved lipid
    profile, lower injury and complication rate)
  Anaerobic (high complication rate)
Intensity of exercise
  50–70% $\dot{V}o_2$max (may differ in patients with vascular
    complications and in presence of exercise-induced
    systolic hypertension)
Duration of exercise
  10-minute stretching period
  5–10-minute warm-up period
  20–60-minute exercise at 50–70% $\dot{V}o_2$max period
  5–10-minute warm-down period (i.e., exercise ap-
    proximately 20–30% $\dot{V}o_2$max)
Frequency of exercise
  3–7 times/week minimum for glycemic control
  5–7 times/week minimum for weight reduction

*Increased intensity cannot compensate for decreased
frequency.

tensity to generate metabolic acidosis [51]. More information is required to clarify these issues. At any rate, it appears reasonable to recommend an exercise intensity of 50 to 70% of $\dot{V}o_2$max for most individuals. This can be prescribed in terms of heart rate, which can easily be monitored by patients. An estimate of the target pulse can be obtained using the following formula:

$$\text{Target pulse} = 0.5 \text{ to } 0.7 \text{ (maximal heart rate}$$
$$- \text{ resting heart rate)}$$
$$+ \text{resting heart rate}$$

Resting heart rate should be measured by the patient before getting out of bed in the morning. It should be kept in mind that estimates of maximal heart rate derived from standard tables based on normal populations correlate poorly with maximal heart rates of patients with diabetes mellitus. Estimates of the maximal heart rate are determined from submaximal exercise testing, but this rate is probably decreased in patients with type II diabetes even in the absence of neuropathy or coronary heart disease. Autonomic neuropathy or sympatholytic agents may further impair the maximal heart rate and aerobic exercise performance in such patients.

The exercise program can be initiated at a target pulse corresponding to about 50% of $\dot{V}o_2$max and gradually increased to the desired range over a 3- to 4-week period. Thereafter, the intensity of exercise is slowly increased to maintain the same submaximal target pulse, resulting in a smooth progression of exercise intensity. In addition to heart rate, the blood pressure response to exercise is of importance, especially in patients with evidence of vascular disease. In some normotensive patients, severe systolic hypertension develops during exercise, even at low work intensities. The mechanisms responsible for this phenomenon are poorly understood. It is prudent to limit exercise intensities in most patients to avoid sustained levels of systolic blood pressure of 180 mmHg or more, especially in those with established vascular disease. This should be determined during the initial exercise testing and should be confirmed during a standard exercise session.

Frequency of Exercise

The optimal frequency of exercise regimens in unknown. If transient effects of individual exercise bouts are of paramount importance, it is likely that exercise of greater frequency will result in maximal metabolic benefit. One cannot fully compensate for a decreased frequency of exercise by increasing the intensity of individual exercise sessions and, in general, exercise frequencies of less than three to four times a week do not result in substantial benefits. For many brittle type I patients, a daily exercise regimen will allow for more stable metabolic control.

Time of Day

In general, patient convenience is the major determinant of time of exercise. However, because of the relatively transient effects of exercise on glucose disposal, it is likely that exercise done in the early morning prior to breakfast will have the greatest impact on glycemic excursions throughout the day. In addition, exercise late in the evening carries a higher risk of hypoglycemia at night and the next morning because of the delayed hypoglycemic effect. Patients with type I diabetes mellitus, especially those who have brittle diabetes, require special attention. In these patients, consistency of exercise timing and intensity from day to day may be the most important consideration.

REFERENCES

1. Berger, M., P. Berchtold, H.J. Cupper, et al. Metabolic and hormonal effects of muscular exercise in juvenile type diabetics. *Diabetologia* 13:355–S65, 1977.
2. Bjorntorp, P. Effect of exercise and physical training on carbohydrate and lipid metabolism in man. *Adv. Cardiol.* 18:158–166, 1976.
3. Bogardus, C., E. Ravussin, D.C. Robbins, et al. Effects of physical training and diet therapy on carbohydrate metabolism in patients with glucose intolerance and non-insulin dependent diabetes mellitus. *Diabetes* 33(4):311–318, 1984.
4. Chisholm, D.J., A.B. Jenkins, D.E. James, and E.W. Kraegen. Effect of hyperinsulinemia on glucose homeostasis during moderate exercise in man. *Diabetes* 31:603–608, 1982.
5. Clemow, L.P., S.H. Schneider, D.P. Greenfield, et al. Psychological factors affecting outcomes in diabetes education programs. *Diabetes* 33 (Suppl. 1):27, 7a, 1984.
6. Colwell, J.A., and P.J. Halushka. Platelet function in diabetes mellitus. *Br. J. Haematol.* 44:521–526, 1980.
7. Cullinane, E., S. Siconolfi, A. Saritelli, and P.D. Thompson. Acute decrease in serum triglyceride with exercise: Is there a threshold for the exercise effect? *Metabolism* 31:844–847, 1982.
8. De Feo, P., G. Bolli, G. Perriello, et al. The adrenergic contribution to glucose counterregulation in type I diabetes mellitus: Dependency on A-cell function and mediation through beta-adrenergic receptors. *Diabetes* 32:887–893, 1983.
9. Ducimetiere, P., L. Eschwege, J.L. Papoz, et al. Relationship of plasma insulin levels to the incidence of myocardial infarction and coronary heart disease mortality in a middle-aged population. *Diabetologia* 19:205–210, 1980.
10. Ferriere, M., H. Lachkar, J.L. Richard, et al. Captopril and insulin sensitivity. *Ann. Intern. Med.* 102:134–135, 1985.
11. Galbo, H., N.J. Christensen, and J.J. Host. Catecholamines and pancreatic hormones during autonomic blackade in exercising man. *Acta Physiol. Scand.* 101:428, 1977.
12. Ganguli, S., B. Sterman, P.S. Harris, et al. Modulation of hepatic protein kinase activity by indomethacin. *Metabolism* 33:845–852, 1984.
13. Garcia, M.J., P.M. McNamara, T. Gordon, and W.B. Kannel. Morbidity and mortality in diabetics in the Framingham population. *Diabetes* 23:105–111, 1974.
14. Hagan, R.D., J.F., Marks, and P.A. Warren. Physiologic responses of juvenile-onset diabetic boys to muscular work. *Diabetes* 28:1114–1119, 1979.
15. Hanson, J., B. Tabakin, A. Levy, and W. Nedde. Long-term physical training and cardiovascular dynamics in middle-aged men. *Circulation* 38:783–799, 1968.
16. Holloszy, J.O., J.S. Skinner, G. Toro, and T.K. Cureton. Effects of a six-month program of endurance exercise on the serum lipids of middle-aged men. *Am. J. Cardiol.* 14:753–760, 1964.
17. Joslin, E.P.The treatment of diabetes mellitus. In Joslin, E.P., H.F. Root, P. Shite, and A. Marble (eds.) *Treatment of Diabetes Melliltus.* Philadelphia: Lea and Febiger, 1959, pp. 243–300.
18. Kannel, W.B., D. McGee, and T. Gordon. A general cardiovascular risk profile: The Framingham Study. *Am. J. Cardiol.* 38:46–51, 1979.
19. Kannel, W.B., and P. Sorlie. Some health benefits of physical activity: The Framingham Study. *Arch. Intern. Med.* 139:857–861, 1979.
20. Katsch, G. Die Arbeitstherapie der Zuckerkranken. *Erg. Physikal Diat. Ther.* 1:1–36, 1939.
21. Kemmer, F.W., P. Berchtold, M. Berger, et al. Exercise-induced fall of blood glucose in insulin-treated diabetics unrelated to alterations of insulin mobilization. *Diabetes* 28:1131–1137, 1979.
22. Kemmer, F.W., R. Bisping, H.J. Steingruber, H. Baar, F. Hardtmann, K. Schlaghecke, and M. Berger. Psychological stress and metabolic control in patients with type I diabetes mellitus. *N. Engl. J. Med.* 314:1078–1094, 1986.
23. Kennedy, A.L., T.R.J. Lappin, T.D. Lavery, et al. Relations of high density lipoprotein cholesterol concentration to type of diabetes and its control. *Br. Med. J.* 2:1191–1194, 1978.
24. Koivisto, V.A., V. Soman, P. Conrad, et al. Insulin binding to monocytes in trained athletes: Changes in the resting state and after exercise. *Am. Soc. Clin. Invest.* 64:1011–1015, 1979.
25. Kostis, J., J. Baughman, and P. Kuo. Association of recurrent myocardial infarction with hemostatic factors: A prospective study. *Chest.* 81:571–574, 1982.
26. Kramsch, D.M., A.J. Aspen, B.M. Abramowitz, et al. Reduction of coronary atherosclerosis by moderate conditioning exercise in monkeys on an atherogenic diet. *N. Engl. J. Med.* 305:1483–1489, 1981.
27. Krotkiewski, M., K. Mandroukas, L. Sjostrom, et al. Effect of long-term physical training on body fat, metabolism, and blood pressure in obesity. *Metabolism* 28:650–658, 1979.
28. LeBlanc, J., A. Nadeau, and M. Boulay. Effects of physical training and adiposity on glucose metabolism and I^{125} insulin binding. *J. Appl. Physiol.* 46:235, 1979.
29. Lee, P., P.J. Rooney, R.D. Sturrock, et al. The etiology and pathogenesis of osteoarthrosis: A review. *Semin. Arth. Rheum.* 3:189–218, 1974.

30. Lipman, R., P. Raskin, T. Love, et al. Glucose intolerance during decreased physical activity in men. *Diabetes* 21:101–107, 1972.

31. Lohmann, D., F. Leibold, W. Heilmann, et al. Diminished insulin response in highly trained athletes. *Metabolism* 27:521, 1978.

32. Maehlum, S., and E.D.R. Pruett. Muscular exercise and metabolism in male juvenile diabetes. *Scan. J. Clin. Lab. Inves.* 32:149–153, 1973.

33. Mann, G., H. Garrett, A. Farhi, et alk. Exercise to prevent coronary heart disease. *Am. J. Med.* 46:12–27, 1969.

34. Miller, W.J., W.M. Sherman, and J.L. Ivy. Effect of strength training on glucose tolerance and post-glucose insulin response. *Med. Sci. Sports Med.* 16:539–543, 1984.

35. Mogesen, C.E., C.K. Christensen, and E. Vittinghus. The stages in diabetic renal disease with emphasis on the stage of incipient diabetic nephropathy. *Diabetes* 32 (Suppl. 2):64–78, 1983.

36. Monnier, V.M., R.R. Kohn, and A. Cerami. Accelerated age-related browning of human collagen in diabetes mellitus. *Proc. Natl. Acad. Sci. USA* 81:583–587, 1984.

37. Montoye, H.J., W.D. Block, H. Metzner, et al. Habitual physical activity and glucose tolerance. *Diabetes* 26:172–176, 1977.

38. Montoye, H.J., H. Metzner, J. Keller, et al. Habitual physical activity and blood pressure. *Med. Sci. Sports Exer.* 4:175–181, 1972.

39. Olefsky, J.M. Pathogenesis of insulin resistance and hyperglycemia in non-insulin dependent diabetes mellitus. *Am. J. Med.* 79 (Suppl. 3B): 1–7, 1985.

40. Paffenbarger, R.S., A.L. Wing, R.T. Hyde, et al. Physical activity as an index of heart attack risk in college alumni. *Am. J. Epidemiol.* 108:161–175, 1978.

41. Poussier, P., B. Zinman, E.B. Marliss, et al. Open-loop intravenous insulin waveforms for postprandial exercise in type I diabetes. *Diabetes Care* 6:129–134, 1983.

42. Pyorala, K. Relationship of glucose tolerance and plasma insulin to the incidence of coronary heart disease: Results from two population studies in Finland. *Diabetes Care* 2:131–141, 1979.

43. Robertson, W.B., and J.P. Strong. Atherosclerosis in persons with hypertension and diabetes mellitus. *Lab. Invest.* 18:538–551, 1968.

44. Rollo, J. *Cases of Diabetes Mellitus with the Results of the Trials of Certain Acids and Other Substances in the Cure of the Lues Venerea.* 2nd ed., London, 1798.

45. Rubler, S. Asymptomatic diabetic females: Exercise testing. *NY State J. Med.* 81:1185–1191, 1981.

46. Ruderman, N.B., O.P. Ganda, and K. Johansen. The effect of physical training on glucose tolerance and plasma lipids in maturity-onset diabetes. *Diabetes* 28 (Suppl. 1):89–92, 1979.

47. Saltin, B., F. Lindgarde, M. Houston, et al. Physical training and glucose tolerance in middle-aged men with chemical diabetes. *Diabetes* 28:30–32, 1978.

48. Saltin, B., F. Lindgarde, H. Lithell, et al. Metabolic effects of long-term physical training in maturity-onset diabetes. In Walshausl, W.K. (ed.). Amsterdam: Excerpta Medica, 1980, p. 345.

49. Schiffrin, A., S. Parikh, E.B. Marliss, and M.A. Desrosiers. Metabolic responses to fasting exercise in adolescent insulin-dependent diabetic subjects treated with continuous subcutaneous insulin infusion and intensive conventional therapy. *Diabetes Care* 7:255–260, 1984.

50. Schneider, S.H., L.F. Amorosa, A.K. Khachadurian, and N.B. Ruderman. Studies on the mechanism of improved glucose control during regular exercise in type 2 (non-insulin-dependent) diabetes. *Diabetologia* 26:355–360, 1984.

51. Schneider, S.H., H. Kim, N.B. Ruderman, et al. Effects of exercise and physical training on certain coagulation parameters in diabetes. *Clin. Res.* 30(2):403A, 1982.

52. Schneider, S.H., A. Vitug, and N.B. Ruderman. Atherosclerosis and physical activity. *Diab./Metab. Rev.* 1(4):513–553, 1986.

53. Seals, D., J. Hagberg, W. Allen, B. Hurley, et al. Glucose tolerance in young and older athletes and sedentary men. *J. Appl. Physiol.* 56:1521–1528, 1984.

54. Skor, D., J. Gavin, J. Hagberg, et al. The effects of acute and chronic exercise on insulin sensitivity in non-insulin dependent diabetes mellitus. *Diabetes* 32(Suppl. 1):64A, 1983.

55. Stout, R.W. Overview of the association between insulin and atherosclerosis. *Metabolism* 34 (Suppl. 1):7–12, 1985.

56. Sushruta, S.C.S. *Vaidya Jadavaji Trikamji Acharia,* 11/11, 12, 13, Rev., 3rd ed. Bombay: Nirnyar Sagar Press, 1938, (Original book published in 500 B.C.)

57. Tonino, R.P., W.H. Nede, D.C. Robbins, and E.S. Horton. Effect of physical training on insulin resistance of aging. *Clin. Res.* 34(2):557A, 1986.

58. Vranic, M., and M. Berger. Exercise and diabetes mellitus. *Diabetes* 28:147–167, 1979.

59. Waine, H., D. Nevinny, J. Rosenthal, et al. Association of osteoarthritis and diabetes mellitus. *Tufts Fol. Med.* 7:13–19, 1961.

60. Wallberg-Henriksson, H., R. Gunnarsson, J. Henriksson, et al. Increased peripheral insulin sensitivity and muscle mitochondrial enzymes but unchanged blood glucose control in type I diabetics after physical training. *Diabetes* 31:1044–1050, 1982.

61. Welborn, T.A., and K. Wearne. Coronary heart disease incidence and cardiovascular mortality in Busselton with reference to glucose and insulin concentrations. *Diabetes Care* 2:154–160, 1979.

62. White, N.H., D.A. Skor, P.E. Cryer, et al. Identification of type I diabetic patients at increased risk for hypoglycemia during intensive therapy. *N. Engl. J. Med.* 308:485–491, 1983.

63. Wilhelmsen, L., K. Suardsudd, K. Korsan-Bengtsen, et al. Fibrinogen as a risk factor for stroke and myocardial infarction. *N. Engl. J. Med.* 311:501–505, 1984.

64. Wood, F., and W. Haskell. The effect of exercise on plasma high density lipoproteins. *Lipds* 14:417–427, 1979.

Chapter 17

EXERCISE AND ENERGY BALANCE IN THE CONTROL OF OBESITY AND HYPERTENSION

Ethan A. H. Sims, M.D.

INTRODUCTION

An abundance of evidence has been presented in this book that people thrive if they stir about. There is also hard-won evidence that they thrive better in the face of diabetes, diseases of the heart and blood vessels, and hypertension as well. In the United States in the 20th century, obesity is increasing, despite the fact that people do not eat more on an absolute basis than they did previously. This suggests that Americans are physically less active. In underdeveloped areas of this hemisphere, the incidence of disorders most associated with obesity, namely, type II diabetes and hypertension, is also increasing. There is much to suggest that movement from labor-intensive farms in the hills to Americanized automated urban communities is a major contributing factor [29].

It is true that today there are many joggers, but the individuals jogging are not always those who would profit most from the exercise. The dominant problem with respect to exercise is not that people do not understand the benefits, but rather that people most in need of those benefits are not motivated. For this reason I plan in this chapter to emphasize the implementation of behavioral change with respect to physical activity, in addition to discussing energy balance and the special problems of the hypertensive obese. First, a number of questions have to be addressed:

1. Is the national increase in obesity over the past 60 years due more to decrease in physical exertion or to dietary change and more readily available food?
2. Does physical activity influence the thermogenic adaptation to excess caloric intake in the lean, and do the obese respond differently?
3. To what degree can increase in physical activity affect the development and course of hypertension and cardiovascular disease?
4. What is the effect of increased physical activity on net energy balance in the lean and the obese?
5. Who stands to gain most from programs of increased physical activity, and what determines success?
6. How can programs of physical activity best be implemented?
7. What are some priorities for research?

IS DECREASED ACTIVITY TO BLAME FOR OUR NATIONAL INCREASE IN WEIGHT?

This question has been considered in detailed by Brownell and Stunkard [7] and by Stern [34].

Draft statistics in the successive wars of this country and other data all indicate that as a nation we have become heavier and presumably fatter during this century. Since per capita caloric intake has decreased over the same period (by 7%, according to 1970 figures [9, 34], it is argued that the cause of the increased weight gain must necessarily be decreased energy expenditure from increasing mechanization. Surveys between the years 1978 and 1984 suggest that two-thirds of North Americans do not exercise on a regular basis, and 28 to 45% do not exercise at all [17]. Many studies of physical activity of infants, school children, and adults suggest that relative inactivity may be a prime cause of obesity [7, 34]. It cannot be quite this simple, however, since, the proportion of calories taken in as fat increased 25% during this century and, as Danforth [9, 31] has recently emphasized, the efficiency of energy storage increases with the percent of fat in the diet because of lessened cost of storage and a reduced thermogenic response.

Brownell and Stunkard [7] have recently reviewed studies in which the level of activity of overweight children and adults has been compared with that of normal subjects and studies in which attempts have been made to quantitate the energy expenditure. In general, obese children tend to be as active or more active than nonobese children. On the basis of activity measurement, adults with obesity tend to be less active, although, as Brownell and Stunkard pointed out, energy expenditure and the greater cost of movement for the obese have not been measured in studies to date.

A major problem is that one subtype of obesity may bear a different relationship to physical activity than another type. Critical studies of fully characterized subjects have not yet been done. For example, very likely an obese child in whom so-called maturity-onset diabetes of youth (MODY) develops might be relatively inactive, while a child with familial obesity could be a dynamo. The same may be true of the adult with obesity of central distribution and early non-insulin-dependent diabetes, as opposed to one with a relatively "healthy" form of obesity.

Sophisticated techniques are now available for measurement of energy expenditure. Schutz et al. in Jequier's laboratory at Lausanne have used the Doppler principle and a radar device in an open-circuit respiratory chamber to quantitate and calibrate the cost of physical activity above the basal level [reviewed in 29]. Extrapolating to zero the plot of percent activity versus oxygen consumption, it is possible to estimate the cost of activity above the resting metabolic rate. Later use of a similar technique by Ravussin and Bogardus [22] in the new National Institutes of Health respiratory chamber at Phoenix, Arizona, has indicated that small spontaneous movements of the body, which these investigators haver termed "fidgeting," even within the confines of the chamber can account for as much as 75 to 790 kcal/day. Thus, individuals may differ in their level of spontaneous activity. This is a factor that may well be independent of environmental factors, such as labor-saving devices. Some years ago Rose and Williams [23] compared easy-gaining students with those who could apparently "eat like a horse" without gaining. The most discriminatory of a battery of measurements was the rate of their walking when asked to carry out an assigned task. When given the opportunity, obese adults choose the physically less demanding course in their daily life. Brownell, Stunkard, and Albaum [8] found that when both escalators and adjacent stairs were available, the obese chose the former more often. However, if the lean were carrying an equivalent amount of body weight, they might also choose the escalator. If output of energy is reduced by use of mechanical devices and weight is gained, a vicious cycle of increasing inactivity and increasing weight gain is set up. In our Vermont study [29] of experimental obesity, we and the work supervisors of our prison volunteers noted that when they had gained weight by their monumental efforts at overeating, they were less energetic and had less initiative in their work assignments. It is true that even quite vigorous physical activity above the basal level amounts to only a relatively small proportion of the overall energy expenditure. However, small changes in the energy equation are cumulative in the long run.

The Pima Indians of Arizona on the reservation at Sakaton show the effects of a survival trait that now is a liability. Originally they subsisted by irrigating crops along the banks of the Gila River and may well have suffered periodic crop failures and famine. Ancient survival mechanisms may promote inactivity when food is in abundance. Neel has suggested that the tendency to become obese may be the result of a "thrifty gene [29]." Those who have a strong component of the thrifty gene will tend to be less active when they have stored excess energy; by conserving their energy stores they are more apt to survive a subsequent famine. The Gila River is now dammed to the east of Sakaton and at times is nearly a dry bed. Today there is little incentive for the Indians to work for food, since it is supplied in part by the government, and boredom is endemic. Obesity is almost universal, and diabetes is prevalent. Again, however, decreased physical activity cannot be pinpointed as the major cause of the obesity, since increased percent of fat in the diet may also be an important factor.

In summary, the evidence that decreased need for physical work is a major contributor in excess gain in weight is strongly suggestive, but not conclusive. We do know, however, that the way to fatten cattle for market, in addition to providing ample food, is to confine them in a pen. The demands of modern living too frequently confine us in pens of our own making.

RELATION OF EXERCISE TO OBLIGATORY AND FACULTATIVE THERMOGENESIS

The time has passed when we can take a simplistic view of energy balance. The equation

$$\text{Energy stored} = \text{energy in} - \text{energy expended}$$

still must apply, but we can no longer assume a constant figure for the cost of mechanical work or for the effect of particular caloric excess or deficit. We cannot assume that there is a linear relationship between caloric excess or deficit and body fat stores based on a fixed ratio of 3500 kcal/lb of fat tissue. We must consider the composition of a diet and the thermogenic response as well. It has long been known that animals and humans can vary their rate of heat production on exposure to cold. Certain metabolic functions, such as the absorption, transport, and interconversions of substrates, have an obligatory thermogenic cost. We are justified in using the term "facultative" when thermogenesis is modulated in the interests of heat production or conservation, or in the interests of decreasing or increasing the efficiency of utilization of foodstuffs during overnutrition or undernutrition. Small animals can increase their wasting of energy as heat when they are forced to eat an excess of food of poor quality, and may thus obtain adequate essential nutrients. This has obvious survival value in avoiding the handicap of obesity. A major part, but not all, of this adaptation in animals is accomplished by stimulation of brown fat by the sympathetic nervous system. During starvation, the resting metabolic rate declines, and this again has obvious survival value. The degree to which such adaptations persist and serve to stabilize the weight of industrialized humans, in spite of artificial insulation against temperature extremes and famine, has been a matter of intense investigation over the past two decades. Results have often been contradictory, but important information is emerging. The interested reader is referred to two recent reviews from our group for further documentation and background of statements included in this chapter [29a, 31]. The present discussion is limited to the direct effects of exercise on resting metabolic rate and on response to overfeeding and to catecholamine stimulation.

Increase in Metabolic Rate Following Exercise

There remains considerable uncertainty as to the degree and duration of the increase in resting metabolic rate (RMR) following a bout of acute exercise. Freedman-Akabas et al. [12] at Columbia and coworkers failed to demonstrate a sustained increase. Bielinski et al. [2] used the respiratory chamber in Jequier's laboratory at Lausanne to study the thermic response of normal young athletes to mixed meals at various intervals after 3 hours of exercise at high intensity. Under these strenuous conditions there was a greater contribution of lipid oxidation when the meal followed the exercise. The RMR declined during sleep, but was elevated an average of 4.7% the following morning, 15 hours after the exercise. There was, however, much individual variation, and the exercise was demanding. Devlin and Horton [10] measured the thermic response in lean subjects to infused insulin at two concentrations while plasma glucose was kept constant during a euglycemic clamp procedure 12 to 16 hours following exercise to exhaustion the previous evening. They found a 3 to 7% increase in basal energy expenditure, with increase of lipid oxidation and decrease in oxidation of glucose. The thermic effect of insulin at both physiological and elevated concentrations was potentiated. In contrast, LeBlanc et al. [see review in 29] found that highly physically trained women have a lesser diet-induced response to a meal than only moderately active or sedentary persons. They attributed this to the lesser sympathetic nervous response to eating in these in-

dividuals and to their physiological favoring of deposition of glucose as glycogen over more costly metabolic routes. Later studies by the same laboratory [29] indicated that the super-trained subjects had a lower insulin and catecholamine response than sedentary subjects. Periods of measurement were limited to 2 hours, but the data suggest that the differences would remain significant over longer periods.

Relatively small differences in the total RMR are involved, and further work is required to put these differences in perspective. A sustained increase in thermogenesis and in the thermic response to subsequent meals could have a clinical significance.

Effect of a Preceding Meal on the Thermic Response to Exercise

It was Miller, Mumford, and Stock who first called attention to the increase in cost of exercise following a meal in overfed subjects [reviewed in 29]. Segal and Gutin [26] have reported that when food is taken before a bout of exercise, the thermic response to the exercise is increased over the response to the exercise alone. This effect was considerably less in obese as opposed to lean women. The actual amount of exercise was carefully matched to the aerobic threshold of the subjects. In a similar series of studies [27], Segal et al. compared the response to exercise with or without an antecedent meal in men matched for age, weight, and height, but differing in percent of body fat (10 vs. 30%). The two groups had comparable RMRs in relation to fat-free mass. But due to their greater fat-free mass, the lean had a 15 to 17% greater rate of oxygen uptake, either total or in relation to body weight. The thermic response of the lean subjects to the meal alone was increased over that of the obese. Presumably this would also be true of sedentary subjects of comparable weight. The thermic response to exercise after a 750-kcal meal was also considerably greater in the lean, either during or following a 30-minute bout of exercise. These results contrasted sharply with those of the LeBlanc studies of super-trained women. However, the differing results may be related to differing effects of the types of physical training, aerobic by the avid runners, skiers, and cyclists as opposed to anaerobic by the iron-pumping body builders.

A number of factors may explain the potentiating effect of a previous meal. One involves the substrate cycling across a step or steps in a biochemical pathway that are enzymatically controlled in both directions. This was once termed "futile" cycling, but, as emphasized by Newsholme [29], such cycling is important in affecting the rapidity and intensity of response to a stimulus. This is analogous to increasing the rate of idling of a car prior to making a rapid start at a traffic light. Thus, a preceding meal or bout of exercise might be expected to increase the response to a subsequent bout of exercise or a meal.

Another is the degree of insulin response and sympathetic stimulation. As discussed below, there is reason to believe that the facultative response to a meal or to exercise is modified by the degree of sympathetic nervous response, which in turn is influenced by insulin action.

Effect of Physical Training on Plasma Norepinephrine Concentrations and Turnover

Studies of the role of catecholamines in exercise and in various thermogenic responses have often given conflicting results. This may be partly because consideration of plasma concentrations of the catecholamines alone may be misleading. Measurement of the rate of appearance and clearance (the spillover or turnover rate) by the technique recently developed by Esler provides more meaningful results. O'Dea and others in Esler's laboratory [29] have shown that both norepinephrine appearance and clearance are increased by overfeeding, and that under-

feeding results in their reductions. There were parallel changes in serum thyroid hormones. Thus, these two hormones mediate a facultative response to moderate the effects of changes in food intake. Schwartz and colleagues [25] have recently used this technique to study the effects of a 3-month walk-jogging program in eight normal young subjects. There was a correlation between the appearance and clearance, and hence the turnover, of norepinephrine with the training effect, as indicated by maximal oxygen uptake ($\dot{V}o_2$max).

Brown Fat in Adult Humans

In animals, in many situations an increase in nonshivering thermogenesis is mediated mainly by brown fat, with its unique capacity to uncouple oxidation of substrate and formation of adenosine triphosphate (ATP). Much of the brown fat of the newborn human infant is lost during later years. Protective clothing, housing, and a relatively smaller surface area minimize the stimulation by cold of this tissue in humans. However, humans are capable of retaining or forming brown fat. Huttunen *et al.* [29] in Finland found that brown fat, identified by its enzymatic characteristics, is plentiful in outdoor workers but minimal in sedentary office workers. This might suggest that lowering the thermostat, sleeping with the windows open, and indulging in sports involving exposure to cold may be particularly good for long-term health.

Relative Importance of Facultative Increase in Thermogenesis in Weight Control

The maximum increase in metabolic rate that can be produced by overfeeding is perhaps 10%. The effect of strenuous bouts of exercise or of physical training are relatively short-lived. However, the accumulated effects of even small differences in thermic response to over-ample meals can be considerable, and a vicious cycle can be set up in increasing body fat, increasing insulin resistance, and blunted sympathetic response.

Studies employing the euglycemic hyperinsulinemic clamp technique have helped to clarify the underlying mechanisms. In obese subjects there is a diminished disposal rate of glucose and a diminished thermogenic response to insulin and glucose, and this is more marked when there is increased insulin resistance associated with glucose intolerance or frank non-insulin-dependent diabetes [29]. If enough insulin is infused to overcome the insulin resistance and increase glucose disposal to normal, the thermogenic response becomes normal. This, however, is not the situation in a free-living obese or non-insulin-dependent diabetic person, and thus it is likely that the reduced thermogenic response is important in the development and perpetuation of obesity. One cannot conclude, however, that because of the reduced thermogenic response obese persons expend less total energy. The RMR, related both to total weight and to fat-free mass, is usually increased as a result of the cost of increased splanchnic glucose production, mainly in the form of hepatic gluconeogenesis. As will be discussed, physical training can reduce the splanchnic glucose production toward normal.

There is a decrease in RMR in animals and humans subjected to caloric deprivation, another compensatory mechanism with obvious survival value [29]. This is associated with a decrease in plasma insulin concentrations, in free triiodothyronine, and, as already noted, in catecholamine turnover rate. It explains in part the frustrating tendency of the rate of loss of weight to decrease or plateau during attempts at weight loss by caloric restrictions.

In summary, both acute bouts of exercise and long-term moderate physical training may enhance the facultative thermogenic mechanisms that contribute to stabilization of body weight, through increasing the thermogenic responses.

DIFFERENCES IN THE EFFECT OF EXERCISE ON INTAKE OF FOOD IN THE LEAN AND OBESE

To date the relation between physical activity and spontaneous intake of food has been examined in many studies (see reviews by Brownell and Stunkard [7], Sims [29], and Stern [34]. Variables such as adequacy of the measurements of intake and expenditure of energy, sex of the subjects, and stores of body fat all affect the conclusions. Except at the extremes of physical exertion, lean animals and humans adjust intake to activity and maintain body weight. Woo and Pi-Sunyer [40] found this to be true in lean women. In the very sedentary range, intake is not proportionally reduced, and weight is gained. On the other hand, the obese as a general group tend not to compensate for increased activity with a proportional increase in intake of food. Recent precise studies by Woo, Garrow, and Pi-Sunyer [38] in Garrow's laboratory have shown this to be true of obese women during 19-day periods in which expenditure was increased to 110 and 125% of the basal level and intake of food was covertly monitored. More prolonged increase in physical activity was also studied by Woo, Garrow, and Pi-Sunyer [39]. Three obese women, ranging in age from 17 to 46 years, increased their activity by 25% above sedentary level. Their weight averaged 187% above the supposed ideal. One had hypertrophy of adipocytes and the other two had hyperplasia as well. They differed in distribution of fat and in age of onset and severity of the obesity. Their usual activity level, however, was comparable to that of lean, age-matched control subjects (R. Woo, personal communication, 1986). In spite of this heterogeneity, the prolonged treatment failed to elicit a compensatory response in intake, and all had substantial loss of weight, 89% of which was fat. Whether subjects with other subtypes of obesity would all react in similar manner is not yet known.

An important study by Wood, Terry, and Haskell [41] at Stanford University addressed the same question in free-living sedentary, middle-aged men in an uncontrolled 2-year program of physical conditioning. The men were simply asked to run as much as they were able, and were not given instructions regarding diet. They progressively reached an average of 12 miles/week of running during the second year and gained a training effect, and were thus typical of the low-level joggers now frequenting our streets and trails. Body fat decreased from 21.6 to 18% and there was a small increase in lean body mass. Average caloric intake increased from 2380 to 2750 cal by the second year. Most important, they spontaneously increased their intake of carbohydrate 30%. There was also significant improvement in serum lipids.

Possible Role of Beta-Endorphin

The relation of the endogenous opioids to physical activity and the intake of food in the lean and the obese is as yet incompletely resolved. The endorphin opioids stimulate food intake, apparently by central action, in both animals and humans [29]. A striking hyperendorphinemia in obese children and adults, comparable to that in Prader-Willi syndrome, has recently been reported by Genazzani [13]. Exercise increases immunoreactive beta-endorphin in the plasma in normal subjects, and this may partly explain the euphoria and even occasional addiction to running of the avid jogger. Thus, the opioids might well mediate the compensatory hyperphagia in the normal person following increased physical activity. However, the response of beta-endorphin in the obese person following exercise has not yet been studied. A relatively reduced response in the obese could explain the fact that they do not increase their food intake following exercise. That the obese are indeed less responsive in one respect is indicated by recent studies of the effect of opioid inhibitors. Cohen and colleagues have shown that the opioid antagonist naloxone, at a dosage

of 2 mg/kg, reduces food intake in normal persons [29]. However, in a controlled study of 27 women 30 to 100% overweight, Malcolm and co-workers could find no effect on food intake of the long-acting oral opioid antagonist, naltrexone [29].

PHYSICAL ACTIVITY, HYPERTENSION, AND CARDIOVASCULAR DISEASE

A pronouncement by John Dryden is particularly relevant to the management of essential hypertension (quoted by R. Paffenberger):

Better to hunt the Fields, for Health unbought,
Than fee the Doctor for a nauseous Draught.
The Wise, for Cure, on Exercise depend;
God never made his Work, for man to mend
      From *Fables Ancient and Modern*, 1700

In 1980, a stimulating first international meeting of the Association of Obesity and Hypertension was held in Florence [30]. This was at a time when the "first step" in management of hypertension was apt to be a "nauseous draught," which at times interferred with God's work with respect to lipids and electrolytes. At this meeting it was emphasized that the endocrine-metabolic derangements often seen in the obese could contribute to hypertension. Increased sympathetic tone and insulin resistance with hyperinsulinemia are both common to obesity and to hypertension, and the two can interact. Insulin, at least acutely, promotes the reabsorption of sodium by the kidney. Overfeeding and an increase in plasma insulin level increase sympathetic nervous system tone by their central action, and norepinephrine also increases renal tubular reabsorption of sodium.

It is also quite possible that some subtypes of essential hypertension may be related to a disturbance of steroid metabolism. The association of obesity of central distribution with hypertension is well established [36]. In women with the central, android, or cushingoid type of obesity there are associated abnormalities of the android group of steroids. It seems quite possible that both the distribution of body fat and the hypertension are secondary to derangements of steroid metabolism yet to be elucidated.

Overnutrition increases the activity of thyroid hormones, and this plays a permissive role in relation to sympathetic activity. "Hunting the fields" and various other forms of exercise can of course strikingly reduce insulin resistance and other abnormalities of the overweight. Krotkiewski *et al.* [15] have shown that the most marked lowering of blood pressure by physical training occurs in hypertensive subjects who are hyperinsulinemic and hyperlipidemic. Björntorp [4] has emphasized the reduced activity of the sympathetic nervous system that accompanies reduction of blood pressure in the normal person and in the overweight. This may be brought about by an adaptation in the central sympathetic nervous system and, secondarily, by an increased sensitivity of the peripheral system.

Obesity is common in the hypertensive population. There must also be many of the "physiologically obese" persons described by Ruderman *et al.* [24]. They are not obese by the usual criteria, but have an increased ratio of fat to muscle, and may have an increase in the size of adipocytes. Such individuals may be hyperinsulinemic, insulin resistant, and hyperlipidemic and thus may respond metabolically like the overtly obese. They stand to benefit from programs of exercise and may have a better chance of taking part successfully than those handicapped by overt obesity.

Increased physical activity was incorporated in the Chicago Coronary Prevention Evaluation Program [30] with apparent benefit, but to date this variable has not been evaluated in a large-scale controlled clinical trial. Such a trial must include identification of subgroups that may or may not respond to nonpharmacological management. It is also important that nonpharmacological management be fully evaluated, since a number of the commonly employed antihypertensive

agents increase the risk factors of hyperlipidemia and hyperglycemia [30] and may produce impotence. The very long-term effects of the drugs are, of course, not yet known.

Paffenbarger *et al.* [19] have reviewed the relation of physical activity to the mortality and longevity of 16,936 Harvard graduates, whom they admit may not be typical subjects. The death rate of these subjects was half that of the general population, but they committed suicide twice as often. The authors admitted that the possible influences of disease on physical activity patterns, and vice versa, were not addressed in this study. Nevertheless, the evidence was strong that maintaining an active life-style is beneficial. The death rate showed a steady decline with reported exercise expenditure increasing from 500 to 3500 kcal/week and was one-quarter to one-third lower in those expending 2000 or more kcal/week. Survival was also increased in those at increased risk from hypertension, smoking, or a family history of early parental death. For what it is worth, by age 80 the additional years of life attributable to adequate exercise was 1-2 years. Former varsity athletes who exercised at expenditures less than 500 or more than 2000 kcal/week in their later years had *higher* death rates than those who reported moderate exercise of 500 to 2000 kcal/week. The authors concluded that inheritance of a sturdy constitution, as in varsity athletes, is less important to longevity than continuation of adequate exercise over the lifetime. Of interest would have been a request for subjects to report abdomen/thigh circumferences as an index of central distribution of body fat.

The Joint National Committee on Detection, Evaluation and Treatment of High Blood Pressure in its most recent recommendation has modified the stepped-care program to give more emphasis to calorie restriction and increased physical activity as initial therapy.

In summary, John Dryden might well have gone on to write, for benefit of the hypertensive:

He who on nauseous Draught for years depends
must face the Risk the Drug his Powers will
end,
while Fat his Vessels all are clogging,
This Same he might prevent by Jogging."

CONTRIBUTION OF EXERCISE TO DIETARY REGIMENS

Sporadic bouts of exercise provide relatively so little additional energy expenditure above the basal expenditure that to rely on them for weight loss is usually not rewarding. It is better not to eat the plum pudding than to run the miles to burn off its caloric equivalent. However, one of the greatest potential benefits of exercise is the improvement in sense of well-being and morale and in ability to adhere to other aspects of a regimen for control of weight.

Exercise gives other benefits when added to a dietary regimen for management of obesity and non-insulin-dependent diabetes or hypertension in the overweight. In the study by Bogardus *et al.* [6] in our laboratory at the University of Vermont, the effect of a program of dietary restriction to 450 kcal/m² body surface area was compared with the effect of the same dietary program with addition of an intensive 3-day/week program of physical training. Both groups of 8 to 10 subjects had comparable and significant reduction in body fat. There was improvement in glucose tolerance accomplished by reduced insulin and C-peptide secretion. The $\dot{V}O_2max$, indicative of a training effect, was increased in the exercising group. There was a reduction in the abnormally high splanchnic glucose production and restoration of its suppression by insulin in both groups. This accounted for a lowering in both groups of the fasting glucose concentration. Total glucose disposal during a euglycemic hyperinsulinemic clamp procedure was increased by 30% in the group given added exercise and was unchanged in the dietary group. By means of simultaneous indirect calorimetry it was possible to separate glucose disposal into oxidative and nonoxidative rates. An important finding was that in the group with added exercise, nonoxidative disposal, presumed largely to represent glycogen deposition in muscle, was increased. Since the glucose intolerance in this type of diabetes is due mainly to decreased apparent carbohydrate storage rather than to oxidation rates, the combined exercise and dietary therapy more directly addresses these defects. Under conditions of the hyperinsulinemic clamp, a major portion of nonoxidative glucose disposal is an increase in muscle glycogen and, as in a trained athlete, this increases the capacity for sustaining acute exercise. In contrast, when weight loss in similar subjects was achieved by use of a protein-supplemented modified fast with minimal intake of carbohydrate, Bogardus *et al.* [5] found depletion of muscle glycogen, and the capacity for sustained severe exercise (75% of $\dot{V}O_2max$) was dismal.

CHARACTERISTICS OF THE OVERWEIGHT MOST IN NEED OF EXERCISE AS A COMPONENT OF WEIGHT CONTROL

Those most in need of an exercise program are those with a family history of cardiovascular disease of early onset. Women with a history of gestational diabetes are also prime candidates, since O'Sullivan [18] found that after 15 years, over 60% of a group of patients with gestational diabetes who were overweight during the pregnancy had become overtly diabetic. Over 40% of those lean during the pregnancy had the same outcome. Primary prevention of obesity and increase in physical activity in this group may reduce this high incidence.

There is now a mass of evidence that persons with obesity of central distribution are at a greater risk for diabetes, hypertension, and cardiovascular disease [28]. Dr. Jean Vague of the University of Marseilles first called attention to central obesity as a risk factor for cardiovascular disease and diabetes. A recent symposium at Marseilles has brought this subject up to date [36]. Simply measuring with a tape measure the ratio of the maximal circumference of the abdomen to that of the hips at the gluteal fold provides a useful index of the distribution of body fat. Recent data of Larsson and coworkers [16] from Sweden indicate that a ratio greater than 1.0 in men and 1.2 in women in significant.

The physiologically obese of Ruderman et al. [24], already mentioned, are equally in need of rehabilitation.

Another category of persons are those at the upper range of the distribution curve for body fat who have a normal family history, are basically healthy, and have a universal distribution of body fat and no detectable metabolic abnormality. For such persons, attempts to reach a supposedly ideal weight derived from data from the population as a whole may be counterproductive. Similarly, it may be counterproductive to try for a supposedly ideal weight in an individual with marked hyperplasia of adipocytes and other body cells.

WHAT DETERMINES THE SUCCESS OF EXERCISE PROGRAMS

Much work has been done both on the psychological and the physiological fronts to learn why programs succeed or fail, what the prognostic factors are for a given individual, and how a program can best be structured. Reports dealing with success rates, usually over the short term, of the effects of physical training in the management of obesity in general are not encouraging. Brownell and Stunkard [7] estimated that 30% or more of obese subjects drop out of the usual physical training programs, while Dishman [11] estimated the dropout rate within 6 months as over 50%. Martin and Dubbert [17] extensively analyzed the factors related to cooperation with such programs and reported an

even more dismal picture. There are few long-term follow-up studies. Jordan and Canavan [14] contacted, after 6 to 10 years, a selected sample of 437 patients who had enrolled in an intensive 20-week behavioral program that included emphasis on physical activity. Of 190 who had lost over 15 pounds originally, 111 responded. They had regained an average of 7 pounds. It would be valuable to know the subtype of obesity and other characteristics of patients who selected themselves out and also of those who were unsuccessful, particularly in relation to their maintenance of increased physical activity.

Our own experience [6] with adding a program of physical training to a program of calorie restriction for middle-aged, overweight subjects with mild to moderate type II diabetes was encouraging in the short term but discouraging in the long term. During a 3-month period, two or three members of the staff met 3 days a week in the University gym for a progressively graded workout with the volunteers. Effects on the diabetes have been described in Chapter 16 of this book; the thermogenic effects have been described previously in this chapter. There was reason to believe that the effects, at least in the exercise group, might be sustained. Detailed information had been obtained through a questionaire of past experience and preferences for exercise and other relevant factors. Arrangements were made for several of the spouses to work out with the subjects. A number of group meetings were held, and the subjects had the feedback reinforcement of monitoring their own weight, their heart rate, and particularly their blood glucose level. The follow-up at 1 1/2 years was encouraging in regard to sustained activity and weight loss. However, 1 year later, only 2 of 18 questionaires were returned, and these were discouraging. I describe this in some detail, because it brings home the need to learn more about how to help people with a problem that may well be managed by nonpharmacological means to incorporate exercise. It may be that a program based more on exercise in the home setting with long-continued group support would be more effective.

Physicians are becoming more aware of the advantages of recommending a program of increased physical activity. An evaluation of the effect of the Clinical Education Program of the American Diabetes Association in relation to exercise in type II diabetes was carried out following the 1984 televised lectures. Prior to the program, 62% of 10,000 physicians who attended wrote that they recommended public exercise programs for 90% of their patients. Following the program, 79% indicated that they now recommend exercise in the management of type II diabetes. In half of their patients the recommendation was apparently effective, at least in the short term (R. Mazze, personal communication, 1985).

Prognostic Factors in the Success of Increased Activity in the Management of Obesity

Wilson [37] offered the discouraging summary that "reliable psychological prognostic factors in the treatment of obesity remain to be identified." He reviewed in some detail the main factors that explain some of the variance, perhaps 60% related to weight loss during the actual period of a program. These include the initial degree of overweight (the major factor), age, sex, spouse's degree of overweight, energy intake, and initial rate of loss. On the other hand, Krotkiewski [15], in Björntorp's laboratory, has reported that over 80% of the variance related to weight loss during the actual treatment period can be explained by the individual's degree of adipocyte hyperplasia and by the metabolic rate prior to treatment. However, when it comes to maintenance of weight loss, as Sjöström [33] pointed out, these two factors explain only about 30% of the variance.

In patients with frank non-insulin-dependent diabetes, there may be factors other than these two affecting adherence. Perlmutter *et al.* [reviewed in 29] have measured

psychological performance of 140 patients 55 to 74 years of age with non-insulin-dependent diabetes. Cognitive function was decreased, in comparison with function of age-, sex-, and weight-matched controls. The authors felt this might complicate adherence to medical regimens. Preventive and rehabilitative programs for the overweight are most likely to be effective if initiated before such impairment develops.

STRATEGIES FOR ACHIEVING THE BENEFITS OF EXERCISE

Goals of a Program of Exercise

The main goal is to provide a basis for long-term gradual progress toward an acceptable level of training and body weight reduction specifically targeted for the individual. A supposedly ideal value for body mass or another index may not be appropriate for a given individual, if there is marked hyperplasia of adiopocytes. There is no evidence to date that fat cells can be made to disappear following weight reduction, although it remains possible that this occurs with very prolonged maintenance of normal weight in patients with lifelong obesity of universal distribution or those who were more than 170% above ideal weight. Thus, an attempt at severe weight reduction may simply produce an angry person with adipocytes containing less than a normal complement of lipid, who is plagued by strong drives to regain the lost stores. However, as Björntorp's group [3] and others have shown, physical training without significant weight loss can be adequate to restore insulin sensitivity, blood lipids, and blood pressure to normal. The needs of each person must be individually evaluated.

Short- and Long-term Adherence

Martin and Dubbert [17] have analyzed the elements influencing adherence for periods of from 6 to 12 months in their own experience and in published reports. They summarized the problem in their description of the "drop-out man" as "an overweight, blue-collar smoker with an inactive job and leisure pursuits, with low self-motivation and a spouse who is indifferent towards his exercise participation, and who lives far away from the exercise facility and who exercises infrequently, alone and at high intensity." On the other hand the "ultra-adherence man" is a "white-collar nonsmoker with an active job and leisure pursuits, higher 'self-motivation' and an actively supportive spouse who lives and works close to the place of exercise, where he exercises at moderate intensity with others." They have not yet characterized the female counterpart, but from our experience the same criteria apply. There may, however, be physiological-metabolic characteristics of both men and women yet to be evaluated that influence a person's response.

Psychological Effects of Exercise in the Overweight

Dishman [11] has further analyzed the psychology of patients as they follow a program of exercise. He described the value of exercise as an antidepressant (another means of achieving health unbought and avoiding nauseous draughts). On the other hand, he also described the hazards of addiction to exhausting exercise, that is, becoming hooked on the opioids. This, in extreme cases, may lead to neglect of social responsibilities, to exceeding normal tolerance for physical stress, and generally to becoming programmed for self-destruction.

The psychological effects of increased well-being and initiative brought about by a state of physical training may be as important as the physiological effects of exercise described in the previous chapters. Exercise can be enjoyable, although the early stages of a training program are stressful for the overweight. The ability to exercise improves self-concept and demonstrates command over the body. These effects may be critical in the success of a weight-loss program.

Attitude Toward the Overweight Person

Jean Mayer emphasized some years ago that in our society the obese share many of the problems of a minority group with respect to such matters as college entrance and employment. This is further demonstrated by unthinking or cruel cartoons and advertisements. No matter how much we may know about the genetic, metabolic, and social problems that run in families plagued by an abundance of Neel's thrifty gene, it is difficult to curb an initial reaction of blame and censure when first encountering a severely overweight person. It is easy to think in terms of their being "grossly" rather than "severely" overweight. Yet, if any sort of satisfactory client relationship is to be developed, this must be overcome. The word "adherence" is preferable to "compliance," as it avoids regarding the patient in a subordinate position. My wife and I [32] have reviewed the relation between metabolic and psychological problems in overweight persons with non-insulin-dependent diabetes.

Establishing a Data Base and Sharing the Health Record

Obesity is a heterogeneous condition, and only rarely can a single etiologic factor or diagnosis be established. Rather, the aim is to characterize the individual so that suggestions may be appropriate for each individual [7, 29, 29B]. To establish the needs and possible approaches for each person, a comprehensive questionnaire covering medical and personal history can be useful. It serves a double purpose in calling the person's attention to particular problems and personal assets and enlisting the individual as an active participant in planning the exercise program. A profile of the usual daily energy expenditure can be recorded initially in graphic form by each individual, as described by Beeken [1]. The distribution of body fat should be noted, for reasons already mentioned. The status of each person's carbohydrate and lipid metabolism and cardiovascular status must be evaluated.

Suitable Types of Exercise for Weight Control and Training

As Brownell and Stunkard pointed out [7], in recommending an exercise program for an overweight or physiologically obese patient one must decide between programmed versus routine activity.

Programmed activities can include aerobic workouts with jogging, swimming, cycling, and so on. These include commercial programs and community programs. Weight Watchers has placed more emphasis than previously on exercise in their programs. The main features of the available commercial programs have been reviewed by Porcello [21]. The possible advantages of such programs may be regularity, supervision, a graded approach to an aerobic level of training, and opportunity for peer support in a group. Such programs usually enjoy an initial gung-ho period, but long-term adherence in spite of, perhaps, boredom, embarrassment, cost, and difficulty in conforming to a regular schedule generally produce a high dropout rate. They may, however, serve to help a person learn to experience how it feels to be reasonably fit.

Routine activities can be modified so as to increase the daily expenditure of energy, preferably in an enjoyable way. Walking is the most available form of exercise, and the amount can be increased in daily activities. Sports stores can provide lead-ballasted gaiters, which inconspicuously add to the training efficiency of walking. Pandolf and Goldman [20] have shown that a pound carried on the feet has the training effect of 10 pounds carried in a shoulder pack. A

trampoline can be purchased for less than $50 and kept in the living room within sight of the TV. It can double as a coffee table, as well as provide a jar-proof assortment of exercises that can be fitted in while watching a TV program or listening to music. Carrying a weight in the hands exercises the whole body. At home we use a 5-pound cannon ball. Exercycles provide exercise mainly for the legs, and often end up in a corner of the cellar. Rowing and swimming both provide total body exercise. Rowing machines are available, and an elegant poor man's version of a racing scull is provided by a relatively inexpensive new device, now commercially available, which can be set into the centerboard slot of a second hand windsurfer. It incorporates a sliding footrest linked to the outriggers which hold the oars, and is a delight to row. It provides at least the equivalent of a sliding seat, so that the whole body can be involved in the stroke. Consideration should be given, however, to possible adverse effects of sustained strenuous pulling in a patient with hypertension. Finally, dancing is also an excellent, pleasurable, and companionable exercise.

Brownell *et al.* [8] have made over 45,000 observations of people at various locations where they must decide between use of an escalator or of an adjacent stairway. Initially, 1.5% of the obese used the stairs while 6.7% of the lean did so. Stair use was considerably increased, particularly in the obese, by an encouraging sign. The effect was sustained while the sign was present, but gradually tapered off on its removal. This shows that behavioral changes can be effected in the natural environment. Perhaps the day will come when users of elevators and escalators will be warned that "The Surgeon General has concluded that use of these devices is dangerous to your health!"

A return to activities that persons enjoyed during their younger years can help to build morale and capitalize on past skills. As training improves, more vigorous exercise can be added. As noted, adding a program of exercise to moderately severe dietary restriction can be beneficial. However, the capacity for acute, vigorous exercise rather than endurance exercise is sharply reduced when any regimen involving severe restriction of dietary carbohydrate is used [5].

The techniques of *behavior modification* have of course been extremely useful. This is a field in which Storlie and Jordan have been pioneers [35]. The techniques are important, since exercise for the overweight is often a misery at first, and the health benefits seem remote. Direct feedback reflecting progress is useful. The heart rate during standardized exercise, such as the Harvard step test, provides an index of training. Laboratory results, such as blood lipid levels, can be shared with the patient; for the person with diabetes, on-the-spot blood glucose self-monitoring demonstrates the immediate effect of exercise in lowering the blood sugar level. Simultaneous measurement of plasma glucose and insulin levels may serve to emphasize the point that exercise both reduces insulin resistance and the demands on a person's ability to produce insulin. Keeping a running record, preferably in the form of a graph [1], provides further encouragement. Formal contracts or refundable deposits are a stimulus to persistence in a given program.

Undue emphasis should *not* be placed on body weight. The rate of loss is apt to be discouraging, as more dense muscle replaces body fat. Also, rapid weight loss of body fat may be masked by retention of fluid. Furthermore, the beneficial effects of training can be obtained with no loss of weight at all.

The Role of the Family and Friends

Group programs can provide valuable peer support, as can a regular schedule of exercise with a friend. Involving the entire family can also be rewarding, and the interest and support of a spouse is critical. Occasionally one encounters an insecure husband who is acutely concerned when his wife launches on a program of streamlining herself. He may place obstacles in her way as she gains independence and assurance.

The Silent and Unrecognized Successful Ones

Studies of various programs for weight loss are apt to include a high proportion of problem cases with emphasis on those who have failed repeatedly. Many people have worked out their own programs and have successfully combatted their inheritance. They are the exercisers and the restrained eaters. If these people can be persuaded to assist in a weight control program, their example and participation can be of value.

THE RISKS OF EXERCISE IN THE OBESE

Initiating a program of increased physical activity for the overweight or the psychologically obese may be hazardous for some individuals. Careful attention to any history or laboratory findings suggesting underlying cardiovascular disease is in order. A stress test may be indicated, but provides no absolute guarantee against a vascular accident. Since the overweight are particularly susceptible to injury to joints and soft tissues during exercise, a history of such problems should be included in the data base, and consultation obtained, if indicated. The rate of progression of an exercise program must be tailored to the individual. Against the hazards of physical exertion one must, however, weigh the potential risks of a sedentary way of life.

PRIORITIES FOR RESEARCH IN MAKING AVAILABLE BENEFITS OF EXERCISE FOR THOSE WITH OBESITY AND ITS COMPLICATIONS

The various types of obesity and the associated disorders—hypertension, non-insulin-dependent diabetes, and hyperlipid-emias—constitute a major national health problem. Our success in prevention and treatment of obesity remains poor. Increased physical activity alone can reduce spontaneous intake of food, can favorably modify composition of the diet, and can help in stabilizing weight at a more optimal level. We need to learn more about implementation.

We need to learn whether chronic, stable exercise of moderate intensity is more beneficial than intermittent exercise of higher intensity, both for the former college athlete and for his or her less competitive peer. Can the stress of competition offset the benefits of activity? For reducing weight and maintaining normal optimal weight, what is the optimal mix of caloric restriction, dietary composition, and added physical activity?

We are far from a consensus regarding the importance of facultative thermogenesis in maintenance of normal weight and the mechanisms that may be involved.

Measures that might be successful for a subtype of the overweight with a particular metabolic problem might well be futile in another. To help in interpreting clinical and metabolic studies and in planning others, there is need to develop techniques that characterize individual subjects more fully [29B].

Clinical investigators and basic scientists have learned much about the mechanisms underlying obesity, while psychologists, psychiatrists, and sports medicine experts have worked with varying degrees of success at achieving adherence to regimens that we know could be of benefit. There is need for the various disciplines to share their knowledge and to combine their efforts.

CONCLUSIONS

The overall conclusions are, first, that both decreased demands for physical work and changes in diet have contributed to our current health problems, and second, that exer-cise is such a potent adjunct to helping with the problems of the obese and associated disorders that more attention should be given to its implementation.

In brief, John Dryden was right.

ACKNOWLEDGMENT

The preparation of this chapter was aided by U.S. Public Health Service grants NIADDKD AM 10254 (Dr. Sims) and GCRC RR 109 (General Clinical Research Center).

REFERENCES

1. Beeken, R.K. Initiating exercise programs for patients with non-insulin-dependent diabetes. *Diab. Care* 3:627–628.
2. Bielinski, R., Y. Schutz, and E. Jequier. Energy metabolism during the postexercise recovery in man. *Am. J. Clin. Nutr.* 42:69–82, 1985.
3. Björntorp, P. Hypertension and exercise. *Hypertension* 4 (Suppl. III):56–59, 1982.
4. Björntorp, P., P. Berchtold, B. Lindholm, H. Sanne, G. Tibblin, and G. Grimby. Effects of physical training on glucose tolerance, plasma insulin, and lipids and on body composition in men after myocardial infarction. *Acta Med. Scand.* 192:439–442, 1972.
5. Bogardus, C., B.M., LaGrange, E.S. Horton, and E.A.H. Sims. Comparison of carbohydrate-containing and carbohydrate-restricted diets in the treatment of obesity. *J. Clin. Invest.* 68:399–404, 1981.
6. Bogardus, C., E. Ravussin, D.C. Robbins, R.R. Wolfe, E.S. Horton, and E.A.H. Sims. Effects of physical training and diet therapy on carbohydrate metabolism in patients with glucose intolerance and non-insulin-dependent diabetes mellitus. *Diabetes* 33:311–318, 1984.
7. Brownell, K.D., and A.J. Stunkard. Physical activity in the development and control of obesity. In Stunkard, A.J. (ed.). *Obesity*. Philadelphia: J.B. Saunders, 1980, pp. 300–324.
8. Brownell, K.D., A.J. Stunkard, and J.M. Albaum. Evaluation and modification of exercise patterns in the natural environment. *Am. J. Psychiatry* 137:1540–1545, 1980.
9. Danforth, E., Jr. Diet and obesity. *Am. J. Clin. Nutr.* 41:1132–1145, 1985.
10. Devlin, J.T., and E.S. Horton. Effects of prior high-intensity exercise on glucose metabolism in normal and insulin-resistant men. *Diabetes* 34:973–979, 1985.
11. Dishman, R.K. Compliance/adherence in health-related exercise. *Health Psychol.* 3:237–267, 1982.

12. Freedman-Akabas, S., E. Colt, H.R. Kissileff, and F.X. Pi-Sunyer. Lack of sustained increase in Vo_2 following exercise in fit and unfit subjects. *Am. J. Clin. Nutr.* 41:545–549, 1985.

13. Genazzani, A.R., F. Facchinetti, F. Petaglia, C. Pintor, and R. Corda. Hyperendorphinemia in obese children and adolescents. *J. Clin. Endocrinol. Metab.* 62:36–40, 1986.

14. Jordan, H.A., and A.J. Canavan. Patterns of weight change: The interval 6 to 10 years after initial weight loss in a cognitive-behavioral treatment program. *Psychol. Rep.* 57:195–203, 1985.

15. Krotkiewski, M., K. Mandroukas, L. Sjostrom, L. Sullivan, H. Wetterqvist, and P. Björntorp. Effects of long-term physical training on body fat, metabolism, and blood pressure in obesity. *Metabolism* 28:650–658, 1979.

16. Larsson, B., K. Svardsudd, L. Welin, L. Wilhelmsen, P. Björntorp, and G. Tibblin. Abdominal adipose tissue distribution, obesity, and risk of cardiovascular disease and death: 134-year followup of participants in the study of men born in 1913. *Br. Med. J.* 288:1401–1404, 1984.

17. Martin, J.E., and P.M. Dubbert. Adherence to exercise. *Exer. Sports Sci. Rev.* 13:137–167, 1985.

18. O'Sullivan, J.B, Body weight and subsequent diabetes mellitus. *JAMA* 248:397, 1982.

19. Paffenbarger, R.S., R.T. Hyde, A.L. Wing, and C-c. Hsieh. Physical activity, all-cause mortality, and longevity of college alumni. *N. Engl. J. Med.* 314:605–613, 1986.

20. Pandolf, K.B., and R.F. Goldman. Physical conditioning of less fit adults by use of leg weight loading. *Arch. Phys. Med. Rehab.* 56:255–261, 1975.

21. Porcello, L.A.P. Characteristics of professional weight control programs. In Hirsch, J., and T.B. Van Itallie (eds.). *Recent Advances in Obesity Research: IV.* London: John Libbey, 1983, pp. 281–293.

22. Ravussin, E., and C. Bogardus. "Fidgeting": A significant component of 24 hour energy expenditure in man. Presented at Joint Conference on Obesity and Non-Insulin-Dependent Diabetes. Toronto, Oct. 1985.

23. Rose, G.A., and R.T. Williams. Metabolic studies on large and small eaters. *Br. J. Nutr.* 15:1–9, 1961.

24. Ruderman, N.B., S.H. Schneider, and P. Berchtold. The "metabolically obese" normal-weight individual. *Am. J. Clin. Nutr.* 34:1617–1621, 1981.

25. Schwartz, R.S., R.C. Veith, L.F. Jaeger, C.A. Bevan, and J.B. Halter. Effect of aerobic training on norepinephrine kinetics. *Clin. Res.*, in press.

26. Segal, K.R., and B. Gutin. Thermic effects of food and exercise in lean and obese women. *Metabolism* 32:581–589, 1983.

27. Segal, K.R., B. Gutin, A.M. Nyman, and F. Xavier Pi-Sunyer. Thermic effect of food at rest, during exercise, and post-exercise in lean and obese men of similar body weight. *J. Clin. Invest.* 76:1107–1112, 1985.

28. Sims, E.A.H. The characterization of obesity and the importance of fat distribution: Blood pressure and physical activity in the HANES I survey. In *Metabolic Complications of Human Obesities* Vague, J., P. Björntorp, B. Guy-Grand, Rebuffe, Scrive, M., and P. Vague, (eds.). Excerpta Medica, International Congress Series 682, pp. 39–48, 1985.

29a. Sims, E.A.H. Energy balance in human beings: Problems of plenitude. In Auerbach, G.D., and D.B. McCormick, (eds.). *Vitamins and Hormones,* Vol. 43. New York: Academic Press, 1986.

29b. Sims, E.A., and L.B., Weed. The 1987 Herman Award Lecture. A plea for an integrated approach to characterization and management of obesity, type II diabetes, the hyperlipidemias and hypertension: A role for the personal computer? *Am. J. Clin. Nutr.* 46:726–733, 1987.

30. Sims, E.A.H., and P. Berchtold. Obesity and hypertension: Mechanisms and implications for management. *JAMA* 247:49–52, 1982.

31. Sims, E.A.H., and E. Danforth Jr. Expenditure and storage of energy in man. (Perspective) *J. Clin. Inves.* 79:1019–1026, 1987.

32. Sims, E.A.H., and D.F. Sims. Living with non-insulin-dependent diabetes: The interplay of physiologic, cultural, and emotional factors. In Davidson, J.K. (ed.). *Clinical Diabetes.* New York: Thieme-Stratton, 1986.

33. Sjöström, L. Can the relapsing patient be identified? In Hirsch, J., and T.B. Van Itallie (eds.). Recent Advances in Obesity Research IV. London/Paris: John Libbey, 1983.

34. Stern, J. Diet and exercise. In Greenwood, M.R.C. (ed.). *Obesity.* New York: Churchill Livingstone, 1983, p. 65.

35a. Storlie, J., and H.A. Jordan (eds.). *Behavioral Management of Obesity.* New York: S.P. Medical and Scientific Books, 1984.

35b. Stuart, R.B., and B. Davis. Slim chance in a fat world. Champaign Il.: Research Press Co., 1972.

36. Vague, J., P. Björntorp, B. Guy-Grand, and J. Vague (eds.). *Metabolic Complications of Human Obesities.* International Congress Series 68. Amsterdam: Excerpta Medica, 1985.

37. Wilson, G.T. Psychological prognostic factors in the treatment of obesity. In *Recent advances in obesity research:* IV. J. Hirsch and T.B. Van Itallie (eds.). John Libbey, London pp. 301–311, 1983.

38. Woo, R., J.S. Garrow, and F.X. Pi-Sunyer. Effect of exercise on spontaneous caloric intake in obesity. *Am. J. Clin. Nutr.* 36:470–477, 1982.

39. Woo, R., J.S. Garrow, and F.X. Pi-Sunyer. Voluntary food intake during prolonged exercise in obese women. *Am. J. Clin. Nutr.* 36:478–484, 1982.

40. Woo, R., and F.X. Pi-Sunyer. Effect of increased physical activity on voluntary intake in lean women. *Metabolism* 34:836–841, 1985.

41. Wood, P.D., R.B. Terry, and W.L. Haskell. Metabolism of substrates: Diet, lipoprotein metabolism, and exercise. *Fed. Proc.* 44:358–363, 1985.

INDEX

A

Acetaminophen, 203
Acetyl coenzyme A, 72
Actomyosin ATPase, and energy demand, 32−33, *See also* Myosin ATPase
ADP (adenosine diphosphate)
  control of respiration, 53
  regulating PFK, 52
AMP (adenosine monophosphate) deamination, 67
Adipocyte, hyperplasia, 252
Aerobic capacity, maximal, 3*t*
  limiting factors, 5−6
Alanine, 93, 101
Alcohol, 204−205
Aldosterone, 207
Alpha-adrenergic agents, 207
American Dietetic Association, 187
Amenorrhea, 205
Amiloride, 207
Amino acids, 90−97
  branched-chain, oxidation of, 93
  fluxes, 93
  metabolism, 93
  release and uptake, during exercise, 93
S-Aminolevulinate synthetase
  training, 126
Ammonia production
  training, 128
Amphetamines, 209
Anabolic steroids, 209
Analgesics, 201−203, 202*t*
Anemia, folate-induced, 205
Antacids, 196−99, 198*t*
  nonsystemic, 197−98
  systemic, 197−98
Antiarrhythmias, 208−209
Apolipoproteins
  identification and function, 214−215*t*
  physical activity, 220−21
Association of Obesity and Hypertension, 248
Aspirin, 201
  intolerance to, 201

Atherosclerosis, 230−34
  effect of training on, 230−31
  effect of training in diabetics on, 230−31
  in diabetes, 230−34
Autonomic neuropathy, 235

B

Basal metabolic rate, 1
Behavior modification, 255
Beta-adrenergic blockers, 207−208, 235
  metabolic effects, 66
Beta-endorphin, 248
Blood in stools,
  influence of exercise, 160
Body composition,
  lipoprotein metabolism, 224
Brown fat, 244, 246
Busselton, Australia study, 231

C

Caffeine, 203−204
  plasma free fatty acids, 80
Calcium antagonist, 208
Calcium carbonate, 198
Caloric intake, 243
Captopril, 208
Carbohydrate
  dietary source, 46
  in diet, and glycogen storage, 48−49
  ingestion, during exercise, 145−46
    rationale, 141
  loading, muscle, 139
  metabolism
    energy from, 49−50
    heavy exercise, 56−57
    light exercise, 54
    moderate exercise, 54−56
Cardiac muscle, 40−41

Carnitine acyl transferase, deficiency, 75—76
Cathartics, 199—201
Catecholamines, 246
Chicago Coronary Prevention Evaluation Program, 249
Chloride loss, during exercise, 155
Cholesterol, HDL, *See* lipoprotein cholesterol, high
 density
Cholesterol metabolism, 215—16
Cholesterol, plasma, and physical activity, 216—17
Cholesterol synthesis, and LDL degradation, 216
Chromium, 182—83*t*, 188—90, 192
 deficiency, 188
 excretion, 189
 requirement, 188—89
 sources, 188
 status, 189
  effect of exercise, 190
Cimetidine, 199
Citrate,
 regulating PFK (phosphofructose kinase), 52
Clinical Education Program of the American Diabetes
  Association, 252
Coagulation abnormalities, in diabetes, 233
 effect of exercise training, 233
Cocaine, 209
Colonic motility, during exercise, 164
Contraction-relaxation cycle, factors requiring energy,
  32
Copper, 182—83*t*, 185—88, 192
 blood concentrations, effect of exercise, 186—87
 deficiency, 185—86
 excretion, 187
 requirement, 186
 sources, 186
 status, effect of exercise, 187—88
Cori cycle, 101
Corticosteroids, 209
Creatine
 control of respiration, 53
 kinase reaction, 33
Cytochrome c, and training, 126

D

Degenerative joint disease, 237
Defecation, influence of exercise, 159
Dehydration
 body temperature, 153
 exercise performance, 153—54
 extracellular fluid volume, 153
 intracellular fluid volume, 152—53
 maximal oxygen consumption, 153
 voluntary, during exercise, 154
Detraining, effect on mitochondrial enzymes, 127—28
Diabetes
 gestational, 250
 Type I, 229—30, 234—40
  effect of regular exercise in, 229—30

Type II, 230—40
 effect of regular exercise in, 230
Diarrhea, following exercise, 168
Diet
 composition, and energy metabolism, 66
 high-fat
  exercise performance, 85
  muscle 3-hydroxyacyl CoA dehydrogenase, 85
 intake, 7
 regimen, and exercise, 250
 requirements, 96—97
  protein, 96—97
Digitalis, 208
Diuretics, 205—206
Doppler principle, 243
Dryden, John, 248

E

Electrolyte,
 loss during exercise, 154—56
  replacement, 157
 in urine, 156
 transport, and vasoactive intestinal polypeptide,
  167—68
Elite distance runners, and muscle fiber type, 125
Embden-Meyerhof pathway, 49
Endergonic processes, 31
Endurance performance, limiting factors, 6
Energy balance equation, 244
Energy expenditure, 243—56
 extreme in, 3
 running, 2
 swimming, 3
 walking, 2
Energy-rich phosphate compound, 31
Energy stores in body
 carbohydrate, 135—36*t*
 fat, 135
 protein, 136—37*t*
Erythrocyte glutathione reductase activity coefficient,
  175
Estrogen, 205
Exercise
 capacity
  in diabetes, 234
  McArdle's disease, 62
  PFK (Phosphofructose kinase) deficiency, 58
  phosphorylase deficiency, 58
 complications, in diabetes, 234—37
 guidelines, for insulin-dependent diabetics, 235—36,
  233*t*
 performance
  caffeine and, 147
  carbohydrate in diet and, 138—39
  carbohydrate ingestion during exercise, 145—46
  elevated plasma free fatty acids and, 146—47
 prescription, for diabetes, 238—40, 239*t*

frequency of exercise, 239
intensity and duration of exercise, 238–39
time of day, 239–40
type of exercise, 238
programs, 251–254
adherence, 253
for obese, 254
goal, 252
psychological effects in obese, 253
selection of participant, 237–38
success rates, 251
stimulus for lipoprotein change, 223
training, *See* Training
Extracellular volume expansion, 156

F

Fasting
effect on glucose metabolism, 112–14
effect on liver glycogen content, 140
Fat, *See also* Lipid
storage, 74
as a metabolic fuel
characteristics, 73
Fat oxidation, during exercise
based on R-values, 76–77
Fatigue
muscle glycogen and, 62
muscle pH and, 62
Fiber type, muscle. *See* Muscle fiber type
Flavoprotein dehydrogenases, 175–76
Fluid absorption, and exercise intensity, 156
Fluid ingestion
fluid osmolality, 156–57
influence of temperature, 156
Folate status, 176
Food intake, effect of exercise on, 247–48, 300–301
Framingham study, 231
Free fatty acids
fat cells
growth hormone, 79–80
sympathetic influence, 79
oxidation
energy yield and, 76
plasma free fatty acids concentration, and, 120
process of, 75
plasma concentrations, 133
during exercise, 79
elevation with heparin, 80
oxidation and, 120
glycogen depletion and, 119
toxicity, 73
transport, 74
uptake in muscle, 80–81, 113, 119
during fasting, 113
Fructose, 46
Fructose ingestion
blood lactate, 143

prior to exercise, 143–44
response to, 64–65
Futile cycling, 246

G

Gastric acid secretion, during exercise, 165
Gastric emptying, during exercise, 163–64
Gastrin, during exercise, 166
Gastroenteropancreatic (GEP) hormones, 166–68
stimulus for release during exercise, 166–67
Gastrointestinal bleeding, 159–60, 199
exercise and, 159–60
Gastrointestinal hemorrhagic lesions, 163
Glucagon, during exercise, 166
Gluconeogenesis, 48
energy source during exercise, 57
hepatic, 101–102
liver glycogen content, 140
Glucose
concentrations, blood, central nervous system, 63
homeostasis, 228–29
ingestion
during exercise, 64
metabolic effects, 172
pre-exercise, 63–64
prior to exercise, 142–43
intolerance, 229
production by liver. *See* Hepatic glucose production
tolerance, 229–30
turnover, 46
uptake, muscle, 102–106
blood flow, effect of, 103
during fasting, 113
exercise duration, effect of, 103–104
exercise intensity, effect of, 102–103
recovery following exercise, 109–112
regulation during exercise, 104–106
uptake, with heavy exercise, 63
utilization, liver release, 58
utilization, plasma
during exercise, 135
during postabsorptive state, 100–101
Glucose-alanine cycle, 101
Glucose-fatty acid cycle, and training, 118–19
Glucose-l-phosphate, 49
Glucose-6-phosphate, 49
Glycerol-phosphate shuttle, 121
Glycogen
characteristics, 46–47
debranching enzyme, 49
depletion, and plasma free fatty acids concentration, 119
hepatic depletion during exercise, 106–107
muscle
influence of diet, 137
utilization during exercise, 133–34
resynthesis
diet effect, 137–38

Glycogen, resynthesis (*Cont.*):
    following exercise, 137—38
  sparing, 64
    training, 67
  storage, and water retention, 49, 140
  supercompensation, 48
  synthase, 47—48
  utilization, 4
    aerobic/anaerobic energy provision, 59—60
    fructose ingestion, 143—44
    relation to glucose uptake, 58
Glycogenolysis, hepatic, 101—102
Glycolysis
  control of, 50—51
    effect of training on, 128—29
  muscle pH, 61—62
Gut peristalsis, and migrating motor complex, 164—65

H

Harvard, longevity study of graduates, 249
Harvard step test, 255
Heat balance, and exceptional situations, 150
Heat exchange
  conduction, 150
  convection, 150
  radiation, 150
Hemostasis abnormalities, in diabetes, 233
Hepatic glucose production, 100—102, 106—10,
    112—13, 140—41, 228—29, 235
  during exercise, 106—109, 140—41
  during fasting, 112—13
  hormonal factors, 102
  recovery following exercise, 110—12
  regulation during exercise, 107—109
    hormonal, 107—109
    nervous activation, 109
Hepatic glycogen, *See* Glycogen, hepatic
Hepatic lipase
  HDL metabolism and, 222
  physical activity and, 222
Helsinki policemen study, 231
Hexokinase, 34—35
HDL. *See* Lipoprotein composition
High-density lipoprotein cholestrol. *See* Lipoprotein
    cholesterol, high density
Hormonal response, during recovery from exercise,
    111—12
Hyperglycemia, 231—34
  effect of exercise on, 236
Hyperinsulinemia, 229, 231—32
Hyperlipidemia, 232
Hyperlipidemia, in diabetes
  effect of training, 232
Hypertension, 233, 248—50
  effect of physical training on, 233
Hypertension, in diabetes, 233
  effect of physical training on, 233

Hypoglycemia, 234—35
  exercise induced, 235, 236
  effect of medication on, 235

I

Ibuprofen, 203
Indomethacin, 203
IMP (inosine monophosphate) production, and training,
    128
Institute of Nutrition of Central America and Panama,
    89
Insulin
  glycogen metabolism, 47—48
  heavy exercise, 63
  response to fructose ingestion, 65
Insulin sensitivity, 229
  effect of physical training on, 229
  triglyceride reduction with training and, 222
Isometric exercise, 57

J

Joint National Committee on Detection, Evaluation and
    Treatment of High Blood Pressure, 429

K

Keshan disease, 190
Ketosis, effect of exercise on, 236

L

Lactate
  influence on plasma free fatty acids, 80
  metabolism, 23—24
  oxidation, during exercise, 61
Lactate production
  aerobic conditions, 59
  control of, 59
  muscle fiber type and, 59
  muscle pH and, 60
Lactate threshold, 24
  endurance performance and, 122—23
Laxatives, 199—201, 200*t*
LDL. *See* Lipoprotein composition
Lecithin-cholesterol acyltransferase, activity during
    exercise, 222
Leucine, 93
Lipid. *See also* Fat
Lipid synthesis, 73—74
Lipoprotein
  cholesterol, high density
    adipose tissue distribution, 222—23
    from VLDL, 216

physical activity, 218—19
plasma triglycerides, 218
production, 216
smoking-exercise interaction, 224
subfractions and exercise, 219
training duration, 219
cholesterol, low-density
physical activity, 217
subspecies and exercise, 217
composition (HDL, LDL, VLDL), 214*t*
lipase
activity during exercise, 221
training, 221
triglyceride removal, 221
metabolism
body composition, 224
exercise stimulus for change, 223—24
nutrient intake, 224
profile
androgen, 223
estrogen, 223
Low-density lipoprotein cholesterol. *See* Lipoprotein
cholesterol, low density

M

Magnesium loss during exercise, 155
Malate-aspartate shuttle, 121
Malnutrition, 174
Mayer, Jean, 253
McArdle's syndrome, 62, 92
Metabolic rate, resting, 244—45
following exercise, 245
3-methyl histidine, 95—96
Metoprolol, 196
Migrating motor complex, during exercise, 165
Mitochondrial respiration
control of, 53, 128
cytosolic phosphorylation potential, 37
free ADP and, 36
muscle ADP
training effect, 128
Motilin, during exercise, 166, 168
Muscle. *See also* Muscle, skeletal
blood flow, 19
control of, 20
buffer capacity, 60
capillarization increase and metabolite exchange,
83—84
fiber type conversion, 124—25
Muscle adaptations, and oxidative capacity, 22—23
Muscle contraction (tetanus), and energetics, 28—29
Muscle contraction
inorganic phosphate, 30
intracellular pH, 30
phosphocreatine, 30
Muscle fiber transformation, 17
Muscle fiber type. *See also* Muscle, skeletal

blood flow capacity, 21
contraction energetics, 29—30
glycogen depletion, 21—22
Muscle free fatty acid uptake. *See* Free fatty acid
uptake, muscle
Muscle function/design
relationship, 39—40
Muscle glycogen. *See* Glycogen, muscle
Muscle growth, 89—90
effect of denervation on, 89
effect of immobilization on, 89
Muscle pH
glycolysis, 61—62
maximal exercise, 60
Muscle, skeletal
fast-twitch red, 12—13
fast-twitch white, 12—13
fiber type
characteristics, 11, 13—14
classification, 11—12*t*
distribution, 13—14
oxidative capacities, 17—18
motor unit, 9—10
rate coding, 16
'size principle', 16
motor unit recruitment, 14—15
motor unit spacial recruitment, 15—16
oxidative capacity activity/inacitivity, 18
slow-twitch red fibers, 12, 13
Muscle, smooth, economy of tension maintenance, 41
Muscle spindles, 16
Muscle triglyceride. *See* Triglyceride, muscle
Myofibrillar ATPase, 12
Myoglobin, and training, 126—27
Myokinase reaction, 33—34
Myosin ATPase, 12. *See also* Actomyosin ATPase

N

NADH, and mitochondria, 121
Naloxone, 248
Naltrexone, 248
National Institutes of Health, Phoenix, Arizona, 243
National Research Council, 92
Nitrates, 208
Nitrogen balance, 209
Norepinephrine, 246
Norepinephrine turnover, effect of overfeeding and
underfeeding, 246
Nutrient, gastrointestinal absorption, 196
Nutrient intake, and lipoprotein metabolism, 224
Nutritional deficiencies, 172—73

O

Obesity, 232—33, 242—56

Obesity (*Cont.*):
  and activity levels, 243
  attitude toward, 253
  central, 251
  "physiological", 249, 251
  potential risks of exercise, 255
Opioid, endogenous, 248, 253
Oral contraceptives, 205
Oxidative capacity, 12
Oxygen consumption, maximal (VO$_2$max), 3t, 18

P

Pancreatic secretion during exercise, 165−66
Paris study, 231
Peripheral neuropathy, 237
PFK. *See* Phosphofructokinase
Pharmacological agents, 196−210
Phenylbutazone, 202−203
Phosphate potential, and control of respiration, 53
Phosphocreatine hydrolysis, and muscle buffer, 60
Phosphofructokinase, 35, 50
  muscle pH, 61−62
  regulatory factors, 52
Phosphorylase, 34 −35, 49
  activation of, 51−52
Phosphorylase a, during contractions, 51−52
Physical training. *See* Training
Pima Indians, 244
Postabsorptive state, 100−102
  glucose utilization during, 100−101
Potassium loss, during exercise, 155
Potassium redistribution during exercise, 155−56
Prader-Willi syndrome, 248
Progestin, 205
Propranolol, 196
Protein
  degradation, 95−96
  metabolism, 89−97
    during exercise, 135
    endocrine influences, 89
    measurement of, 92, 95
  sparing, effect of exercise on, 89
  synthesis, during exercise, 93−95
    isotonic and isometric, 94−95
Proteinuria, 237
Psychological stress, in diabetes, 233−34
Pyruvate dehydrogenase, 35−36
Pyruvate metabolism, 49

R

R-value. *See* Respiratory exchange ratio
Rectal temperature, and exercise intensity, 150
Renal complications, 236−37
Research priorities, exercise and obesity, 255−56

Respiratory control. *See also* Mitochondrial respiration
  adenine nucleotide translocase, 38
  near-equilibrium hypothesis, 37−38
  smooth muscle, 42
Respiratory exchange ratio (R-value), 45
  substrate oxidation, 117
Respiratory quotient, 1
  definition, 54
Riboflavin, 205
Rochester State Hospital, 173
Runners' diarrhea, 177

S

Salicylate, 201−203
Sarcoplasmic reticulum ATPase, 32
Secretin, during exercise, 166
Selenium, 182−83t, 190−91, 193
  deficiency, 190, 191
  requirement, 190
  sources, 190
  status, effect of exercise, 191
Sex hormones, and lipoprotein profile, 223
Skeletal muscle. *See* Muscle, skeletal
Skin temperature
  ambient temperature and, 150
  exercise intensity and, 150
Small intestine transit time, during exercise, 164
Smoking cigarettes, and high-density lipoprotein
    cholesterol, 224−25
Smooth muscle. *See* Muscle, smooth
Sodium bicarbonate, 198
Sodium loss, during exercise, 155
Somatostatin, during exercise, 166
Spironolactone, 207
Splanchnic circulation
  anatomy, 160
  'autoregulatory escape', 161
  blood flow redistribution, 162
  influence of exercise, 160−63
  reduced perfusion pressure, 163
  sympathetic influence, 161−63
Splanchnic glucose production, 247
Stanford University, 247
Steroid metabolism, 248−49
Stomach emptying, and fluid composition, 156
Substrate
  reserves, 90−91
  utilization, determined from R-values, 132
  utilization, during exercise
    carbohydrate, 91
    lipid, 91
    protein, 91−92
Sucralfate, 199
Symmorphosis, 24
Sympathomimetic amines, 208
Sweat, and electrolyte content, 154
Sweat heat loss formula, 152

Sweat loss, rates of, 152
Sweating, intracellular fluid volume, 153

T

Theophylline, 204
Thermogenesis, facultative, 244–47
Thermogenesis, nonshivering, 246
Thiazides, 205–206
Training
  adaptations to, 82–83
  adrenergic mediated glycogenolysis and, 118
  blood glycerol concentration and, 119–20
  cardiovascular adaptations to, 116
  effect on glycolytic rate, 66
  fatty acid oxidation, influence of cardiac output
      change, 83
  free fatty acid oxidation mitochondrial content, 129
  glucose-fatty acid cycle, 118–19
  glycerophosphate shuttle, 126
  glycogen depletion during exercise, 117
  glycogen sparing, 67
  glycolytic pathway enzymes, 127
  HDL cholesterol, 218–19
  hexokinase, 127
  increased fatty acid oxidation benefit, 82
  lactate dehydrogenase, 127
  LDL cholesterol, 217
  malate-aspartate shuttle, 126
  metabolic control, 83
  mitochondrial protein synthesis, 126
  muscle lactate, 123
  muscle mitochondria, 125
  muscle triglycerides, 120
  plasma free fatty acid concentrations, 84, 119
  plasma ketone bodies, 84
  plasma total cholesterol, 216–17
  stimulus for lipoprotein change, 223–24
Triacylglycerol (*see* Triglyceride)
Triglyceride
  hydrolysis, cyclic AMP and, 80
  lipolysis, muscle sympathetic influence on, 79
  muscle stores
    influence of exercise, 77–78
    utilization, estimates based on glycerol release,
        78–79
  plasma
    physical activity and, 220
    uptake into muscle during exercise, 81

U

Ultramarathon, and hyponatremia, 157

Urea production, during exercise, 92

V

Vascular complications, 236–37
Vasoactive intestinal polypeptide (VIP)
  during exercise, 166–68
  intestinal ischemia, 167
Vermont study, 244
Very-low density lipoprotein triglycerides, and exercise
      training, 220
Vitamins, 172–78
  B, 173–75
  B_6, 205
  B_{12}, 205
  C, 177
  deficiencies, 172–73, 174–75
  E, 176–77
  K, 205
  nicotinamide, 173
  pantothenic acid, 173
  pyridoxine, 173
  riboflavin, 173
  thiamin, 173
Vitamins, malabsorption of, 204
  in alcoholics, 204
Vitamins, supplements, 176–77
Vitamin requirements, 175–76
  for athletes, 177
  for physical activity, 177
VLDL. *See* Lipoprotein composition
von Liebig, Justus, 91

W

Weight control, 246–47
Weight Watchers, 254
White-muscle disease, 191

Z

Zinc, 180–81, 182–83*t*, 184–85, 192
  blood, change with exercise, 181
  excretion, effect of exercise, 184
  requirements, 181
  sources, 181
  status, effect of exercise, 184
  supplements
    hypercholesterolemia, 185
    with exercise, 184–85